# Burn Rehabili

*Editor*

KAREN KOWALSKE

# PHYSICAL MEDICINE AND REHABILITATION CLINICS OF NORTH AMERICA

www.pmr.theclinics.com

*Consulting Editor*
BLESSEN C. EAPEN

November 2023 • Volume 34 • Number 4

ELSEVIER

1600 John F. Kennedy Boulevard • Suite 1800 • Philadelphia, Pennsylvania, 19103-2899

http://www.theclinics.com

PHYSICAL MEDICINE AND REHABILITATION CLINICS OF NORTH AMERICA Volume 34, Number 4
November 2023 ISSN 1047-9651, 978-0-443-13041-0

Editor: Megan Ashdown
Developmental Editor: Nitesh Barthwal

*Reprints.* For copies of 100 or more of articles in this publication, please contact the Commercial Reprints Department, Elsevier Inc., 360 Park Avenue South, New York, NY 10010-1710. Tel.: 212-633-3874; Fax: 212-633-3820; E-mail: reprints@elsevier.com.

*Physical Medicine and Rehabilitation Clinics of North America* (ISSN 1047-9651) is published quarterly by Elsevier Inc., 360 Park Avenue South, New York, NY 10010-1710. Months of issue are February, May, August, and November. Business and Editorial Offices: 1600 John F. Kennedy Blvd., Suite 1800, Philadelphia, PA 19103-2899. Customer Service Office: 3251 Riverport Lane, Maryland Heights, MO 63043. Periodicals postage paid at New York, NY and additional mailing offices. Subscription price per year is $342.00 (US individuals), $722.00 (US institutions), $100.00 (US students), $388.00 (Canadian individuals), $950.00 (Canadian institutions), $100.00 (Canadian students), $491.00 (foreign individuals), $950.00 (foreign institutions), and $210.00 (foreign students). Foreign air speed delivery is included in all *Clinics* subscription prices. All prices are subject to change without notice. **POSTMASTER:** Send address changes to *Physical Medicine and Rehabilitation Clinics of North America*, Customer Service Office: Elsevier Health Sciences Division, Subscription Customer Service, 3251 Riverport Lane, Maryland Heights, MO 63043. **Customer Service: 1-800-654-2452 (US). From outside of the United States, call 314-447-8871. Fax: 314-447-8029. E-mail: JournalsCustomer Service-usa@elsevier.com (for print support); JournalsOnlineSupport-usa@elsevier.com (for online support).**

*Physical Medicine and Rehabilitation Clinics of North America* is indexed in *Excerpta Medica, MEDLINE/PubMed (Index Medicus), Cinahl,* and *Cumulative Index to Nursing and Allied Health Literature.*

# Contributors

### CONSULTING EDITOR

**BLESSEN C. EAPEN, MD**
Chief, VA Greater Los Angeles Health Care System, Associate Clinical Professor, Division of Physical Medicine and Rehabilitation, Department of Medicine, David Geffen School of Medicine at UCLA, Los Angeles, California, USA

### EDITOR

**KAREN KOWALSKE, MD**
Professor, Department of Physical Medicine and Rehabilitation, University of Texas, Southwestern Medical Center, Dallas, Texas, USA

### AUTHORS

**SHYLA KAJAL BHARADIA**
Research Assistant, Cumming School of Medicine, University of Calgary, Foothills Medical Centre, Calgary, Alberta, Canada

**TRUDY BOULTER, OTR/L, CHT, BT-C**
Children's Hospital Colorado Burn Center, Aurora, Colorado, USA

**LINDSAY BURNETT, RN, BScN, MN, NP**
Alberta Health Services, Adjunct Clinical Assistant, University of Calgary, Foothills Medical Centre, Calgary, Alberta, Canada

**AUDRA T. CLARK, MD**
Assistant Professor, Department of Surgery, University of Texas Southwestern Medical Center, Dallas, Texas, USA

**CRAIG G. CRANDALL, PhD**
Professor of Internal Medicine, Division of Cardiology, Department of Internal Medicine, University of Texas Southwestern Medical Center, Institute for Exercise and Environmental Medicine (IEEM), Texas Health Presbyterian Hospital Dallas, Dallas, Texas, USA

**HUAN DENG, PhD**
Assistant Professor, Department of Physical Medicine and Rehabilitation, Spaulding Rehabilitation Hospital, Harvard Medical School, Boston, Massachusetts, USA

**CELESTE C. FINNERTY, PhD**
Associate Professor, Department of Surgery, Division of Surgical Sciences, University of Texas Medical Branch, Galveston, Texas, USA

**JOSH FOSTER, PhD**
Postdoctoral Research Fellow, Department of Internal Medicine, University of Texas Southwestern Medical Center, Institute for Exercise and Environmental Medicine (IEEM), Texas Health Presbyterian Hospital Dallas, Dallas, Texas, USA

**VINCENT GABRIEL, MD, MSc, FRCPC**
Assistant Professor, Departments of Clinical Neurosciences and Surgery, University of Calgary; Medical Director, Calgary Firefighters Burn Treatment Centre, Foothills Medical Centre, Calgary, Alberta, Canada

**TIMOTHY J. GENOVESE, MD, MPH**
Resident Physician, Department of Physical Medicine and Rehabilitation, Spaulding Rehabilitation Hospital, Harvard Medical School, Boston, Massachusetts, USA

**MATTHEW GODLESKI, MD**
Assistant Professor, Department of Physical Medicine and Rehabilitation, Sunnybrook Health Sciences Centre, University of Toronto, St. John's Rehab, Toronto, Ontario, Canada

**ALISON HARUTA, MD**
Surgical Critical Care Fellow, Department of Burns, Trauma, Acute, and Critical Care Surgery, UT Southwestern, Dallas, Texas, USA

**DANIKA HINES, DPT**
Physical Therapist, Burn Therapy, Arizona Burn Center, Valleywise Health, Phoenix, Arizona, USA

**STEPHANIE JEAN, MD, MSc, FRCPC**
Assistant Professor, Department of Physical Medicine and Rehabilitation, Institut de Réadaptation Gingras-Lindsay de Montréal (Darlington), Université de Montréal, Montréal, Québec, Canada

**SAMUEL P. MANDELL, MD, MPH**
Associate Professor, Section Chief of Burn Surgery, Medical Director of Parkland Burn Center, Medical Director of Parkland Surgical Quality, Department of Burns, Trauma, Acute, and Critical Care Surgery, UT Southwestern, Dallas, Texas, USA

**DEREK MURRAY, MSPT**
Physical Therapist, Master of Science, Physical Therapy, Burn Therapist, Certified, Supervisor of Burn Rehabilitation, Burn Therapy, Arizona Burn Center, Valleywise Health, Phoenix, Arizona, USA

**BROOKE MURTAUGH, OTD, OTR/L, BT-C**
Department of Rehabilitation Programs, Madonna Rehabilitation Hospitals, Lincoln, Nebraska, USA

**KIRAN K. NAKARMI, MBBS, MS, MCH**
Associate Professor of Plastic Surgery, Director of Hand and Microsurgery Fellowship, Nepal Cleft and Burn Center at Kirtipur Hospital, National Academy of Medical Sciences, Kathmandu, Nepal

**JOHANNA H. NUNEZ, MD**
Resident, University of Texas Southwestern Medical Center, Dallas, Texas, USA

**AUDREY O'NEIL, DPT**
Burn Therapist, Certified, Certified Wound Specialist, Physical Therapist III – Team Leader of Research / Advanced Clinical Specialist, Burn Rehabilitation Services; Eskenazi Health, Richard M Fairbanks Burn Center, Indianapolis, Indiana, USA

**JOHN PORTER, MD**
Medical Director for Physical Medicine and Rehabilitation, District Medical Group, Valleywise Health, Trauma and Burn Services, Associate Professor, Department of Surgery, University of Arizona, Creighton University, Phoenix, Arizona, USA

**ERIC RIVAS, PhD**
Program Manager, Microgravity Research, In-Space Solutions, Axiom Space Headquarters, Houston, Texas, USA

**KIMBERLY ROATEN, PhD**
Professor, The University of Texas Southwestern Medical Center, Dallas, Texas, USA

**DIANA M. ROBINSON, MD**
Assistant Professor, The University of Texas Southwestern Medical Center, Dallas, Texas, USA

**KATHLEEN S. ROMANOWSKI, MD, MAS, FACS, FCCM**
Associate Professor of Clinical Surgery, Department of Surgery, University of California, Davis and Shriners Children's Northern California, Sacramento, California, USA

**JEFFREY C. SCHNEIDER, MD**
Medical Director, Trauma, Burn and Orthopedic Program, Department of Physical Medicine and Rehabilitation, Spaulding Rehabilitation Hospital, Associate Professor, Harvard Medical School, Rehabilitation Outcomes Center at Spaulding, Massachusetts General Hospital, Harvard Medical School, Boston, Massachusetts, USA

**CLIFFORD C. SHECKTER, MD**
Assistant Professor of Plastic and Reconstructive Surgery, and Surgical Critical Care, The Burn Center at Santa Clara Valley Medical Center, Stanford University, CA

**BARCLAY T. STEWART, MD, PhD**
Assistant Professor of Trauma, Burn, and Critical Care Surgery, UW Medicine Regional Burn Center at Harborview Medical Center, University of Washington, Seattle, Washington, USA

**OSCAR E. SUMAN-VEJAS, PhD**
Professor, Department of Surgery, Division of Surgical Sciences, University of Texas Medical Branch, Galveston, Texas, USA

**CODY THORNBURG, DPT**
Physical Therapist, Certified Lymphedema Specialist, Burn Therapy, Arizona Burn Center, Valleywise Health, Phoenix, Arizona, USA

**LORI TURGEON, PT, DPT**
Director of the Therapeutic Services, Shriners Children's Boston, Boston, Massachusetts, USA

**EMMA TURNER, BA**
The University of Texas Southwestern Medical Center, Dallas, Texas, USA

**MARIA TWICHELL, MD**
Assistant Professor, Department of Physical Medicine and Rehabilitation, School of Medicine, University of Pittsburgh, Pittsburgh, Pennsylvania, USA

**RENEE WARTHMAN, MS, OTR/L, BT-C, CHT**
Arizona Burn Center, Valleywise Health Medical Center, Phoenix, Arizona, USA

**CHRISTOPHER WHITEHEAD, PT**
Shriners Children's Texas, Galveston, Texas, USA

**EMILY WIRDZEK, DPT**
Physical Therapist, Burn Therapy, Arizona Burn Center, Valleywise Health, Phoenix, Arizona, USA

**MIRANDA YELVINGTON, MS, OTR/L, BT-C**
Occupational Therapist, Department of Rehabilitation, Arkansas Children's Hospital, Little Rock, Arkansas, USA

# Contents

Alison Haruta and Samuel P. Mandell

Burn injuries can affect patients from all walks of life and represent a significant healthcare problem globally. The skin is the largest organ of the body
and consequences of injury range of minor pain to severe end-organ dysfunction and even death. The acute assessment and management of
burn-injured patients is a critical part of their short-term and long-term outcomes and often benefit from specialty, multidisciplinary care. Local wound
care and appropriate excision and grafting are important parts of managing
the functional, cosmetic, and physiologic derangements caused by burn injuries. Large burns also require judicious fluid resuscitation. Electrical, chemical, and inhalational injuries are less common than thermal burns but require
additional care and are often associated with increased morbidity.

Johanna H. Nunez and Audra T. Clark

Following severe burns, patients have unique metabolic derangements
that make adequate nutritional support imperative for their survival and recovery. Patients with burns have persistent and prolonged hypermetabolic
states that lead to increased catabolism following injury. During rehabilitation, catabolism leads to increased muscle wasting and cachexia. Failure
to adequately meet the patient's increased nutritional requirements can
lead to poor wound healing, increased infections, and overall organ dysfunction. Because of these risks, adequate assessment and provision of
nutritional needs are imperative to care for these patients.

Audrey O'Neil, Danika Hines, Emily Wirdzek, Cody Thornburg, Derek Murray,
and John Porter

Rehabilitation therapies in the burn acute care environment continue to
evolve. Immediate access to therapy is considered standard, and therapy
is a key component of the transprofessional care team. Early positioning,
edema management, and therapy care in the intensive care unit (ICU) environment can limit later complications; mobility in the ICU can be engaged
safely using a systems-based approach in the absence of nondirectable
agitation. Later in the course of acute care, early ambulation is an appropriate intervention that can improve outcomes.

> This article presents information on the benefits of exercise in counteracting the detrimental effects of bed rest, and/or severe burns. Exercise is key for maintaining physical function, lean body mass, metabolic recovery, and psychosocial health after major burn injuries. The details of an exercise training program conducted in severely burned persons are presented, as well as information on the importance of proper regulation of body temperature during exercise or physical activity. The sections on exercise and thermoregulation are followed by a section on the role of exercise in scarring and contractures. Finally, gaps in the current knowledge of exercise, thermoregulation, and contractures are presented.

> Burns are the fifth leading cause of non-fatal childhood injuries. Physiological differences between children and adults lead to unique considerations when treating young burn survivors. In addition to the physical and psychological concerns which must be considered in adult burn rehabilitation, pediatric burn rehabilitation must also consider the developmental stage of the child, preexisting developmental delays, and the impact of scaring on growth and motor skill attainment. Treatment of pediatric burn survivors requires a multidisciplinary approach centered around caring for not only the child but also for their parents, siblings, and other caregivers. For children who sustain burns early in life, long-term follow-up is essential and should be conducted under the guidance of a burn center for the early identification of needed interventions during periods of growth and development. This article considers pediatric-specific factors, which may present during the rehabilitation of a child with a burn injury.

> The number of older people is increasing and as a result so will the number of older adult patients who present with a burn injury. There are distinct differences between older and younger burn patients, particularly with respect to skin anatomy and physiology and frailty. These are 2 important factors that influence the rehabilitation efforts with respect to older adult burn patients. There has been minimal work done studying the specific rehabilitation of older adult burn patients. More work is needed to fully understand the rehabilitation needs of older adult burn patients.

> Psychological distress is common following a burn injury, and many burn survivors have pre-morbid psychiatric illnesses including mood and trauma-related disorders, and substance and alcohol use. This article is intended to be used by all interdisciplinary health care team members to improve the identification and treatment of common psychological concerns experienced by survivors and is organized to follow the general recovery timeline.

Burn injury commonly causes long-term physical impairments and psychosocial limitations that impact survivorship. This article uses the World
Health Organization (WHO) International Classification of Functioning, Disability and Health (ICF) framework to summarize burn rehabilitation outcomes related to body functions and structures and how they relate to
activities and participation within the social context. This article will contribute to a better understanding of burn recovery, facilitate the identification of specific and meaningful issues common to burn survivorship that
may be under-reported in prior investigations and guide future rehabilitation to advance long-term burn outcomes.

More than 11 million burn injuries occur each year across the world. Many
people with burn injuries, regardless of injury size, develop hypertrophic
scar, contracture, unstable scar, heterotopic ossification, and disability resulting from these sequelae. Advances in trauma systems, critical care,
safe surgery, and multidisciplinary burn care have markedly improved
the survival of people who have experienced extensive burn injuries.
Burn scar reconstruction aims to improve or restore physical function,
confidence, and body image. Like acute burn care, burn scar reconstruction requires thoughtful, coordinated approaches along the continuum of
burn injury, recovery, and rehabilitation.

# PHYSICAL MEDICINE AND REHABILITATION CLINICS OF NORTH AMERICA

**FORTHCOMING ISSUES**

*February 2024*
**Disorders of Consciousness**
Sunil Kothari and Bei Zhang, *Editors*

*May 2024*
**Innovations in Stroke Recovery and Rehabilitation**
Joel Stein and Joan Stilling, *Editors*

*August 2024*
**Traumatic Brain Injury Rehabilitation**
Amy Hao and Blessen C. Eapen, *Editors*

**RECENT ISSUES**

*August 2023*
**Post-Covid Rehabilitation**
Monica Verduzco-Gutierrez, *Editor*

*May 2023*
**Shoulder Rehabilitation**
Thomas (Quin) Throckmorton, *Editor*

*February 2023*
**Orthobiologics**
Michael Khadavi and Luga Podesta, *Editors*

---

**SERIES OF RELATED INTEREST**

*Orthopedic Clinics*
*https://www.orthopedic.theclinics.com/*
*Neurologic Clinics*
*https://www.neurologic.theclinics.com/*
*Clinics in Sports Medicine*
*https://www.sportsmed.theclinics.com/*

---

**VISIT THE CLINICS ONLINE!**
Access your subscription at:
www.theclinics.com

# Foreword

# Burn Rehabilitation

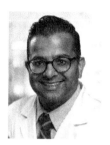

Blessen C. Eapen, MD
*Consulting Editor*

The skin is the largest organ in the body and the main protective barrier against external stimuli. The skin is involved with regulation of body temperature, immunologic response, sensation, endocrine and exocrine activity, and other regulatory functions. The skin is the first barrier to the environment and can be susceptible to burn injuries caused by thermal, chemical, electrical, or radiation contact. Burn injuries can vary in severity from mild superficial burns to full-thickness burns. While superficial burns can often be treated in the outpatient setting, there is a subset of partial- or full-thickness burns that may require acute hospitalization and additional management in specialized burn treatment units.

Burn rehabilitation is a specialized area of physical medicine and rehabilitation that starts at the date of injury, to prevent long-term complications, such as scarring, neuropathies, and contractures, and to maximize nutritional status and promote early mobilization. Burn rehabilitation focuses on a holistic approach to treatment and management of burn injuries, including medical, physical, functional, and psychological recovery of individuals who have suffered burn injuries. Burn rehabilitation typically involves an interdisciplinary team approach and may include a physiatrist, pain medicine physician, wound care nurses, physical therapists, occupational therapists, psychologists, nutritionist, social workers, and other specialists, depending on the specific needs of the patient.

Burn rehabilitation is a comprehensive and patient-centric process with individualized goals and interventions, which may vary depending on the severity of the burn, the location of the injury, associated medical comorbidities, and the unique needs and goals of the patient and caregiver. The rehabilitation course can last from months to years, thus requiring continuous care and support to maximize outcomes and well-being. Burn rehabilitation treatment paradigms have expanded over the last decade and continue to evolve and grow. We want to thank Dr Kowalske and the expert

Phys Med Rehabil Clin N Am 34 (2023) xiii–xiv
https://doi.org/10.1016/j.pmr.2023.07.004
1047-9651/23/© 2023 Published by Elsevier Inc.

team of clinicians, who contributed their time and effort to sharing their valuable clinical experience and expertise with the physical medicine and rehabilitation community!

Blessen C. Eapen, MD
Physical Medicine and Rehabilitation Service
David Geffen School of Medicine at UCLA
VA Greater Los Angeles Health Care System
11301 Wilshire Blvd
Los Angeles, CA 90073, USA

*E-mail addresses:*
Beapen@mednet.ucla.edu; Blessen.eapen2@va.gov

# Preface

# Evolution of Burn Rehabilitation

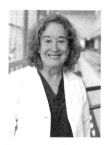

Karen Kowalske, MD
*Editor*

It has been 12 years since the last issue of *Physical Medicine and Rehabilitation Clinics of North America* on Burn Rehabilitation. During that time, acute care of burn injury has improved with the expansion of available antibiotics and wound coverage products. Most notably, there has been a dramatic shift toward acknowledging and addressing the experiences of burn survivors. The American Burn Association established the Aftercare and Integration Committee, a joint effort with the Phoenix Society for Burn Survivors. This group provides education at the annual meeting about issues associated with living with a burn injury, including returning to work, social activities, and family life after acute treatment. The Burn State of the Science Meetings now includes burn survivors in each area of discussion.

From a research perspective, there has been a significant increase in studies examining the incidence of complications and predicting outcomes. We now know that one-third of patients with a major burn leave the hospital with a contracture,[1] and delirium is a common complication especially for those in the ICU and on a ventilator.[2] Half of burn survivors report muscle weakness and fatigue at more than a decade post injury.[3] Psychiatric symptoms and illnesses are also common among burn survivors, and research has shown that at 6 months post injury 55% of burn survivors met criteria for at least one psychiatric condition.[4] It is established that skin issues persist after the original injury, but recent research suggests that medical issues associated with burn injury, such as kidney injury, endocrine changes, lung scarring, and bone loss, can lead to persistent challenges as the survivor ages and underscores the importance of long-term monitoring and education for providers. There is also increased recognition of the role of inpatient rehabilitation in facilitating positive outcomes, such as return to work.[5]

The rehabilitation community is now shifting toward a focus on intervention trials to identify and create effective treatments. This is well demonstrated throughout the issue, including new practice guidelines, early mobilization and exercise, utilization of nonpharmacologic pain control adjuncts, and many other advances.

Phys Med Rehabil Clin N Am 34 (2023) xv–xvi
https://doi.org/10.1016/j.pmr.2023.06.031
1047-9651/23/© 2023 Published by Elsevier Inc.

The next important steps are more closely addressing all aspects of burn recovery, including psychological and social wellness is now the standard of care, including early treatment of psychological distress, and better addressing the long-term medical and psychosocial issues associated with burn injury recovery.

Facilitating optimum outcomes after a major burn injury requires knowledge across multiple domains, including wound and scar management as well as rehabilitation techniques, such as exercise, medication management, and understanding the range of available support services. Knowledge of common complications and evidence-based interventions is essential for providing top-quality care for burn survivors.

Karen Kowalske, MD
Department of Physical Medicine and Rehabilitation
University of Texas
Southwestern Medical Center
5323 Harry Hines Boulevard
Dallas, TX 75390-9055, USA

*E-mail address:*
Karen.Kowalske@UTSouthwestern.edu

## REFERENCES

1. Goverman J, et al. Adult contractures in burn injury: a burn model system national database study. J Burn Care Res 2017;38(1):e328–36.
2. Agarwal V, et al. Prevalence and risk factors for development of delirium in burn intensive care unit patients. J Burn Care Res 2010;31(5):706–15.
3. Holavanahalli RK, Helm PA, Kowalske KJ. Long-term outcomes in patients surviving large burns: the musculoskeletal system. J Burn Care Res 2016;37(4):243–54.
4. Palmu R, et al. Mental disorders after burn injury: a prospective study. Burns 2011; 37(4):601–9.
5. Espinoza LF, et al. Postacute care setting is associated with employment after burn injury. Arch Phys Med Rehabil 2019;100(11):2015–21.

# Assessment and Management of Acute Burn Injuries

Alison Haruta, MD*, Samuel P. Mandell, MD, MPH

## KEYWORDS

• Acute burn • Burn assessment • Early burn management

## KEY POINTS

- Burn injuries are a global problem that can result in significant functional, cosmetic, and physiologic derangements.
- The acute assessment and management of burn-injured patients is a critical part of their short-term and long-term outcomes and often benefit from specialty, multidisciplinary care.
- Judicious fluid resuscitation for large burns and diligent local wound care is important to the survival of the patient and success of the future skin grafts.

## INTRODUCTION

Over 450,000 burn injuries occur each year in the United States requiring medical attention with an estimated 4000 resulting in death.[1] Globally, burn injuries are also a significant healthcare problem, with an estimated 180,000 deaths annually.[1] These injuries are caused by a variety of mechanisms such as scalds, flame, chemicals, or electricity in settings from the home to the workplace resulting in significant pain, physical disability, psychosocial disorders, and in some cases, death. Minimizing the impact of burn injury begins with prevention. This includes education about safe practices for handling flammable substances, using protective gear when working with hot materials, installing smoke detectors and fire extinguishers in homes and workplaces, and supervising children around cooking, fires, outlets, and other hazards.

When prevention fails, rapid assessment and management of acute burn injuries are essential to improving patient outcomes. Initial management of acute burns involves the principles of Advance Burn Life Support (ABLS)[2] and the primary survey, which provide guidance for the management of the initial burn up to 24 hours postinjury.

Department of Burns, Trauma, Acute, and Critical Care Surgery, UT Southwestern, 5323 Harry Hines Boulevard, Dallas, TX 75390-9005, USA
* Corresponding author.
E-mail address: aharuta@uw.edu

Phys Med Rehabil Clin N Am 34 (2023) 701–716
https://doi.org/10.1016/j.pmr.2023.06.019

In cases where mechanical trauma is present with the burn injury, Advanced Trauma Life Support (ATLS)[3] should also be followed.

Effective management of burn injuries requires a multidisciplinary team including prehospital providers, burn surgeons, nurses, physical and occupational therapists, psychologists, nutritionists, and family support. Here we focus on the provider assessment and initial management of acute burns.

## PATIENT EVALUATION

Acute burn injuries are defined as tissue damage caused by thermal, chemical, electrical, or radiation exposure. They are classified according to the mechanism, depth of injury, location, and total body surface area (TBSA) affected. Patient factors may contribute to the overall severity of the burn including medical comorbidities, concomitant trauma, presence of inhalational injury, and age.

Life-threatening injuries should be identified and treated in the primary survey. The primary survey evaluates the airway, breathing, circulation, disability, and exposure. Large-bore peripheral IVs should be secured and may be placed through burns; Intraosseous access should be used if peripheral IVs cannot be obtained rapidly. Initial fluids should be started during this time for large burns which will be discussed further in the resuscitation section later in discussion. Once immediate life threats are addressed, we proceed with the secondary survey which includes a complete physical exam and detailed burn assessment including history, depth, and size. It is important to remove jewelry which may a tourniquet effect as the patient becomes edematous and be mindful of hospital bands.

### Burn Mechanism

The mechanism describes the inciting agent leading to the burn. It may be scald, flame, contact, electrical, radiation, or chemical. Each may give clues to other potential injuries, such as a flame burn in an enclosed area increasing the risk for inhalational injury, or an electrical injury increasing the risk of other traumatic injuries such as fracture or dislocation. It is also important to understand the circumstances under which the injury occurred, for example, when the reported mechanism does not match the injury, this may raise the concern for abuse or neglect in vulnerable populations.

### Burn Depth

Depth is determined by the temperature, duration of contact, and skin thickness of the exposed area (**Fig. 1**). Superficial burns, also known as first-degree burns, involve only the epidermis and usually heal without scarring in 3 to 4 days. They are characterized by erythema and are painful to the touch but do not blister. A classic example of a first-degree burn is a sunburn (**Fig. 2**A). These are not included in the calculation of burn size. Treatment includes symptom control and topical moisturizers. Partial-thickness burns, or second-degree burns, involve the epidermis and part of the dermis, leaving some epithelial elements (**Fig. 2**B). They can further be subdivided into superficial and deep. Superficial partial thickness burns are painful and blister with the underlying wound maintaining moisture and a blanching pink color; typically, these take 2 to 3 weeks to heal. Deep partial thickness burns are painful, paler pink that may progress to white; typically, these take 3 to 9 weeks to heal and may result in severe scarring and loss of function. Many deep partial thickness burns benefit from excision and grafting to accelerate wound closure.[4–6] Full-thickness burns (previously third-degree burns), extend through the epidermis and

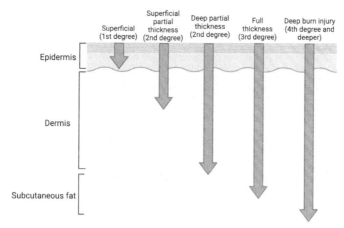

Fig. 1. Burn depth. (Created with Biorender.com.)

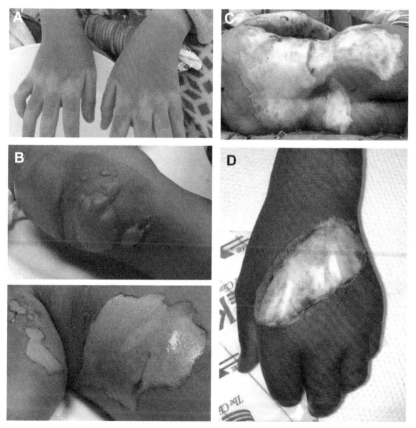

Fig. 2. Clinical examples of different burn depth. (A) Superficial burn. (B) Partial thickness burn. (C) Full-thickness burn. (D) Very deep burn injury. (Photo credit [A–C] Ashley Sanders, PA-C; [D] Alison Haruta, MD.)

dermis (**Fig. 2**C). They are insensate, non-blanching wounds that may appear white or deep red under eschar that may be black. There may be initial blistering but the underlying skin is dry. These are often seen with flame burns and grease burns and are typically treated with excision and grafting. Very deep burn injuries (4th-6th degree), extend into the subcutaneous tissue and sometimes down to muscle or bone. These burns can be seen with electrical injuries or deep thermal burns to areas with thinner skin (**Fig. 2**D).

### Burn Size

Burn size accounts for the surface area of burn that is partial thickness and deeper. For smaller burns, the size may be estimated using the patient's palm and fingers which represents 1% TBSA (**Fig. 3**). One method to estimate the size of larger burns is by using the rule of nines, which divides the body into regions, each representing 9% or multiples of 9% TBSA (**Fig. 4**). The Lund and Browder chart considers the age of the patient since body proportions change over time (with children having relatively

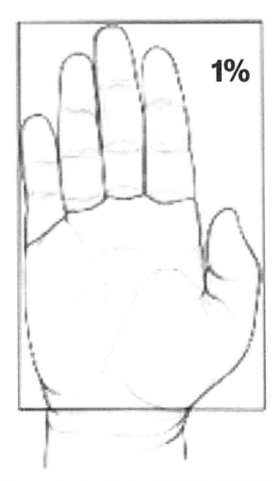

**Fig. 3.** Palm and finger method for estimating %TBSA.[2] (Credit: 2018 American Burn Association, ABLS provider manual.)

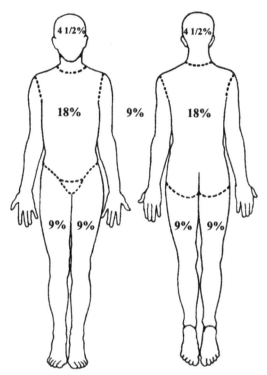

**Fig. 4.** Rule of 9's.[2] (Credit: 2018 American Burn Association, ABLS provider manual.)

larger heads and smaller lower extremities compared to adults) and subdivides body parts into smaller units to aid in more accurate calculations (**Fig. 5**). Newer tools include software such as Pixamed and smartphone apps which aim to rapidly and accurately calculate %TBSA.[7,8]

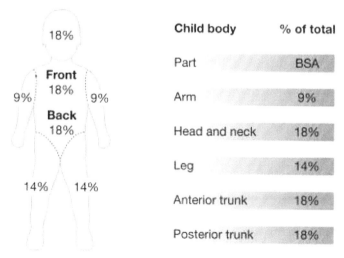

**Fig. 5.** Lund and Browder Chart.[2] (Credit: 2018 American Burn Association, ABLS provider manual.)

## TRANSFER TO SPECIALTY BURN CARE

The American Burn Association (ABA) has established verification criteria for burn centers to ensure that verified burn centers provide high-quality specialty burn care. Some burns can safely be managed outside of these centers and the ABA has established criteria to transfer (**Table 1**).[1] The patient should be stabilized with any life-threatening injuries addressed. The wounds can be covered with clean dressings and the patient should be kept warm. For larger burns, IV access should be secured and a foley catheter placed to closely monitor urine output. For longer transport times, a plan should be in place for adjusting resuscitation fluid rates (see later in discussion).

## RESUSCITATION

Early and appropriate volume resuscitation is crucial. Burn injury leads to increased vascular permeability beginning at the time of injury, peaking around 8 to 10 hours post burn, and persisting for about 24 hours post burn. The capillary leak allows fluid to pass into the extravascular space, and the degree of leak is proportional to the % TBSA.[9,10] Burns involving more than 20% TBSA in adults or 15% TBSA in children require fluid resuscitation as the capillary leak is no longer localized but becomes systemic. The goal of fluid resuscitation in burn-injured patients is to replace the intravascular volume and prevent shock. Under resuscitation leads to hypotension and organ dysfunction, while over resuscitation leads to pulmonary compromise, compartment syndromes, and other complications.

### Fluid Rates

In the prehospital or emergency department setting, a patient may have a large burn but an exact %TBSA is not yet available. During the primary survey, we use standard initial fluid rates based on age until a %TBSA is calculated in the secondary survey. The American Burn Association recommends starting lactated ringers at 125 cc/h

| Table 1 ABA burn referral criteria[1] | |
| --- | --- |
| | **Immediate Consultation with Consideration for Transfer** |
| Thermal Burns | • Full thickness burns<br>• Partial thickness $\geq$ 10% TBSA<br>• Any deep partial or full thickness burns involving the face, hands, genitalia, feet, perineum, or over any joints<br>• Patients with burns and other comorbidities<br>• Patients with concomitant traumatic injuries<br>• Poorly controlled pain |
| Inhalation Injury | • All patients with suspected inhalation injury |
| Pediatrics ($\leq$14 y, or < 30 kg) | • All Pediatrics burns may benefit from burn center referral due to pain, dressing change needs, rehabilitation, patient/caregiver needs, or non-accidental trauma |
| Chemical Injuries | • All chemical injuries |
| Electrical Injuries | • All high voltage ($\geq$1,000V) electrical injuries<br>• Lightning injury |

American Burn Association. Guidelines for Burn Patient Referral, 2022. https://ameriburn.org/resources/burnreferral/.

for children 5 years and younger, 250 cc for children age 6 to 13 years, and 500 cc/h for patients 14 years and older.

Once a specific %TBSA has been determined calculate predicted fluid requirements using an estimate such as the Parkland formula, Modified Brooke formula, or ABA consensus formula (**Box 1**).[1,11] These calculate the expected 24-hour fluid requirement with the first half being given in the first 8 hours and the second half given over the next 16 hours.

Regardless of the starting rate, fluids are titrated hourly to urine output with a goal of 0.5 mL/kg/h (30–50 cc/h) in adults and 1 to 1.5 cc/kg/h in children. We increase fluids by about 10% if the urine output is not at goal for the previous hour. We use the Burn Navigator for the first 24 hours postburn as an adjunct to help guide resuscitation. The Burn Navigator is a clinical decision tool that uses the patient age, weight, and burn size to calculate a starting fluid rate and recommends hourly changes based on the prior hour's urine output. It also identifies patients that may be "non responders" and should be considered for other interventions. Early results demonstrate lower overall fluid volumes as well as decreased incidence of burn shock.[12–14] While this tool can be helpful to guide resuscitation, it is not a replacement for bedside evaluation and clinical judgment. We bolus for evidence of hypovolemic shock, such as hypotension, but not for low urine output. Other endpoints such as POCUS, lactate, and advanced noninvasive monitoring may be helpful in patients with signs of shock. If the urine output is at goal, the fluids should be down titrated; providers must be diligent to minimize the burden of fluid overload by decreasing excess fluid administration. After the initial 24 hours postburn has passed, we decrease fluids as able by about 10% per hour until a weight-based maintenance rate is reached.

### Pediatric Considerations

Pediatric patients around 30 kg or smaller have higher volume to surface area and lower glycogen storage, so they require maintenance fluids in addition to their calculated resuscitative rate as well as dextrose supplementation. We recommend adding D5LR at a weight-based maintenance rate that remains constant throughout the acute phase.

---

**Box 1**
**ABA consensus resuscitation formula**

- 2 to 4 mL/kg/% TBSA for the first 24 h postburn
  - Give 1/2 over the first 8 hours postburn
  - Give 1/2 over the next 16 hours postburn

- Adults: 2 mL/kg/% TBSA

- Children: 3 mL/kg/% TBSA

- Electrical: 4 mL/kg/% TBSA

In adults:
- Adjust fluid rate hourly for goal urine output 0.5 mL/kg/h

In children:
- Adjust fluid rate hourly for goal urine output 1 mL/kg/h
- If < 30 kg, add dextrose containing fluid at weight based maintenance rate in addition to the resuscitative fluids.

Created in Word by Ali Haruta, MD.

## FAILING RESUSCITATIONS

Early identification of a failing resuscitation is important to promptly initiate rescue therapies and identify nonresponders. Failure can occur anytime during the resuscitation, so frequent reassessment is essential. While there is no clear definition, concerning signs include fluid requirements in excess of the predicted rate, persistent oliguria, worsening acidosis, and hypotension despite fluid escalation.[15] It should also raise concern if at any point the estimated fluid volume exceeds the Ivy index, or 250 mL/kg, as this has independently been associated with increased mortality[16,17] Some reasons for failure include the underestimation of burn size, delayed presentation, concurrent inhalation injury, electrical injury, or trauma.

### Albumin

One adjunct for a difficult resuscitation is albumin, which in theory increases the oncotic pressure to decrease fluid leakage, though clinical utilization is variable.[18,19] Colloids have a long history in burn resuscitation, but use declined as crystalloids provided effective resuscitation. A 1998 review noted higher risk of death in patients who received albumin.[19,20] In 2000, the problem of over resuscitation, termed "fluid creep," was described which renewed an interest in colloid use.[21] Currently, it is used by most as a "rescue" adjunct to failing resuscitations and several studies suggest that this improves outcomes.[22–24] The *Acute Burn Resuscitation Multicenter Prospective Trial* (ABRUPT), a prospective observational study again demonstrated the variability of albumin use with 2/3 of the enrolled patients receiving albumin at 15h ± 8.4 h postburn; it also showed albumin rescue was used most frequently in older patients, larger/deeper burns, and patients with more severe organ dysfunction at presentation, improving the in/out balance in patients whose crystalloid volumes were in excess of predicted.[25] *The Acute Burn Resuscitation Multicenter Prospective Trial (ABRUPT2) is a prospective randomized trial currently enrolling to look at early albumin vs crystalloid only resuscitation.* In our practice, we typically use albumin as an adjunct in patients not responding to resuscitation at 8 to 12 hours postburn, starting at a rate 1/3 of the crystalloid rate.

### Fresh Frozen Plasma

FFP is an effective volume expander, decreasing fluid volumes and improving clinical outcomes when added to resuscitation,[26,27] however cost, availability, risk of bloodborne disease transmission, and its association with the development of transfusion-related lung injury has limited its widespread clinical use. Animal models have demonstrated that the endotheliopathy of trauma, mediated by damage to the endothelial glycocalyx, is partially reverses by FFP, but not by LR or albumin, to mitigate the vascular permeability in animal hemorrhage models.[28–30] Similarly, the endotheliopathy of burns appears to occur via the same mechanism, suggesting that plasma may mitigate the capillary leak and improve outcomes when used as a resuscitation fluid. The Plasma Resuscitation without Lung Injury (PROPOLIS) trial is a prospective, randomized control trial currently enrolling to evaluate plasma versus crystalloid based burn resuscitation, however there is not presently a standard protocol for plasma use in burns.

### Blood Purification

Plasma exchange can also be used as an adjunct to resuscitation. It is thought to remove the inflammatory mediators of burn shock. There is some retrospective data that demonstrate a benefit to plasma exchange as a rescue therapy with a subsequent decrease in fluid rates, decrease in lactate, and increase the urine output and blood pressure[31–33] though prospective data is lacking.

Another method of clearance is high volume hemofiltration (HVHF) which may have a role in failing burn resuscitation, though data here is also limited. In burn patients with septic shock, it was found to reverse the shock and improve organ dysfunction, though there was no difference in mortality and this was not studied during the initial resuscitation phase as a rescue adjunct.[34]

### Ultra-Early Eschar Excision

Typically, the tangential excision occurs after the patient is resuscitated so as not to worsen the physiologic derangements of the burn injury with the stress and consequences of operation. However, the burn eschar is a source of ongoing inflammatory burden, so in the face of refractory shock, early excision within the first 24 hours has been described and may benefit the patient's physiology.[15]

## WOUND MANAGEMENT

Initial wound care includes the debridement of the dead tissue and coverage with a dressing until the area heals or can be excised and grafted. The wound should be cleansed thoroughly with soap and water. There are many topical options and dressing materials; there is no perfect dressing, but the goal is to promote healing, prevent infection, and provide comfort to the burned area. They should have antibacterial properties, provide moisture, and keep the wound clean and covered without restricting range of motion. As the wound or graft heals, it will contract, so mobilization and specialized therapy should begin early to minimize loss of function.

### Compartment Syndrome and Escharotomies

Compartment syndrome can develop, usually in areas of circumferential full-thickness burn, as the tissue swells, and the burn constricts the area. This can compromise perfusion, as seen in the distal extremities with increasingly tight compartments and diminishing pulses. It can also restrict chest wall and abdominal wall motion which can worsen oxygenation and ventilation manifesting as increased airway pressures. **Fig. 6** demonstrates the typical locations escharotomies are performed but they need not be perfectly located if the pressure is released from the compartment through burned skin. It is more important to avoid nonburned skin and avoid going too deep; escharotomies should be performed just through the eschar to release the dermal bands, but should not go into the subcutaneous fat. Going too deep may lead to bleeding, excess tissue excision, poor graft take, and muscle herniation.

Muscle compartment syndrome may be seen with electrical burns even when the surface injury does not appear as severe. Compartment syndrome is a clinical diagnosis with the patient demonstrating tense compartments, pain out of proportion, and pain with passive motion. Pulselessness, paresthesia, and weakness are late findings. Treatment is with fasciotomies.

### Excision and Coverage

Deeper burns typically require excision and grafting. Tangential excision is the standard method used to remove the nonviable tissue to provide a perfused wound bed for grafting. Current consensus recommends excision before the 6th day postburn, and most undergo initial excision within 2 to 5 days postburn. A recent retrospective cohort study across almost 900 US centers found that early excision within 48 hours postburn was associated with fewer complications, shorter ICU stays, and shorter hospital stays.[35]

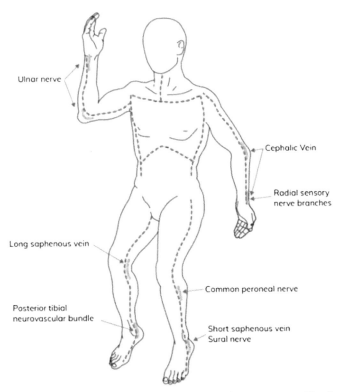

**Fig. 6.** Escharotomy Incisions and Adjacent Neurovascular Structures. (Credit: Butts CC, Holmes JH, Carter JE. Surgical Escharotomy and Decompressive Therapies in Burns. *J Burn Care Res.* Feb 19 2020;41(2):263-269. https://doi.org/10.1093/jbcr/irz152.)

Large burns sometimes require staged excision as the eschar removal must be balanced against operative time, blood loss, and hypothermia. Many patients require blood transfusions perioperatively. Extremity excisions may be done under tourniquet to mitigate some of this. In contrast, fascial excision removes the skin and subcutaneous tissue down to a relatively avascular fascial plane which often leads to decreased blood loss but may remove more tissue than necessary, resulting in more deformities and functional loss.

### Autograft

Excised wounds will usually need an autograft, though the timing depends on the patient's clinical picture, donor sites available, and viability of the wound bed. Most areas are covered with split-thickness skin grafts (STSG) which include the epidermis and partial dermis from the donor site whereas full-thickness skin grafts harvest the epidermis and dermis. STSGs are harvested using a dermatome set to 0.006 to 0.014 inches. These grafts can be placed on the wound bed as a sheet, which we commonly use to cover cosmetic areas such as the neck, hands, and feet (**Fig. 7**A), or meshed to various degrees (**Fig. 7**B). Donor site selection depends on what skin is available, color match, and what will heal with the best cosmesis and least amount of pain. In general, we avoid crossing joints and avoid arms below the elbow and legs below the knee if alternate grafts sites are available; in large burns this is not avoidable,

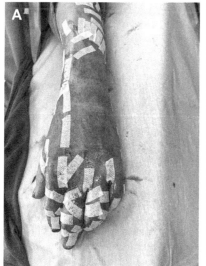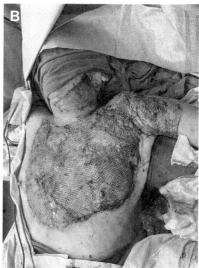

**Fig. 7.** Grafted Burn Wounds. (*A*) Sheet graft. Photo credit: Sam Mandell, MD. (*B*) Meshed Graft. (Photo credit: Sam Mandell, MD.)

and these areas do provide adequate STSG. The scalp provides good color match for face/neck though may be more difficult to harvest due to the convexity of the scalp.

Grafts are covered with a dressing that is left in place for typically 2 to 5 days depending on the area to minimize shear forces and encourage graft incorporation.

### Skin Substitutes

If the wound bed or patient is not ready for autografting, there are temporary coverage options to protect the wound bed and minimize insensible losses. Allograft, donated human cadaver skin, is commonly used for temporary grafting or on top of a widely meshed graft to protect it and confer a coverage benefit. In the latter example, the allograft is allowed to separate and slough off as the autograft heals in. If only allograft is covering the wound bed, these patients typically need another operation in about 1 to 2 weeks for repeat excision and autografting. Acellular fish skin xenografts may be a future option for temporary coverage.[00]

Myriad biologic and synthetic options are also on the market which we use on a case by case basis. They may provide temporary coverage to a large or poorly vascularized wound bed, act as a scaffolding for the dermal matrix formation, or be used in conjunction with an STSG to accelerate revascularization and healing. This is not meant to be a comprehensive review of these products but rather to mention that alternatives are being developed for coverage of wounds that may be too deep, too large, or otherwise not ready for autografting.

### Epidermal Autografts

Epidermal Autografts, (RECELL, Valencia, CA), or "spray on skin," utilizes a small sized STSG which is enzymatically and mechanically processed to suspend epidermal cells is a buffer. These are then applied to the prepared wound bed. We selectively use this method to cover partial thickness burns if healthy dermis appears present after excision. Current data suggests decreased donor site requirements and faster healing with less scarring, fewer procedures to wound closure, and shorter lengths of stay for small burns.[37-39] It can also be used in combination with meshed autografts to help fill in the interstitial spaces and accelerate healing.

## CONSEQUENCES OF HYPERMETABOLISM

Large burn injuries lead to a profound alteration in metabolism with high rates of protein catabolism leading to muscle wasting and end-organ dysfunction. It is thought to be due in part to a prolonged stress response leading to sustained and increased expression of stress-related hormones including catecholamines and glucocorticoids.[40] Initially patients have decreased metabolic rates in the first 48 hours postburn; this gradually increases until around 5 days postburn where it plateaus and can persist for up to 3 years.[41] Care of the burn-injured patient aims to address this response and mitigate negative side effects.

### Nutrition

Adequate nutrition is an important component of burn care. Many patients are able to tolerate oral intake but because of their high caloric needs, patients with greater than 20% TBSA burns usually require supplementation with tube feeding. Dietician consultation is recommended and tube feeds should be started early. This will be discussed further in a later article.

### Stress Ulcer Prophylaxis

Burn-injured patients are at increased risk for stress ulcers as the systemic response leads to splanchnic hypoperfusion causing gastrointestinal ischemia and mucosal atrophy which decreases mucosal healing and increases the risk of ulceration. Gastric tube feeding/oral intake decreases this risk and we treat with an H2 blocker for prophylaxis in large burns as well as in intubated patients, similar to other critically ill populations.

## SPECIAL CONSIDERATIONS

There are some specific cases that require special management and may increase the volume of fluids a patient needs during resuscitation compared to what is expected.

### Inhalation Injury

Inhalation injury can add significant mortality to a burn-injured patient. There are three main mechanisms of injury.

#### Supraglottic injury
Upper airways can suffer thermal damage as hot gases are inhaled and cooled; this is most common in patients who were in an explosion or unconscious in an enclosed fire. This leads to upper airway edema which typically peaks 24 to 48 hours postburn, so these patients often need intubation until the swelling decreases, and they have a cuff leak. We do not recommend routine steroids in these cases.

#### Subglottic injury
Lower airway inhalation injury can lead to lower airway mucosal damage, triggering an inflammatory cascade that worsens pulmonary function, fluid requirements, and overall metabolic demands. Typically these patients have a history of being trapped in an enclosed space fire or inhaled chemical. Singed nasal hairs and facial burns are less indicative of a true inhalational injury without the right history. Admission labs include carboxyhemoglobin levels which are concerning if > 10. Bronchoscopy may be used

to grade the severity of injury as higher grades are associated with higher morbidity and mortality.[42,43] The treatment is supportive care with aggressive pulmonary toilet and inhaled triple therapy with inhaled heparin to decrease the fibrin plug and airway cast formation, albuterol for bronchodilation, and N-acetylcysteine to combat the free radical damage from the high oxygen concentrations. These patients often need intubation and may go on to develop complications such as ARDS and pneumonia.

### Systemic poisoning

Carbon monoxide (CO) is an odorless, colorless gas created by incomplete combustion of carbon-containing materials. It has an affinity for hemoglobin over 200 times that of oxygen which can lead to profound and sometimes irreversible hypoxic damage. The oxygen saturation on the pulse oximetry may be falsely elevated so carboxyhemoglobin levels should be measured. Treatment is with 100% oxygen as it decreases the half-life of CO from about 4 hours to about 1 hour.

Smoke inhalation injury may also lead to hydrogen cyanide poisoning which binds cytochrome oxidase and inhibits cellular respiration. It rarely occurs without smoke inhalation and high levels of carboxyhemoglobin may be a clue to its presence. Treatment is empiric with hydroxocobalamin, which binds the cyanide and increases the rate of excretion. We recommend treating with hydroxocobalamin in patients with a clinical history of smoke inhalation, GCS less than 10, carboxyhemoglobin greater than 10%, and lactate greater than 10 mmol/L.[44]

### Electrical Burns

Management of electrical burns partly depends on whether the exposure was low voltage (<1000V) or high voltage (>1000V). This is a convenient division to identify cases where exposure to high doses of electrical current is likely. In both cases, the patient may have cutaneous injuries known as contact points that may give clues to the path of the current. Low-voltage electrical burns, such as those caused by most household exposures, typically have minimal deep tissue injury and contact points may or may not need local wound care depending on the size and location. These patients should get an EKG and if normal, with no loss of consciousness, and manageable symptoms from the burn, can often discharge. One case of note is oral commissure injury for electrical cords in the mouth. These patients have attention to mouth position and range of motion, and watched for bleeding; characteristically around 7 to 10 days postburn the labial branch of the facial artery may bleed. It is managed with direct pressure inside the cheek.

High voltage electrical injuries carry a risk of deeper tissue destruction regardless of the size of the cutaneous wound. These patients should be admitted with cardiac monitoring; we typically observe them in the ICU for at least 24 hours postburn and serially evaluate for compartment syndrome. Due to the risk of neurologic symptoms and cataracts, we also recommend a neurologic exam and an ophthalmic exam during the admission. They are also at risk for rhabdomyolysis from the tissue destruction, so the urine color should be noted to assess for myoglobin; if the urine appears brown or red, we increase the IV fluid rate to target a urine output of 50 to 100 cc/h until the pigment clears. These patients often have an associated trauma and should be examined and evaluated for other injuries.

### Chemical Burns

Chemical burns account for about 3% of admitted burn patients.[1] If the chemical exposure is a liquid, it should be irrigated with large volumes of water for at least 30 minutes. If the chemical exposure is dry, this should be brushed off the patient prior to irrigation. Additional chemicals should not be used to neutralize the substance. Hydrofluoric acid burns lead to hypocalcemia so these patients are treated with topical calcium gluconate to the wound bed as well as IV calcium gluconate for symptomatic hypocalcemia. Refractory hypocalcemia may necessitate emergent excision.[45] Tar burns are managed by first cooling the tar to solidify it and dissipate the heat, then removed with a solvent, such as Neosporin ointment, to dissolve it and prevent further damage from removal.

### Non-accidental Trauma

Providers and burn care team must evaluate the burn pattern for consistency with the history of injury to evaluate for NAT, especially in vulnerable populations such as children and the elderly. If this is suspected, it should be reported in accordance with local laws and regulations.

## SUMMARY

Burn injuries affect a wide range of patients and are a significant burden on the healthcare system. Prevention is a cornerstone of decreasing this, however once an acute burn arrives at your center, a rapid, multidisciplinary approach is needed to improve outcomes for the patients. Transfer to a burn specialty center may be indicated in some patients given the unique surgical and physiologic management they often require.

## CLINICS CARE POINTS

- If accurate %TBSA has not yet been calculated for adult burns >20% TBSA, start fluids at 500cc/hr and titrate hourly based on urine output and vital signs rather than delaying resuscitation.
- The goal of burn resuscitation is to prevent shock rather than react to it so we titrate the fluid rates based on urine output and boluses should be utilzied when there are signs of shock such as hypotension.
- Fluids are a necessary part of the early management of large burn injuries but early recognition of a non-responder is important to mitigate over administartion of non beneficial fluid volume.
- Understanding the mechanism of the burn is important to raise suspicion for additional injuries that require assessment and treatment such as inhalation injury, non-accidental trauma, or concomitant traumatic injuries.

## DISCLOSURES

The authors have nothing to disclose.

## REFERENCES

1. American Burn Association-Burn Incident Fact Sheet. 2023.
2. Advanced Burn Life Support Course. Accessed April 1, 2023. https://ameriburn.org/wp-content/uploads/2019/08/2018-abls-providermanual.pdf.
3. Advanced Trauma Life Support. Accessed April 1, 2023. https://www.facs.org/quality-programs/trauma/education/advanced-trauma-life-support/.
4. Deitch EA, Wheelahan TM, Rose MP, et al. Hypertrophic burn scars: analysis of variables. J Trauma 1983;23(10):895–8.

5. Johnson RM, Richard R. Partial-thickness burns: identification and management. Adv Skin Wound Care 2003;16(4):178–87, quiz 188-9.

6. Engrav LH, Heimbach DM, Reus JL, et al. Early excision and grafting vs. nonoperative treatment of burns of indeterminant depth: a randomized prospective study. J Trauma. Nov 1983;23(11):1001–4.

7. Pixamed-Wound Care Management Solution. Accessed April 29, 2023. pixamed.com.

8. Cheah AKW, Kangkorn T, Tan EH, et al. The validation study on a three-dimensional burn estimation smart-phone application: accurate, free and fast? Burns Trauma 2018;6:7.

9. Rowan MP, Cancio LC, Elster EA, et al. Burn wound healing and treatment: review and advancements. Crit Care 2015;19:243.

10. Kaddoura I, Abu-Sittah G, Ibrahim A, et al. Burn injury: review of pathophysiology and therapeutic modalities in major burns. Ann Burns Fire Disasters 2017;30(2): 95–102.

11. Vercruysse GA, Alam HB, Martin MJ, et al. Western trauma association critical decisions in trauma: preferred triage and initial management of the burned patient. J Trauma Acute Care Surg 2019;87(5):1239–43.

12. Arcos Burn Navigator. Accessed April 10, 2023. https://us.burnnav.net/.

13. Salinas J, Chung KK, Mann EA, et al. Computerized decision support system improves fluid resuscitation following severe burns: an original study. Crit Care Med 2011;39(9):2031–8.

14. Rizzo JA, Liu NT, Coates EC, et al. Initial results of the american burn association observational multicenter evaluation on the effectiveness of the burn navigator. J Burn Care Res 2022;43(3):728–34.

15. Brownson EG, Pham TN, Chung KK. How to recognize a failed burn resuscitation. Crit Care Clin 2016;32(4):567–75.

16. Ivy ME, Atweh NA, Palmer J, et al. Intra-abdominal hypertension and abdominal compartment syndrome in burn patients. J Trauma 2000;49(3):387–91.

17. Chung KK, Wolf SE, Cancio LC, et al. Resuscitation of severely burned military casualties: fluid begets more fluid. J Trauma 2009;67(2):231–7, discussion 237.

18. Greenhalgh DG. Burn resuscitation: the results of the ISBI/ABA survey. Burns 2010;36(2):176–82.

19. Cartotto R, Greenhalgh D. Colloids in acute burn resuscitation. Crit Care Clin 2016;32(4):507–23.

20. Reviewers CIGA. Human albumin administration in critically ill patients: systematic review of randomised controlled trials. BMJ 1998;317(7153):235–40.

21. Pruitt BA. Protection from excessive resuscitation: "pushing the pendulum back". J Trauma 2000;49(3):567–8.

22. Park SH, Hemmila MR, Wahl WL. Early albumin use improves mortality in difficult to resuscitate burn patients. J Trauma Acute Care Surg 2012;73(5):1294–7.

23. Cochran A, Morris SE, Edelman LS, et al. Burn patient characteristics and outcomes following resuscitation with albumin. Burns 2007;33(1):25–30.

24. Dulhunty JM, Boots RJ, Rudd MJ, et al. Increased fluid resuscitation can lead to adverse outcomes in major-burn injured patients, but low mortality is achievable. Burns 2008;34(8):1090–7.

25. Greenhalgh DG, Cartotto R, Taylor SL, et al. Burn resuscitation practices in north america: results of the acute burn resuscitation multicenter prospective trial (ABRUPT). Ann Surg 2023;277(3):512–9.

26. O'Mara MS, Slater H, Goldfarb IW, et al. A prospective, randomized evaluation of intra-abdominal pressures with crystalloid and colloid resuscitation in burn patients. J Trauma 2005;58(5):1011–8.

27. Choi J, Cooper A, Gomez M, et al. The 2000 moyer award. the relevance of base deficits after burn injuries. J Burn Care Rehabil 2000;21(6):499–505.

28. Torres Filho IP, Torres LN, Salgado C, et al. Plasma syndecan-1 and heparan sulfate correlate with microvascular glycocalyx degradation in hemorrhaged rats after different resuscitation fluids. Am J Physiol Heart Circ Physiol 2016;310(11):H1468–78.

29. Pati S, Peng Z, Wataha K, et al. Lyophilized plasma attenuates vascular permeability, inflammation and lung injury in hemorrhagic shock. PLoS One 2018;13(2):e0192363.

30. Gurney JM, Kozar RA, Cancio LC. Plasma for burn shock resuscitation: is it time to go back to the future? Transfusion 2019;59(S2):1578–86.

31. Klein MB, Edwards JA, Kramer CB, et al. The beneficial effects of plasma exchange after severe burn injury. J Burn Care Res 2009;30(2):243–8.

32. Mosier MJ, DeChristopher PJ, Gamelli RL. Use of therapeutic plasma exchange in the burn unit: a review of the literature. J Burn Care Res 2013;34(3):289–98.

33. Neff LP, Allman JM, Holmes JH. The use of theraputic plasma exchange (TPE) in the setting of refractory burn shock. Burns 2010;36(3):372–8.

34. Chung KK, Coates EC, Smith DJ, et al. High-volume hemofiltration in adult burn patients with septic shock and acute kidney injury: a multicenter randomized controlled trial. Crit Care 2017;21(1):289.

35. Ramsey WA, O'Neil CF, Corona AM, et al. Burn excision within 48 hours portends better outcomes than standard management: a nationwide analysis. J Trauma Acute Care Surg 2023. https://doi.org/10.1097/TA.0000000000003951.

36. Luze H, Nischwitz SP, Smolle C, et al. The use of acellular fish skin grafts in burn wound management-a systematic review. Medicina (Kaunas) 2022;58(7). https://doi.org/10.3390/medicina58070912.

37. Holmes JH, Molnar JA, Shupp JW, et al. Demonstration of the safety and effectiveness of the RECELL. Burns 2019;45(4):772–82.

38. Holmes Iv JH, Molnar JA, Carter JE, et al. A Comparative study of the recell® device and autologous spit-thickness meshed skin graft in the treatment of acute burn injuries. J Burn Care Res 2018;39(5):694–702.

39. Kowal S, Kruger E, Bilir P, et al. Cost-effectiveness of the use of autologous cell harvesting device compared to standard of care for treatment of severe burns in the united states. Adv Ther 2019;36(7):1715–29. https://doi.org/10.1007/s12325-019-00961-2.

40. Jeschke MG. Post-burn hypermetabolism: past, present and future. J Burn Care Res 2016;37(2):86–96.

41. Jeschke MG, Gauglitz GG, Kulp GA, et al. Long-term persistance of the pathophysiologic response to severe burn injury. PLoS One 2011;6(7):e21245.

42. Mosier MJ, Pham TN, Park DR, et al. Predictive value of bronchoscopy in assessing the severity of inhalation injury. J Burn Care Res 2012;33(1):65–73.

43. Sutton T, Lenk I, Conrad P, et al. Severity of inhalation injury is predictive of alterations in gas exchange and worsened clinical outcomes. J Burn Care Res 2017;38(6):390–5.

44. Sheckter CC, Mandell S. Say no to cyanokit. Pause at the 10, 10 threshold. Burns 2022;48(6):1516–8.

45. Wang X, Zhang Y, Ni L, et al. A review of treatment strategies for hydrofluoric acid burns: current status and future prospects. Burns 2014;40(8):1447–57.

# Burn Patient Metabolism and Nutrition

Johanna H. Nunez, MD[a], Audra T. Clark, MD[b],*

KEYWORDS

• Burn • Nutrition • Metabolism • Critical care

KEY POINTS

- Nutritional support plays a unique and vital role in the survival and rehabilitation of burn patients.
- Patients suffering from severe burns experience a radically increased metabolic rate for months to years following the injury.
- Burn energy expenditure fluctuates significantly throughout the patient's rehabilitation and can lead to underfeeding in times of early high-energy expenditure and overfeeding later in the treatment course.
- Micronutrients play a vital role in burn patients' wound healing and immune responses.

## INTRODUCTION

Nutritional support plays a unique and vital role in the survival and rehabilitation of patients with burns. Following severe burn injury, patients experience a significant and sustained increase in their metabolic rate up to two times baseline.[1] This hypermetabolic state leads to severe catabolism, causing both immune dysfunction and the loss of lean body mass.[2] To counteract the damage caused by a sustained hypermetabolic state, significant nutritional support is needed to meet the demands of increased energy expenditure. Nutritional assessments and feeding regimens vary from center to center, and many questions remain concerning the optimal route, nutritional composition, and volume of diet for patients with burns following injury. Here, the authors review the current understanding of burn hypermetabolism and nutritional requirements following burn injuries.

## NUTRITION AND THE HYPERMETABOLIC RESPONSE

Patients suffering from severe burns experience a radically increased metabolic rate for months to years following the injury. There are two stages that burn patient

[a] University of Texas Southwestern Medical Center, Dallas, TX, USA; [b] Department of Surgery, University of Texas Southwestern Medical Center, E05514B, 5323 Harry Hines Boulevard, Dallas, TX 75390, USA
* Corresponding author.
E-mail address: audra.clark@utsouthwestern.edu

Phys Med Rehabil Clin N Am 34 (2023) 717–731
https://doi.org/10.1016/j.pmr.2023.06.001
1047-9651/23/Published by Elsevier Inc.

metabolism goes through following injury. The first is the "ebb" state, which happens immediately after the burn in which patients have a decrease in metabolism and overall reduced tissue perfusion. Immediately following this stage is the "flow" state in which patients have hyperdynamic circulation and hypermetabolic rates up to two times normal[3] (**Fig. 1**).

When resting energy expenditure (REE) is increased by 10%, patients are considered hypermetabolic. Patients who have a 40% total body surface area (TBSA) burn have an REE between 40% and 100% above baseline.[4] Although not yet fully understood, hypermetabolism at the cellular level is caused by increased whole-body oxygen consumption, leading to increased adenosine triphosphate (ATP) turnover and thermogenesis. In addition to ATP turnover, mitochondrial oxygen consumption plays a role in the hypermetabolic response. This is thought to be due to the uncoupling of mitochondrial respiration from ATP formation, which results in heat.[5]

Investigation of the hypermetabolic response has led to several studies indicating catecholamines as the primary mediators of hypermetabolism.[6,7] Elevation of epinephrine, cortisol, and glucagon levels are known to inhibit lipogenesis and protein synthesis. Patients experience skeletal muscle cachexia with long-term imbalances between protein synthesis and breakdown, which can last 1 to 3 years after severe burn injury.[8,9]

Adequate nutrition following severe burn injuries is vital to prevent long-term complications. Animal models have shown that early nutrition mitigates burn-induced hypermetabolism and catabolism, but this has not been observed in human trials.[10,11] Although early enteral feeding has not been shown to decrease the hypermetabolic state in burn patients, it is still universally recommended owing to its many benefits, including improved muscle mass maintenance, mucosal integrity, improved wound healing, and shorter intensive care unit stays.[12,13]

## PARENTERAL VERSUS ENTERAL NUTRITION

Early treatment of burn patients up until the 1970s focused on parenteral nutrition (PN). This was soon after transitioned to enteral nutrition (EN), as PN was found to be associated not only with overfeeding, liver dysfunction, and an impaired immune response but also three times normal mortality.[14,15] Since the switch to EN, many benefits have been discovered including preservation of bowel mucosal architecture and function, increased blood flow, improved gut-associated immune function, decreased bacterial translocation, and decreased hyperglycemia.[16,17] All these benefits lead to EN being the preferred choice of nutrition administration in severely burned patients.

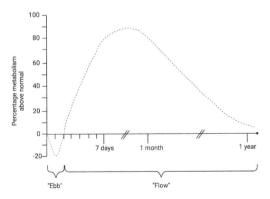

**Fig. 1.** Burn hypermetabolism timeline.

Enteral feeds can be delivered either via gastric or post-pyloric feeding. Gastric feeding tubes are larger in diameter, allowing for bolus feeding and have decreased clogging, but are associated with ileus in the stomach following burns. The post-pyloric tube's smaller diameter makes them more prone to clogging; they can be used intraoperatively without an increased risk of aspiration and are more comfortable for the patient.[18] Recent studies have confirmed the safety and nutritional benefits of intraoperative feeding in both pediatric and adult populations and may move practitioners to opt for post-pyloric feeding.[19,20]

## NUTRITIONAL SUPPORT INITIATION

Early and adequate nutritional support is vital for patient survival after burn injuries. Severely burned patients experience decreased nutrient absorption due to intestinal mucosal damage and increased bacterial translocation.[16] Previous animal studies showed that early enteral feeding of Guinea pigs following burns led to a decrease in metabolic rate 2 weeks following the burn compared with those fed at 72 hours.[10] When tested in humans early feeding has been shown to decrease catecholamine, glucagon, and cortisol levels while preserving mucosal integrity, motility, and perfusion.[11,17,21,22] In addition to these physiologic responses, early feeding has also been shown to improve wound healing, help with muscle mass maintenance, decrease Curling ulcers, and shorten the length of stay in the ICU.[12,13]

## CALORIC REQUIREMENTS

Finding a balance between fulfilling increased requirements due to the hypermetabolic state while not overfeeding the patient is difficult. Many formulas have been developed to estimate the caloric needs of burn patients, with one of the earliest examples being the Curreri formula.[23,24] Early formulas tended to lead to patient overfeeding; therefore, new, more comprehensive formulas with different variables have been proposed to better calculate burn patient nutritional needs (**Table 1**).[25] Despite the newly proposed formulas, a study of 46 different formulas found that none correlated well with the patients' measured energy expenditure.[1] Burn energy expenditure fluctuates significantly throughout the patient's rehabilitation, and these formulas can lead to underfeeding in times of early high-energy expenditure and overfeeding later in the treatment course.

The gold standard for the measurement of energy expenditure is indirect calorimetry (IC). IC machines work by calculating consumption ($VO_2$) and carbon dioxide production ($VCO_2$) determine thee respiratory quotient and metabolic rate[26] and can detect underfeeding or overfeeding.[23] The respiratory quotients change depending on the substrate being metabolized. Normal metabolism yields an respiratory quotient (RQ) in the range 0.75 to 0.9. During starvation, when fat is the main source of energy, RQ less than 0.7. An RQ greater than 1.0, it indicates overfeeding. In critically ill patients, overfeeding needs to be avoided because it causes several issues, including ventilator weaning difficulties.[27] Despite concerns regarding overfeeding, a pediatric burn study demonstrated that a high-carbohydrate diet led to decreased muscle wasting, no respiratory complications, and RQs less than 1.05.[28]

## SUBSTRATES

Although many nutrients are important for the metabolic process, the metabolism of carbohydrates, proteins, and lipids provides the main energy source for burn patients via different metabolic pathways (**Fig. 2**). Carbohydrates are the macronutrients of

**Table 1**
Formulas used to calculate caloric needs for burn patients

| Adult Formula | Kcal/day | Comments |
|---|---|---|
| Harris Benedict | *Men:*<br>66.5 + 13.8 (weight in kg) + 5 (height in cm) − 6.76 (age in years)<br>*Women:*<br>655 + 9.6 (weight in kg) + 1.85 (height in cm) − 4.68(age in years) | Estimates basal energy expenditure<br>Can be adjusted by both activity and stress factor<br>Multiply by 1.5 for common burn stress adjustment |
| Toronto Formula | −4343 + 10.5 (TBSA) +0.23 (calorie intake in last 24 h) + 0.84 (Harris Benedict estimation without adjustment) + 114 (temperature) − 4.5 (number of postburn days) | Useful in acute stage of burn care<br>Must be adjusted with change in monitoring parameters |
| Davies and Liljedahl | 20 (weight in kg) + 70 (TBSA) | Overestimates caloric needs for large injuries |
| Ireton-Jones | *Ventilated patient:*<br>1784−11 (age in years) + 5 (weight in kg) + (244 if male) + (239 if trauma) + (804 if burn)<br>*Non-ventilated patient:*<br>629−11 (age in years) +25 (weight in kg) − (609 if obese) | Complex formula which integrates variables for ventilation and injury status and obesity |
| Curreri | Age 16–59 y: 25 (weight in kg) + 40 (TBSA)<br>Age>60 y: 20 (weight in kg) + 65 (TBSA) | Often overestimates caloric needs |
| *Pediatric formulas* | | |
| Galveston | *0–1 y:*<br>2100 (body surface area) + 1000 (body surface area × TBSA)<br>*1–11 y:*<br>1800 (body surface area) + 1300 (body surface area × TBSA)<br>*12–18 y:*<br>1500 (body surface area) + 1500 (body surface area × TBSA) | Focuses on maintaining body weight |
| Curreri Junior | <1 y: recommended dietary allowance + 15 (TBSA)<br>1–3 y: recommended dietary allowance + 25 (TBSA)<br>4–15 y: recommended dietary allowance + 40 (TBSA) | Commonly overestimates caloric needs |

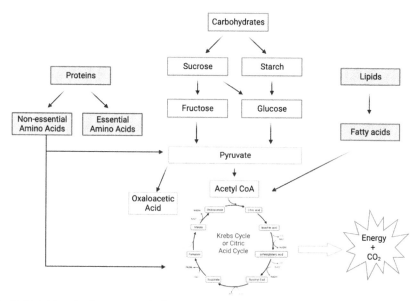

**Fig. 2.** Nutritional substate metabolism.

choice for burn patients, as high-carbohydrate diets have been shown to have a protein-sparing effect and promote wound healing.[29] An randomized controlled trial (RCT) on severe pediatric burns showed that children receiving a high-carbohydrate diet, instead of a high-fat diet, had significantly less proteolysis.[29] Although carbohydrates are vital in the diet of burn patients, patients can only oxidize glucose at a rate of 7 g/kg/day[30,31] In some patients, this rate is less than the caloric amount required to prevent lean body mass loss. If patients are administered excess glucose, hyperglycemia can occur, leading to dehydration, respiratory problems, and maladaptive conversion of glucose into fat.[32]

Owing to the hormonal imbalance in burn patients during acute injury, many patients require supplemental insulin to help regulate glucose. Insulin administration has also been shown to assist in burn patients' wound healing and muscle protein synthesis.[33] Multiple studies have shown that severely burned patients who received insulin infusions with a high-carbohydrate, high-protein diet had increased lean body mass and bone density, improved donor site healing, and decrease hospital length of stay.[34,35]

## FATS

Fats are important nutrients to prevent essential fatty acid deficiency but are only recommended in limited amounts in the burn diet.[36] Following burn injury, the use of lipids for energy is greatly decreased owing to suppressed lipolysis. Although increased beta-oxidation of fat can provide energy in the hypermetabolic state, only 30% of free fatty acids are used. In addition to its limited use as an energy source, multiple studies have found that high-fat diets can adversely affect a patient's immune function.[10,37] This has been taken into consideration when formulating formulas for burn patient EN, with many formulas having less than 15% of total calories from lipids.

The type of lipid administered to patients must be considered following burn injury. Many common formulas use omega-6 fatty acids, which contain precursors to pro-inflammatory cytokines, such as prostaglandin E2. However, formulations enriched with omega-3 fatty acids can be metabolized without promoting pro-inflammatory molecules. "Immune enhancing diets" that have increased omega-3 fatty acids and decreased omega-6 fatty acids have been shown to improve patient outcomes in part by reducing hyperglycemia and enhancing immune function.[38,39]

## PROTEIN

Following severe burn injury, proteolysis is significantly increased, and protein supplementation is required to meet ongoing demands. Protein is used as an energy source under catabolic conditions, and giving excess calories will only lead to overfeeding and not increased protein synthesis. Although catabolism is not reduced by supernormal doses of protein, it facilitates protein synthesis and can reduce the negative nitrogen balance.[40] The current recommendations of protein for burned adults is 1.5 to 2.0 gm/kg/day and 2.5 to 4.0 gm/kg/day for pediatric patients with a nonprotein calorie to nitrogen ratio of 1:50 for small burns and 1:100 for large burns.[41] Despite supplementation, most severely burned patients still experience muscle loss due to the associated hormonal and pro-inflammatory responses following injury.

Specific amino acids play unique roles in burn recovery. Following injury, there is an efflux of glutamine, alanine, and arginine, all of which are important for transport, energy supply to the liver, and wound healing.[42] Glutamine is essential for maintaining bowel integrity, as it directly provides fuel for lymphocytes and enterocytes and helps to preserve gut-associated immune function.[43] Glutamine supplementation has been shown to decrease hypermetabolism and increase survival in animal models. Previously, supplementation with 25 g/kg/day of glutamine has been shown to decrease length of hospital stay in burn patients.[44,45] Recent human trials showed that glutamine supplementation decreased the incidence of gram-negative bacteria, improved serum transferrin and prealbumin levels, and decreased patient C-reactive protein levels, but did not decrease mortality.[46,47]

In addition to glutamine, arginine is critical to immune function, as it improves natural killer cell performance, stimulates T lymphocytes, and increases nitric oxide synthesis.[48,49] Although supplementation of arginine in burn patients has been shown to improve wound healing and immune responsiveness,[49] studies in other critically ill populations have shown that arginine is potentially harmful, making current data insufficient to definitively recommend its use.[50]

## MICRONUTRIENTS

Vitamins and trace elements, collectively known as "micronutrients," play a vital role in burn patients' wound healing and immune responses. Severe burns cause high oxidative stress and a continuous inflammatory response, leading to a severe decrease in micronutrient-dependent antioxidant defenses.[51,52] Decreases in vitamins A, C, and D, iron (Fe), copper (Cu), selenium (Se), and zinc (Zn) have been shown to impair immune function and wound healing.[53–55]

Vitamin A improves wound healing by increasing epithelial growth. Vitamin C is necessary for collagen creation and cross-linking.[56] Vitamin D cannot be manufactured in normal quantities in burned skin, leading to derangements in calcium and vitamin D levels. Children can suffer significant dysfunction due to vitamin D deficiency following burn injury as they have increased bone reabsorption and urinary calcium wasting, and are unable to produce normal quantities of vitamin D3.

Trace elements essential for cellular and humoral immunity are lost in large quantities because of exudative burn wound losses.[54] Iron is an important cofactor for oxygen-carrying proteins necessary for healing. Selenium is essential for cell-mediated immunity.[52,57] Zn is essential for protein synthesis, lymphocyte function, and wound healing.[58] Copper is crucial for wound healing and collagen formation and its deficiency has also been associated with decreased immunity, arrhythmias, and worse outcomes. Supplementation of these micronutrients at appropriate doses (**Table 2**) is essential, as it improves patient morbidity following severe burn injury.[52,59–61]

## FORMULAS

Early formulas created for burn patients were simple mixtures that were successful in providing nutrition but were very high in fat. Currently, there is a plethora of commercial formulas with varying percentages of carbohydrates, fats, proteins, and micronutrients, as described in **Table 3**. Because glucose is the preferred energy source for patients with burns, they should be given a high carbohydrate diet.[28,62]

Formula development has steered toward "immune enhancing diets" which are formulas that are enriched with micronutrients to improve immune function and wound healing. This started when omega-3 fatty acid, arginine, histidine, and vitamins A and C were added to pediatric formulas with outcomes showing decreased wound infections and shorter length of stay compared with normal formulas.[63] Follow-up studies have reported varying outcomes in different patient populations. Some studies have shown that the administration of immunonutrition formulas led to improved cardiopulmonary function, neutrophil recruitment, and decreased length of stay in some non-burn populations.[64,65] Other studies performed in patients with sepsis and pneumonia have suggested that immune-enhancing diets could have harmful effects.[50,64] Minimal research exists regarding immune-enhancing diets in the burn population, with one study showing no difference in major outcomes between an immune-enhancing diet versus a high-protein stress formula.[66] Some hypothesize that no differences may be seen due to burn patients receiving sufficient immune-enhancing nutrients from normal formulas due to the high volumes given post-burn injury.

A multitude of formulas and numerous methods for calculating nutritional needs have been used successfully in the burn population, which suggests that no formula or calculation is perfect, but most are adequate to prevent nutritional complications.

**Table 2**
**Micronutrient requirements in non-burned and burned patients**

| Age | 0–13 y | | ≥13 y | |
| --- | --- | --- | --- | --- |
| | Non-burned | Burned | Non-burned | Burned |
| Vitamin A, IU | 1300–2000 | 2500–5000 | 200–3000 | 10000 |
| Vitamin D, IU | 600 | 0 | 600 | 0 |
| Vitamin E, IU | 45093 | 0 | 23 | 0 |
| Vitamin C, IU | 15–50 | 250–500 | 75–90 | 1000 |
| Vitamin K, mcg | 21947 | 0 | 75–120 | 0 |
| Folate mcg | 65–300 | 1000a | 300–400 | 10001 |
| Cu, mg | 0.2–0.7 | 0.8–2.8 | 0.9 | 4 |
| Fe, mg | 0.3–8 | 0 | 45156 | 0 |
| Se, mcg | 15–40 | 60–140 | 40–60 | 300–500 |
| Zn, mg | 44965 | 12.5–25 | 45149 | 25–40 |

**Table 3**
**Enteral feed formula types and composition**

| Formula | Kcal/mL | Carbohydrate g/L (% Calories) | Protein g/L (% Calories) | Fat g/L (% Calories) | Comments |
|---------|---------|-------------------------------|--------------------------|---------------------|----------|
| Impact | 1 | 130 (53) | 56 (22) | 28 (25) | Immune-enhancing diet (IED) with arginine, glutamine fiber |
| Glucerna | 1 | 96 (34) | 42 (17) | 54 (49) | Low carbohydrate, for diabetic patients |
| Osmolite | 1.06 | 144 (54) | 44 (17) | 35 (29) | Inexpensive, isotonic |
| Crucial | 1.5 | 89 (36) | 63 (25) | 45 (39) | IED with arginine, hypertonic |
| Nepro | 1.8 | 167 (34) | 81 (18) | 96 (48) | Concentrated, for patients with renal failure |

A wide range of clinical trials on different nutritional regimens are still being carried out, and a convincing consensus on optimal nutrition for burn patients has not been reached.

## MONITORING NUTRITIONAL SUPPORT

Monitoring the adequacy of nutritional support in patients with severe burns is vital and complex. The overall goal is to supply the patient with sufficient nutrients to gain metabolic equilibrium and to eventually reestablish their normal body composition. This can be measured using several variables, including body weight, serum proteins, nitrogen balance, imaging of lean body mass, and exercise tolerance.

Body weight is not a good measure of nutrition initially, as early fluid resuscitation after severe burns can add up to 20 kg of body weight.[67] The fluid time course is unpredictable and can be compounded by additional fluid shifts associated with ventilator use, infections, and hypoproteinemia. Therefore, using weight is unreliable as total weight can mask the loss of muscle mass that is occurring.[68] Although not very useful alone in the acute burn phase, weight should be closely monitored, as long-term trends during the rehabilitation phase are very valuable.

Traditionally, measurements of serum proteins such as albumin and prealbumin are used to assess nutritional status; however, they have limitations following severe burn injury. The normal metabolic pathways used to create albumin are suppressed after injury, leading to both acute and chronic depression of albumin markers.[69] Prealbumin, which has a shorter half-life of 2 days, is theoretically more sensitive to short-term nutritional changes. However, prealbumin levels fall quickly after burns and are slow to recover, making it potentially unreliable to assess nutritional status.

Nitrogen is a fundamental component of amino acids and can be used as a reliable marker for investigating protein metabolism. A positive nitrogen balance indicates increased total body protein, whereas burns, trauma, and fasting are associated with a negative nitrogen balance. An approximation of the burn patient's nitrogen balance is performed using the following formula.

*Nitrogen Balance = Nitrogen Intake in 24 Hours − [1.25 × (Urine Urea Nitrogen + 4)]*

In severely burned patients, this formula may underestimate nitrogen loss. This is due to the 4 g/dL added to the total urinary nitrogen, possibly being underestimated, and due to burn patients' substantial loss through burn wound protein-rich exudates not being accounted for in the formula.[70,71]

Less commonly used methods of nutritional assessment are bioimpedance analysis and dual-x-ray absorptiometry. Although potentially beneficial, these methodologies are limited by their availability and cost. In 2007, 65 burn centers were surveyed to assess how they monitored burn patient nutrition. The findings from most common to least common were prealbumin level, body weight, calorie count, nitrogen balance, serum albumin level, and transferrin levels.[72] Overall, the clinical picture must be incorporated into the assessment and individualized to the patients' trends, as no individual method is universally reliable for monitoring burn patient nutrition.

## PRE-BURN NUTRITIONAL STATUS EFFECT ON OUTCOMES

Monitoring nutritional support needs can be complicated by the patient's pre-burn nutritional status. Burn patients with a low prognostic nutritional index, a validated tool for nutritional status assessment, were found to have increased major cardiac adverse events after burn surgery and in the elderly population increased 1-year postoperative mortality.[73,74] These conditions need to be considered when calculating the necessary caloric intake in patients with burns and when considering the patient's baseline physiology.

Obesity poses unique conditions that must be considered following burn injury. Obesity is clearly linked with multiple health problems, but in surgical and medical intensive care units, obese patients have been found to have reduced mortality compared with normal weight patents, despite a higher rate of infections and longer length of stays.[75–77] Minimal data exist in the burn population, but a study of the National Burn Repository found a higher mortality for patients listed as obese, although the term was not clearly defined.[78] Studies in pediatric burn populations have demonstrated that obesity leads to longer hospital stays and an increased need for ventilatory support.[79,80]

Obesity has been associated with increased levels of pro-inflammatory cytokines and in burn patients can cause increased hypermetabolism, amplified inflammation, increased insulin resistance, and severe muscle wasting compared with nonobese individuals.[81] Obese patients can also have worsened vitamin D and calcium deficiencies following burns owing to decreased vitamin D3 bioavailability.[82] Nutritional assessment is difficult as obese patients can still be malnourished, despite their weight, and if actual body weight is used in predictive formulas, nutritional needs are overestimated, but if the ideal body weight is used, nutritional needs are underestimated.

Although caloric formulas have been created for obese patients, they have not yet been validated. Non-burn trials of critically ill patients have shown that obese patients on a hypocaloric diet have reduced mortality, improved ventilator weaning, and decreased length of stay.[83,84] Some clinicians therefore endorse low-calorie high-protein diets in an attempt to maintain lean body mass, improve glycemic control, and promote weight loss[85]; however, there are no current data to support this, and more studies are needed before this can be recommended.

## OVERFEEDING

Aggressive nutrition can lead to inadvertent overfeeding as the patient's metabolic rate slows. Overfeeding can lead to complications, such as difficulty in weaning from the ventilator, hepatic steatosis, azotemia, and hyperglycemia. Carbohydrate overfeeding leads to an increase in the respiratory quotient, making ventilator weaning difficult.[25] If patients are overfed, an increase in the deposition of fat in the liver can cause increased mortality and immune dysfunction.[86] Owing to the large amounts of protein administered to burn patients, they can develop significant azotemia, leading to kidney dysfunction. If azotemia is not reduced following hydration, dietary modifications are needed to decrease protein content, and patients should be monitored with blood chemistries to assess metabolic derangements.

Predictive formulas for nutritional needs should be regularly reassessed as the patient's energy requirements change over the course of their rehabilitation. As the patient's healing progresses, other factors, such as the surface area of open wounds and physical and occupational therapy activities, should be considered when estimating the patient's caloric needs.

## NUTRITIONAL SUPPORT DURING POSTHOSPITAL REHABILITATION

Minimal data exist on the optimal diet for burn patients during the later stages of recovery. The hypermetabolic state has been shown to last for up to 2 years following very severe burn injury. Because of this, it is suggested that burn patients increase their caloric intake with a high-protein component for at least a year after injury in children and those with persistent open wounds. In addition to providing adequate caloric intake, resistance exercise is recommended to improve muscle mass. Patients should be followed up by a physician and dietitian and regularly weigh themselves to help determine if they are receiving adequate nutrition. As patients continue to heal, their metabolism slows and the caloric intake that was necessary during the acute burn phase can end up leading to overeating and excessive weight gain. Balanced nutrition and exercise along with continued nutritional assessments are a vital part of healthy burn injury rehabilitation.

## SUMMARY

Balanced nutritional support is a complex and vital component of recovery in burn patients. Adequate nutritional management can lead to enhanced wound healing, decreased complications, and overall improved survival. High-carbohydrate enteral feeds have been shown to be most beneficial but need to be individualized, closely monitored, and appropriately modified as burn patients' hypermetabolism changes over the course of their rehabilitation. To determine the optimal nutritional regimen, further research is needed to validate the most accurate nutritional endpoints and formulas. Continued translational research and prospective RCTs are needed to further analyze the effects of nutritional treatments on burn patient metabolism and long-term outcomes.

## CLINICAL PEARLS

- Enteral nutrition is the preferred choice of nutrition administration in severely burned patients and can be safely given through post-pyloric feeding tubes intraoperatively.
- High-carbohydrate diets are preferred and have been shown to have a protein-sparing effect and promote wound healing.
- Overfeeding must be avoided as it can lead to complications, such as difficulty in weaning from the ventilator, hepatic steatosis, azotemia, and hyperglycemia.

- Monitoring the adequacy of nutritional support in patients with severe burns is vital and complex with goals of gaining metabolic equilibrium and to eventually reestablishing their normal body composition.

- In the outpatient setting, burn patient nutrition and weight should be closely monitored as their metabolism slows and the caloric intake that was originally necessary during the acute burn phase can end up leading to overeating and excessive weight gain.

- Continued translational research and prospective RCTs are needed to further analyze the effects of nutritional treatments on burn patient metabolism and long-term outcomes.

## REFERENCES

1. Dickerson RN, Gervasio JM, Riley ML, et al. Accuracy of predictive methods to estimate resting energy expenditure of thermally-injured patients. JPEN J Parenter Enteral Nutr 2002;26(1):17–29.
2. Suri MP, Dhingra VJ, Raibagkar SC, et al. Nutrition in burns: need for an aggressive dynamic approach. Burns 2006;32(7):880–4.
3. Cuthbertson DP, Angeles Valero Zanuy MA, León Sanz ML. Post-shock metabolic response. 1942. Nutr Hosp 2001;16(5):176–82 [discussion: 175-176].
4. Hart DW, Wolf SE, Mlcak R, et al. Persistence of muscle catabolism after severe burn. Surgery 2000;128(2):312–9.
5. Porter C, Tompkins RG, Finnerty CC, et al. The metabolic stress response to burn trauma: current understanding and therapies. Lancet 2016;388(10052):1417–26.
6. Williams FN, Herndon DN, Jeschke MG. The hypermetabolic response to burn injury and interventions to modify this response. Clin Plast Surg 2009;36(4): 583–96.
7. Jeschke MG, Finnerty CC, Suman OE, et al. The effect of oxandrolone on the endocrinologic, inflammatory, and hypermetabolic responses during the acute phase postburn. Ann Surg 2007;246(3):351–60 [discussion: 360-352].
8. Jeschke MG, Gauglitz GG, Kulp GA, et al. Long-term persistance of the pathophysiologic response to severe burn injury. PLoS One 2011;6(7):e21245.
9. Chao T, Herndon DN, Porter C, et al. Skeletal muscle protein breakdown remains elevated in pediatric burn survivors up to one-year post-injury. Shock 2015;44(5): 397–401.
10. Mochizuki H, Trocki O, Dominioni L, et al. Mechanism of prevention of postburn hypermetabolism and catabolism by early enteral feeding. Ann Surg 1984; 200(3):297–310.
11. Peck MD, Kessler M, Cairns BA, et al. Early enteral nutrition does not decrease hypermetabolism associated with burn injury. J Trauma 2004;57(6):1143–8 [discussion: 1148-1149].
12. Mosier MJ, Pham TN, Klein MB, et al. Early enteral nutrition in burns: compliance with guidelines and associated outcomes in a multicenter study. J Burn Care Res 2011;32(1):104–9.
13. Peng YZ, Yuan ZQ, Xiao GX. Effects of early enteral feeding on the prevention of enterogenic infection in severely burned patients. Burns 2001;27(2):145–9.
14. Ireton-Jones CS, Baxter CR. Nutrition for adult burn patients: a review. Nutr Clin Pract 1991;6(1):3–7.
15. Herndon DN, Barrow RE, Stein M, et al. Increased mortality with intravenous supplemental feeding in severely burned patients. J Burn Care Rehabil 1989;10(4): 309–13.

16. Magnotti LJ, Deitch EA. Burns, bacterial translocation, gut barrier function, and failure. J Burn Care Rehabil 2005;26(5):383–91.
17. Andel D, Kamolz LP, Donner A, et al. Impact of intraoperative duodenal feeding on the oxygen balance of the splanchnic region in severely burned patients. Burns 2005;31(3):302–5.
18. Jenkins ME, Gottschlich MM, Warden GD. Enteral feeding during operative procedures in thermal injuries. J Burn Care Rehabil 1994;15(2):199–205.
19. Pham CH, Fang M, Vrouwe SQ, et al. Evaluating the safety and efficacy of intraoperative enteral nutrition in critically ill burn patients: a systematic review and meta-analysis. J Burn Care Res 2020;41(4):841–8.
20. Hudson AS, Morzycki AD, Wong J. Safety and benefits of intraoperative enteral nutrition in critically ill pediatric burn patients: a systematic review and pooled analysis. J Burn Care Res 2022;43(6):1343–50.
21. Vicic VK, Radman M, Kovacic V. Early initiation of enteral nutrition improves outcomes in burn disease. Asia Pac J Clin Nutr 2013;22(4):543–7.
22. Gottschlich MM, Jenkins ME, Mayes T, et al. The 2002 Clinical Research Award. An evaluation of the safety of early vs delayed enteral support and effects on clinical, nutritional, and endocrine outcomes after severe burns. J Burn Care Rehabil 2002;23(6):401–15.
23. Ireton-Jones CS, Turner WW Jr, Liepa GU, et al. Equations for the estimation of energy expenditures in patients with burns with special reference to ventilatory status. J Burn Care Rehabil 1992;13(3):330–3.
24. Curreri PW. Assessing nutritional needs for the burned patient. J Trauma 1990; 30(12 Suppl):S20–3.
25. Saffle JR, Medina E, Raymond J, et al. Use of indirect calorimetry in the nutritional management of burned patients. J Trauma 1985;25(1):32–9.
26. McClave SA, Snider HL. Use of indirect calorimetry in clinical nutrition. Nutr Clin Pract 1992;7(5):207–21.
27. Graf S, Pichard C, Genton L, et al. Energy expenditure in mechanically ventilated patients: the weight of body weight. Clin Nutr 2017;36(1):224–8.
28. Hart DW, Wolf SE, Zhang XJ, et al. Efficacy of a high-carbohydrate diet in catabolic illness. Crit Care Med 2001;29(7):1318–24.
29. Hart DW, Wolf SE, Herndon DN, et al. Energy expenditure and caloric balance after burn: increased feeding leads to fat rather than lean mass accretion. Ann Surg 2002;235(1):152–61.
30. Sheridan RL, Yu YM, Prelack K, et al. Maximal parenteral glucose oxidation in hypermetabolic young children: a stable isotope study. JPEN J Parenter Enteral Nutr 1998;22(4):212–6.
31. Wolfe RR. Maximal parenteral glucose oxidation in hypermetabolic young children. JPEN J Parenter Enteral Nutr 1998;22(4):190.
32. Rodriguez NA, Jeschke MG, Williams FN, et al. Nutrition in burns: galveston contributions. JPEN J Parenter Enteral Nutr 2011;35(6):704–14.
33. Aarsland A, Chinkes DL, Sakurai Y, et al. Insulin therapy in burn patients does not contribute to hepatic triglyceride production. J Clin Invest 1998;101(10):2233–9.
34. Pierre EJ, Barrow RE, Hawkins HK, et al. Effects of insulin on wound healing. J Trauma 1998;44(2):342–5.
35. Thomas SJ, Morimoto K, Herndon DN, et al. The effect of prolonged euglycemic hyperinsulinemia on lean body mass after severe burn. Surgery 2002;132(2): 341–7.
36. Demling RH, Seigne P. Metabolic management of patients with severe burns. World J Surg 2000;24(6):673–80.

37. Garrel DR, Razi M, Larivière F, et al. Improved clinical status and length of care with low-fat nutrition support in burn patients. JPEN J Parenter Enteral Nutr 1995;19(6):482–91.
38. Alexander JW, Gottschlich MM. Nutritional immunomodulation in burn patients. Crit Care Med 1990;18(2 Suppl):S149–53.
39. Alexander JW, Saito H, Trocki O, et al. The importance of lipid type in the diet after burn injury. Ann Surg 1986;204(1):1–8.
40. Patterson BW, Nguyen T, Pierre E, et al. Urea and protein metabolism in burned children: effect of dietary protein intake. Metabolism 1997;46(5):573–8.
41. ISBI practice guidelines for burn care. Burns 2016;42(5):953–1021.
42. Soeters PB, van de Poll MC, van Gemert WG, et al. Amino acid adequacy in pathophysiological states. J Nutr 2004;134(6 Suppl):1575s–82s.
43. Wischmeyer PE. Can glutamine turn off the motor that drives systemic inflammation? Crit Care Med 2005;33(5):1175–8.
44. Gore DC, Jahoor F. Glutamine kinetics in burn patients. Comparison with hormonally induced stress in volunteers. Arch Surg 1994;129(12):1318–23.
45. Windle EM. Glutamine supplementation in critical illness: evidence, recommendations, and implications for clinical practice in burn care. J Burn Care Res 2006;27(6):764–72.
46. Heyland DK, Wibbenmeyer L, Pollack JA, et al. A randomized trial of enteral glutamine for treatment of burn injuries. N Engl J Med 2022;387(11):1001–10.
47. Wischmeyer PE, Lynch J, Liedel J, et al. Glutamine administration reduces Gram-negative bacteremia in severely burned patients: a prospective, randomized, double-blind trial versus isonitrogenous control. Crit Care Med 2001;29(11): 2075–80.
48. Yu YM, Ryan CM, Castillo L, et al. Arginine and ornithine kinetics in severely burned patients: increased rate of arginine disposal. Am J Physiol Endocrinol Metab 2001;280(3):E509–17.
49. Yan H, Peng X, Huang Y, et al. Effects of early enteral arginine supplementation on resuscitation of severe burn patients. Burns 2007;33(2):179–84.
50. Heyland DK, Samis A. Does immunonutrition in patients with sepsis do more harm than good? Intensive Care Med 2003;29(5):669–71.
51. Gamliel Z, DeBiasse MA, Demling RH. Essential microminerals and their response to burn injury. J Burn Care Rehabil 1996;17(3):264–72.
52. Berger MM. Antioxidant micronutrients in major trauma and burns: evidence and practice. Nutr Clin Pract 2006;21(5):438–49.
53. Gottschlich MM, Mayes T, Khoury J, et al. Hypovitaminosis D in acutely injured pediatric burn patients. J Am Diet Assoc 2004;104(6):931–41 [quiz: 1031].
54. Berger MM, Shenkin A. Trace element requirements in critically ill burned patients. J Trace Elem Med Biol 2007;21(Suppl 1):44–8.
55. Berger MM, Binnert C, Chiolero RL, et al. Trace element supplementation after major burns increases burned skin trace element concentrations and modulates local protein metabolism but not whole-body substrate metabolism. Am J Clin Nutr 2007;85(5):1301–6.
56. Rock CL, Dechert RE, Khilnani R, et al. Carotenoids and antioxidant vitamins in patients after burn injury. J Burn Care Rehabil 1997;18(3):269–78 [discussion: 268].
57. Hunt DR, Lane HW, Beesinger D, et al. Selenium depletion in burn patients. JPEN J Parenter Enteral Nutr 1984;8(6):695–9.
58. Selmanpakoğlu AN, Cetin C, Sayal A, et al. Trace element (Al, Se, Zn, Cu) levels in serum, urine and tissues of burn patients. Burns 1994;20(2):99–103.

59. Rousseau AF, Losser MR, Ichai C, et al. ESPEN endorsed recommendations: nutritional therapy in major burns. Clin Nutr 2013;32(4):497–502.

60. Meyer NA, Muller MJ, Herndon DN. Nutrient support of the healing wound. New Horiz 1994;2(2):202–14.

61. Berger MM, Baines M, Raffoul W, et al. Trace element supplementation after major burns modulates antioxidant status and clinical course by way of increased tissue trace element concentrations. Am J Clin Nutr 2007;85(5):1293–300.

62. Boulétreau P, Chassard D, Allaouchiche B, et al. Glucose-lipid ratio is a determinant of nitrogen balance during total parenteral nutrition in critically ill patients: a prospective, randomized, multicenter blind trial with an intention-to-treat analysis. Intensive Care Med 2005;31(10):1394–400.

63. Gottschlich MM, Jenkins M, Warden GD, et al. Differential effects of three enteral dietary regimens on selected outcome variables in burn patients. JPEN J Parenter Enteral Nutr 1990;14(3):225–36.

64. Heys SD, Walker LG, Smith I, et al. Enteral nutritional supplementation with key nutrients in patients with critical illness and cancer: a meta-analysis of randomized controlled clinical trials. Ann Surg 1999;229(4):467–77.

65. Bower RH, Cerra FB, Bershadsky B, et al. Early enteral administration of a formula (Impact) supplemented with arginine, nucleotides, and fish oil in intensive care unit patients: results of a multicenter, prospective, randomized, clinical trial. Crit Care Med 1995;23(3):436–49.

66. Saffle JR, Wiebke G, Jennings K, et al. Randomized trial of immune-enhancing enteral nutrition in burn patients. J Trauma 1997;42(5):793–800 [discussion: 800-792].

67. Gump FE, Kinney JM. Energy balance and weight loss in burned patients. Arch Surg 1971;103(4):442–8.

68. Zdolsek HJ, Lindahl OA, Angquist KA, et al. Non-invasive assessment of intercompartmental fluid shifts in burn victims. Burns 1998;24(3):233–40.

69. Rettmer RL, Williamson JC, Labbé RF, et al. Laboratory monitoring of nutritional status in burn patients. Clin Chem 1992;38(3):334–7.

70. Konstantinides FN, Radmer WJ, Becker WK, et al. Inaccuracy of nitrogen balance determinations in thermal injury with calculated total urinary nitrogen. J Burn Care Rehabil 1992;13(2 Pt 1):254–60.

71. Milner EA, Cioffi WG, Mason AD, et al. A longitudinal study of resting energy expenditure in thermally injured patients. J Trauma 1994;37(2):167–70.

72. Graves C, Saffle J, Cochran A. Actual burn nutrition care practices: an update. J Burn Care Res 2009;30(1):77–82.

73. Kim HY, Yu J, Kong YG, et al. Prognostic nutritional index and major adverse cardiac events after burn surgery: a propensity score matching analysis. J Burn Care Res 2022;43(4):942–50.

74. Seo YJ, Kong YG, Yu J, et al. The prognostic nutritional index on postoperative day one is associated with one-year mortality after burn surgery in elderly patients. Burns Trauma 2021;9:tkaa043.

75. Akinnusi ME, Pineda LA, El Solh AA. Effect of obesity on intensive care morbidity and mortality: a meta-analysis. Crit Care Med 2008;36(1):151–8.

76. Malnick SD, Knobler H. The medical complications of obesity. QJM 2006;99(9): 565–79.

77. Mullen JT, Moorman DW, Davenport DL. The obesity paradox: body mass index and outcomes in patients undergoing nonbariatric general surgery. Ann Surg 2009;250(1):166–72.

78. Carpenter AM, Hollett LP, Jeng JC, et al. How long a shadow does epidemic obesity cast in the burn unit? A dietitian's analysis of the strengths and weaknesses of the available data in the National Burn Repository. J Burn Care Res 2008;29(1):97–101.
79. Gottschlich MM, Mayes T, Khoury JC, et al. Significance of obesity on nutritional, immunologic, hormonal, and clinical outcome parameters in burns. J Am Diet Assoc 1993;93(11):1261–8.
80. Patel L, Cowden JD, Dowd D, et al. Obesity: influence on length of hospital stay for the pediatric burn patient. J Burn Care Res 2010;31(2):251–6.
81. Jeevanandam M, Young DH, Schiller WR. Obesity and the metabolic response to severe multiple trauma in man. J Clin Invest 1991;87(1):262–9.
82. Klein GL. The interaction between burn injury and vitamin D metabolism and consequences for the patient. Curr Clin Pharmacol 2008;3(3):204–10.
83. Dickerson RN, Boschert KJ, Kudsk KA, et al. Hypocaloric enteral tube feeding in critically ill obese patients. Nutrition 2002;18(3):241–6.
84. McCowen KC, Friel C, Sternberg J, et al. Hypocaloric total parenteral nutrition: effectiveness in prevention of hyperglycemia and infectious complications–a randomized clinical trial. Crit Care Med 2000;28(11):3606–11.
85. Berger MM, Chioléro RL. Hypocaloric feeding: pros and cons. Curr Opin Crit Care 2007;13(2):180–6.
86. Barret JP, Jeschke MG, Herndon DN. Fatty infiltration of the liver in severely burned pediatric patients: autopsy findings and clinical implications. J Trauma 2001;51(4):736–9.

# Early Mobilization, Early Ambulation, and Burn Therapy in the Acute Hospital Setting

Audrey O'Neil, DPT[a,b], Danika Hines, DPT[c], Emily Wirdzek, DPT[c], Cody Thornburg, DPT[c], Derek Murray, MSPT[c,*], John Porter, MD[d,e]

## KEYWORDS

- Early mobility • Early ambulation • Burn positioning • Edema • Burn therapy
- Mobility safety

## KEY POINTS

- Optimized burn rehabilitation requires the commitment and support of multiple disciplines, backed by clear communication.
- Modalities such as positioning, mobility, and compression application can be used to manage multiple domains of impairment concurrently.
- The physiologic impact of burns effects several body systems. This can be severe in the case of larger initial burns or a prolonged course of care.
- Early mobilization is supported for burn survivors.
- Unless exclusion criteria exist, early ambulation after lower extremity autografts can safely commence postoperatively.

## INTRODUCTION

Rehabilitation evaluations and interventions are vital throughout the acute and rehabilitation phase of a burn patient's care and should be initiated within 24 hours of admission. Despite the critical nature of injury for large total body surface area (TBSA) burn patients, early therapy interventions have significant impact on contracture prevention, mobility, and wound healing. Rehabilitation within the critical care setting is rapidly evolving to include not only passive, interventions such as range of motion, splinting,

[a] Burn Rehabilitation Services; [b] Eskenazi Health, Richard M Fairbanks Burn Center, 720 Eskenazi Avenue, 4th Floor, Indianapolis, IN 46202, USA; [c] Burn Therapy, Valleywise, Valleywise Health, 2601 East Roosevelt Street, Phoenix, AZ 85008, USA; [d] Physiatry, Valleywise, Valleywise Health, 2601 East Roosevelt Street, Phoenix, AZ 85008, USA; [e] Trauma and Burn Services, Department of Surgery, University of Arizona, Creighton University, Phoenix, AZ, USA
* Corresponding author.
E-mail address: Derek.Murray@valleywisehealth.org

Phys Med Rehabil Clin N Am 34 (2023) 733–754
https://doi.org/10.1016/j.pmr.2023.06.029
1047-9651/23/© 2023 Elsevier Inc. All rights reserved.

and positioning but also early initiation of mobilization, exercise, and ambulation. Despite the critical nature of burn injuries within the acute care setting, burn rehabilitation must have a strong presence on the care team and initiate specific, progressive therapy interventions because of the potential for significant and long-term effects on the burn survivor.

## DISCUSSION
### Evaluation and Treatment

The foundation of the burn plan of care and burn rehabilitation is built on the initial evaluation. For verified burn centers, this evaluation occurs within the first 24 hours of patient admission. Although there are many components to a complete physical or occupational therapy evaluation, those that focus on the elements of a comprehensive rehabilitation burn plan and can be repeated to assess progress or regression are most useful. Although an ultimate single goal of burn rehabilitation could be that the burned patient demonstrates adequate pliability in their scars to independently perform functional tasks with appropriate speed, strength, endurance, and coordination without pain or discomfort, linear progression toward this goal is not to be anticipated for the burn patient admitted to the intensive care unit (ICU). The elements of a burn rehabilitation plan (**Tables 1** and **2**) are numerous and complex, and baseline patient performance, as well as patient progress, should be documented during the care continuum using several standardized assessments (**Table 3**).

For burn center patients, rehabilitation can be divided into 3 overall phases: the acute rehabilitation phase, the intermediate rehabilitation phase, and the long-term rehabilitation phase. The acute rehabilitation phase is defined as the time from admission until 50% wound closure or grafting has begun; the intermediate phase is defined as the time from initiation of wound closure until complete wound closure; and the long-term phase ranges from wound closure until received maximum benefit from burn rehabilitation to include burn reconstruction.[1] Contracture management should be the primary focus of rehabilitation throughout all phases of care.[2] Burn rehabilitation demands a time commitment for the rehabilitation therapist to support the best possible patient recovery, and patients with both small and large burns benefit from increased rehabilitation time,[3] and increased rehabilitation times lead to better patient outcomes.[4]

### Positioning and Orthotic Management

Positioning is important throughout the entire course of burn rehabilitation and is necessary to counteract potential deformities that contractile forces tend to promote. Goals of positioning include decreasing edema, maintaining joint alignment, promoting wound healing, relieving pressure, and protecting delicate structures.[5] Burn positioning may be most simply described as the positioning of a joint that promotes the most elongated stretch of the integumentary field of skin needed to allow normal range of motion (ROM) of that joint. In 2009, this field of skin was described by Richard and colleagues as the cutaneous functional unit (CFU).[6] Although CFUs are key to understanding how to best position patients to prevent contracture and deformity, standard burn resting positions have been described in the literature predating this concept. **Table 4** describes the ideal burn resting position at most major joints.

The ideal burn position may not always be the best position for a patient, given their habitus, history, concurrent injuries, and medical course of care. A positioning program is designed based on individual patient needs and changed as the patient's

**Table 1**
**Elements of a comprehensive burn evaluation**

| Category | Domain |
|---|---|
| Medical history and interview | Diagnosis |
| | Date of injury |
| | Mechanism |
| | Associated injuries |
| | Previous medical history |
| | Previous surgical history |
| | Physical and psychological health |
| | Social support |
| | Cultural influences |
| | Occupation |
| | Education |
| | Personal interests/hobbies and activities |
| | Pain |
| | Environmental barriers |
| Physical examination | Depth of burn |
| | Distribution of burn and cutaneous functional units involved |
| | Edema |
| | Cognition or mental status |
| | Range of motion |
| | Pain |
| | Strength |
| | Activities of daily living |
| | Coordination |
| | Scar assessment |
| | Skin integrity |
| Mobility assessment | Bed mobility |
| | Posture |
| | Balance transfers |
| | Gait |
| | Endurance |

presentation dictates.[5] **Fig. 1** shows a patient positioned post-cultured epithelial autograft (CEA) placement. Note that while standard positions are maintained at shoulders, elbows, wrists, and knees, adaptations have been made to hips and ankles to protect the CEAs most effectively.

### Range of Motion

Positioning alone will not prevent contracture. Range of motion is a critical intervention throughout all phases of burn rehabilitation, whether done passively when a patient is sedated or actively when the patient is awake. Range of motion need not be lost even

**Table 2**
**Elements of a comprehensive burn rehabilitation plan**

| Positioning | Edema Management | Strengthening | Gait Training | Coordination of Care |
|---|---|---|---|---|
| Range of motion | Pain management | ADLs | Conditioning | Family and caregiver education |
| Orthotics | Wound care | Mobility | Endurance training | Activity reintegration |

**Table 3**
**Assessments utilized in burn rehabilitation**

| Domain | Test or Procedure |
|---|---|
| Cognition | Richmond agitation-sedation scale |
| | Confusion assessment method for the intensive care unit |
| Range of motion | Goniometric measurements in modified position |
| Edema | Circumferential |
| | Figure-of-eight |
| | Volumetric measures |
| Pain | Visual analog scale |
| | Verbal numeric rating scale |
| | Nonverbal pain scale |
| | Critical pain observation tool |
| Mobility | Activity measure for postacute care 6 Clicks |
| | Functional assessment for burns |
| | Functional assessment for burns, intensive care unit |
| | Functional status score for the intensive care unit |
| | Medical Research Council Sum Score |
| | Physical function in intensive care unit test |
| | Functional independence measure |
| | Barthel index |
| | 2-min and 6-min Walk test |
| | Acute care index of function |
| Scar assessment | Vancouver scar scale |
| | Modified Vancouver scar scale |
| Skin integrity and wound | Visual inspection of skin directly |

in the presence of local CFU burn or hypertrophic scar.[2] The burn clinician needs to understand biomechanical principles related to soft tissue to successfully deploy this treatment modality, including successive length induction, tissue creep, and stress relaxation.[7] Because burn scar may develop tightness in as little as 1 to 4 days,[8] ROM frequency of up to 7 days per week may be indicated for burn patients who cannot achieve full ROM independently. Practice recommendations for ROM include early initiation, and duration of more than an hour daily.[9,10] The importance of immediate, focused, and suitably sustained ROM for patients because their transition into the long-term rehabilitation phase cannot be overstated.

### Orthotics

Whether used in conjunction with positioning, in support of ROM, or to protect vulnerable tissue as in the case with autologous grafts or open joints, orthotics have a major role in burn rehabilitation in all phases. Orthotics should be considered as a treatment choice for improving ROM or reducing contracture in all adult patients who have sustained a burn.[11] Orthotics can be classified into the following types: static, static-progressive, or dynamic. In the early acute stages of burn rehabilitation, orthotics are typically of the static type and may need to be modified or refabricated frequently depending on patient presentation. There are many prefabricated orthotic and positioning devices available, reducing the need to fabricate custom orthoses.

### EDEMA

Edema, a common inflammatory response to burn injury, is an important element to manage in the acute phase of a burn injury and throughout the continuum of care.

**Table 4**
**Antideformity positioning**

| Joint or Area | Recommended Position | Comments |
|---|---|---|
| Head | Position above heart | Monitor the occiput routinely and offload if needed to prevent breakdown |
| Neck | Midline rotation and lateral flexion, between 0° and 15° of extension | Limit use of pillows. Screen for cervical spine pathology if able to determine if extension is safe |
| Trunk | Extension, neutral rotation, neutral lateral flexion | |
| Shoulder | Shoulder abduction 90° abduction with 15°–20° of horizontal flexion | Positions above 90° may be poorly tolerated; monitor if able for discomfort |
| Elbow | Within 5°–10° of full extension | Avoid prolonged full extension |
| Forearm | Neutral to 10° of supination | |
| Wrist | Neutral to 10°–15° of extension | Wrist extension will assist with metacarpophalangeal (MCP) flexion due to tenodesis; exception and may position in neutral wrist flexion/extension briefly following dorsal hand and wrist grafts |
| MCP, Digits 2–5 | 70°–90° of flexion | Can aid or facilitate MCP flexion with wrist extension |
| Interphalangeal (IP) Digits 2–5 | Full extension | |
| Thumb | Midway between palmar and radial abduction at the carpometacarpal joint with MCP and IP in extension | |
| Hip | Extension with 10°–15° abduction and neutral rotation | Bed settings critical to maintain position |
| Knee | Within 3°–5° of full extension | Slight flexion prevents capsular tightness with prolonged knee extension |
| Ankle | Neutral to slight dorsiflexion; neutral inversion/ eversion and neutral forefoot supination/pronation | The ankle joint can lose dorsiflexion ROM in critically ill patients even if skin in the ankle CFU is spared and should be stretched routinely |

*Adapted from* Lester ME, Hazelton J, Dewey WS, Casey JC, Richard R. Influence of upper extremity positioning on pain, paresthesia, and tolerance: advancing current practice. *J Burn Care Res.* 2013;34(6:e342-e350.; Serghiou MA, Niszczak J, Parry I, Richard R. Clinical practice recommendations for positioning of the burn patient. *Burns.* 2016;42(2):267-275.

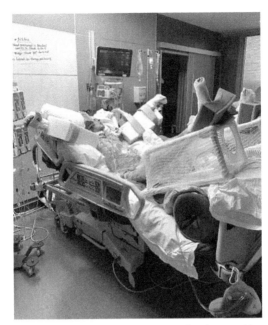

**Fig. 1.** Burn patient positioning post-CEA placement to the chest and legs with dressings off.

Due to the inflammatory process, edema presents in the areas of the injured and burned tissues, as well as systemically, depending on the size and severity of the burn and the age of the individual. **Box 1** lists the threshold for TBSA burns per age range that once crossed can lead to system wide inflammatory response and can present a more complicated critical care phase for edema management and wound care.

*Peripheral Edema*

In large burns, excessive fluid can accumulate in the peripheral tissues of the extremities and may lead to complications (**Box 2**). During the course of care, if edema remains beyond its capacity to be helpful or useful for the burn healing process, it will begin to hinder recovery process.

---

**Box 1**
**Potential compression precautions and contraindications (Torlicasi 2022, Rabe 2020)**

Risk or presence of compartment syndrome (Torlicasi, 2022)

Actively receiving vasopressors

Active infection that is not being treated with antibiotics

DVT that is not actively being treated with anticoagulants

Complete or suspected severe sensory loss in the limb

Suspected or proven severe peripheral arterial disease (Ankle brachial index <0.6)

Late stage or untreated heart failure

*Adapted from* Torlincasi AM, Lopez RA, Waseem M. Acute Compartment Syndrome. In: *StatPearls*. Treasure Island (FL): StatPearls Publishing; August 7, 2022.

> **Box 2**
> **Complications of edema**
>
> Delayed wound healing
>
> Deeper burn conversion
>
> Reduced IV access
>
> Ischemia
>
> Compartment syndrome
>
> Decreased joint ROM
>
> Increased risk of local infection
>
> *Adapted from* Ahmadinejad M, Razban F, Jahani Y, Heravi F. Limb edema in critically ill patients: Comparing intermittent compression and elevation. *International Wound Journal.* 2022;19(5):1085-1091; Rabe E, Partsch H, Morrison N, et al. Risks and contraindications of medical compression treatment – a critical reappraisal. An international consensus statement. *Phlebology:The Journal of Venous Disease.* 2020;35(7): 447-460.

## Interventions and Management

Proper management of acute edema includes noninvasive volume reduction interventions. Interventions generally include a combination of positioning, activity, and compression application—individualized for each specific patient scenario.

## Edema and Positioning

Positioning involves elevation above the level of the heart for affected areas, therefore facilitating movement of fluid from the periphery to the central vasculature.[12] Small area burns will generally need elevation of the affected limb only; however, large area burns may require elevation of all 4 limbs due to the systemic nature of the inflammatory response and fluid balance status.

## Activity and Range of Motion

Active muscle contractions and joint movements act as a muscle "pump" to drive fluid centrally.[13] If the individual is conscious and able to move safely, mobility should be stressed. Mobility should focus on single joint and compound movements involving joints distal and proximal to the injured area. For those that are sedated or unable to mobilize themselves, assisted or passive ROM is important to reduce edema and preserve joint integrity.

## Compression

Applying compression can be an effective tool for managing peripheral edema when taking contradictions into consideration (see **Box 1**). The most common complications due to compression are discomfort and skin breakdown.[14] Compression can be achieved via the following:

- Elastic bandage
- Self-adherent bandage
- Short stretch bandaging
- Tubular elastic compression hose
- Gradient compression hose
- Custom compression garment

Each of these, when applied appropriately, can effectively reduce edema in conjunction with the other interventions previously mentioned.

## CRITICAL CARE MANAGEMENT

Patients experiencing larger TBSA burns will require prolonged time spent in the ICU to heal. Burn rehabilitation should be initiated within 24 hours and continue throughout the critical care phase due to the significant risk of contracture and functional decline.

### Physiologic Effects of Immobility

Patients admitted to the burn ICU frequently require mechanical ventilation either due to inhalation injuries or to support respiratory function due to depression from analgesics and sedatives. Lengthened sedation requirements alongside frequent trips to the operating room can lead to immobility. Prolonged immobility contributes to muscle atrophy (including the diaphragm), deconditioning of the cardiovascular/respiratory systems, and pressure ulcers.[15] Large TBSA burn patients also experience a hypermetabolic response after injury resulting in catabolic erosion of skeletal muscles, increasing the presence of muscle wasting.[15] Psychosocial effects include delirium, anxiety, communication impairments, and depression. Many of these issues can extend past discharge. The International Society for Burn Injuries Practice Guidelines recommend initiation of early mobilization regardless of size TBSA injury and implementation of specific exercises programs, when possible, to achieve preburn ROM, strength, and endurance.[16] **Fig. 2** lists immobility complications, categorized by a modified systems classification approach.

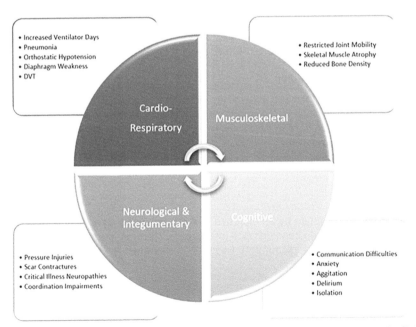

**Fig. 2.** Immobility implications. (Adapted from Cartotto R, Johnson L, Rood JM, et al. Clinical practice guideline: Early mobilization and rehabilitation of critically ill burn patients. J Burn Care Res. 2022;44(1):1-15. doi:10.1093/jbcr/irac008.)

## Coordination of Care

Clear communication with the multidisciplinary team is fundamental for coordination of early mobility and rehabilitative care, and coordinating a specific time for the mobilization to occur that works for all involved staff members and the patient is essential.

## Laboratory Values, Vitals, and Safety

A thorough chart review of the patient's current laboratory values and discussion with the interdisciplinary team before initiating mobility is imperative to patient safety. Understanding the risk of adverse events and anticipating physiologic response when these levels fall into a "critical range" should be at the forefront of each session. Additional precautions may be necessary and detailed monitoring should take place throughout the interventions. **Table 5** briefly outlines major vitals to examine during early mobility and values that indicate need for session modification or termination.

## Intensive Care Unit Equipment: Line and Tube Management

Early mobilization in the ICU requires additional time, consideration, and care to safely maneuver the patient without risking dislodging any medical devices. Disconnection of any possible lines and tubes before mobility is helpful. Properly securing, organizing, and arranging those that cannot be disconnected should be completed before initiating transfers.[17–19] Patients have an average of 8.6 tubes/lines in which staffs spend an average of 12.4 minutes managing during early mobility sessions.[19] Devices often encountered in this setting are grouped by system in **Table 6**. Despite the difficulties of line limitations and airway stability, a recent retrospective analysis demonstrated early mobilization of burn patients on mechanical ventilation to be attainable and safe.[20]

## Pain and Early Mobility

Burn pain poses a unique challenge for providers to control, specifically during rehabilitation as patients' baseline pain is often exacerbated with therapeutic activities.[21–23] American Burn Association Guidelines recommend all patients are provided nonpharmacological pain control adjuncts with the highest evidence include cognitive-behavioral therapy, hypnosis, and virtual reality.[21] Vascular pain in burned extremities with dependent positioning poses a particular challenge in early mobility. Donor site pain is severe and intense in nature, continuing for several days, and frequently

| Table 5 | |
|---|---|
| **Vitals red flags for early mobilization** | |
| **Cardiovascular System** | **Respiratory System** |
| Heart rate (>140 or <50 bpm) | Oxygen saturation (<88%) |
| Systolic blood pressure (>180 or <80 mm Hg) | Respiratory rate (>40 or <5 bpm) |
| Mean arterial pressure (>110 mm Hg or <60) | Asynchrony with mechanical ventilation |
| Arrhythmias | |
| Active bleeding | |
| Symptomatic orthostatic hypotension | |

*Abbreviations:* bpm, beats per minute; mm Hg, millimeter of mercury.
   *Data from* Alaparthi GK, Gatty A, Samuel SR, Amaravadi SK. Effectiveness, safety, and barriers to early mobilization in the Intensive Care Unit. Crit Care Res Pract. 2020;2020:1-14., Conceição TM, Gonzáles AI, Figueiredo FC, Vieira DS, Bündchen DC. Safety criteria to start early mobilization in Intensive Care Units. Systematic review. Rev Bras Ter Intensiva. 2017;29(4).

**Table 6**
**Lines and tubes by systems**

| Respiratory | Cardiovascular | Gastrointestinal/Urinary | Integumentary/Musculoskeletal |
|---|---|---|---|
| Ventilator tubing | Arterial line/bag | Hemodialysis catheter | Wound vacuum |
| ET tube | Electrocardiogram leads | CRRT | JP drain |
| Tracheostomy tube | Blood pressure cuff | Urinary catheter | Temperature probe |
| Airway suction | IV infusion machine | Fecal tube | SCD's |
| Chest tube | Central line | Feeding tube | Restraints |
| Pulse oximeter | Swan Ganz | Nasogastric tubes | |
| BiPAP, CPAP, Nasal Cannula | | | |

*Abbreviations:* BiPAP, bilevel positive airway pressure; CPAP, continuous positive airway pressure; CRRT, continuous renal replacement therapy; JP drain, Jackson Pratt, SCD's, sequential compression devices.

depicted by patients as worse than their initial burn pain.[24] Compression wraps (**Fig. 3**) may help modulate this component of pain.[22,25,26]

Patients with large TBSA injuries require specialized sedation during their stay to facilitate healing and achieve analgesia; however, oversedation can become a major barrier to patient participation in early mobility.[15,22,27] Weaning the ventilator to allow for "sedation vacations or holidays" during mobility is integral, yet particularly challenging with this patient population due to complex pain.[22] Early mobility team members must consider the other factors that affect the perception of pain beyond the nociceptive wound pain itself, including mood and cognition.[22] Without proper dynamic pain control patients are at risk for anxiety and posttraumatic stress associated with the painful period. **Table 7** highlights different types of pain, and their pharmacologic interventions as well as other interventions that may be useful in modulating pain.[22,28]

### Minimizing Anxiety/Agitation

During their first mobilization sessions, patients' anxiety tends to center around feelings of unpreparedness, vulnerability, and instability.[29] Therapists must consider these responses and attempt to reduce them by providing clear instructions, reassurance, and encouragement.[29]

### EARLY MOBILIZATION

Early mobilization, demonstrated in **Fig. 4**, includes a systematic approach to providing physical activity, initiated within at least 14 days of sustaining a burn injury, whereas a patient is still in an ICU setting.[15] General ICU research has been found to not only influence long-term effects of immobility but also contribute to increased functional independence at discharge along with decreased ventilator days, ICU length of stay (LOS), and delirium.[30–34] More recently, burn research and evolutions in practice have also occurred to support early mobilization for burn survivors.[20,35,36]

### Barriers to Early Mobilization

Factors including cardiovascular instability, fluid resuscitation, airway management, sedation management, associated traumas, and surgery that typically occur during the first week of a burn ICU admission greatly limit a patient's availability for

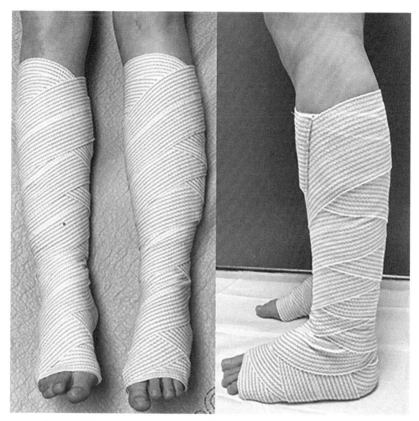

**Fig. 3.** Double ACE-Wrap for management of lower extremity pain management.

| Table 7 Nonopioid pharmacologic and adjunctive therapies for components of burn pain | | |
|---|---|---|
| **Pain Component** | **Pharmacologic Modality** | **Adjunctive Therapies** |
| Background | Ketamine | Music<br>Massage<br>Aromatherapy<br>Cooling<br>Extracorporeal shock wave therapy |
| Neuropathic | Gabapentin<br>Pregabalin | Laser therapy<br>Acupuncture |
| Procedural | Ketamine<br>Intravenous Lidocaine | Music<br>Whole body vibration<br>Jaw relaxation<br>Virtual reality<br>Interactive gaming Console<br>Transcranial direct current stimulation<br>Hypnosis |
| Breakthrough | Acetaminophen<br>Antidepressants | None yet identified |

*Data from* Kim DE, Pruskowski KA, Ainsworth CR, Linsenbardt HR, Rizzo JA, Cancio LC. A Review of Adjunctive Therapies for Burn Injury Pain During the Opioid Crisis. *J Burn Care Res.* 2019;40(6):983-995. https://doi.org/10.1093/jbcr/irz111

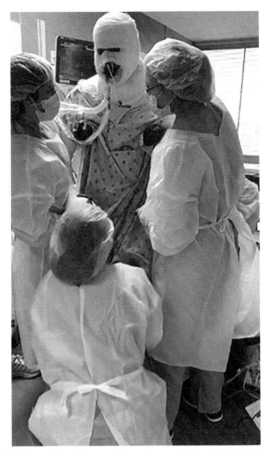

**Fig. 4.** Early mobilization with a burn patient who sustained 85% TBSA injury.

rehabilitation. However, with physician guidance, team coordination, and protocol development, most perceived barriers can be overcome.

Airway security and fear of extubation are challenges when patients are using mechanical ventilation. Security method of the endotracheal (ET) tube should always be considered in planning of the mobility session with inclusion of respiratory therapy and nursing for additional monitoring. Progression out of bed or sustained time upright in a chair may be limited in situations of decreased ET tube security.

Sedation and pain management substantially influence therapy sessions, potentially limiting a patient's ability to participate if oversedated.[37] However, nondirectable agitation can also lead to safety concerns with an increased risk of adverse events. Timing sessions to maximize alertness by coordinating with scheduled sedation interruptions or before dressing changes is crucial for success and safety of early mobilization.

Mobility practices following autograft placement can also be a barrier to early mobilization during the critical care period. Visualizing grafts including location of placement, security method, and adherence is necessary to plan for proper protection during mobility. Compression wraps and support including abdominal binders can be used to bolster postop dressings. Although promoting functional use of extremities is preferred to prevent contracture, splints may need to remain in place to avoid sheer during mobilization. Therapists should always be mindful of hand placement and consider the use of alternative movement patterns for graft protection. For example, if grafts are posterior on the back and buttock, a patient may need to be log-rolled to the edge of the bed then transitioned upright into sitting to avoid scooting, and therefore shear forces to the grafts.

## Treatment Progression

Therapy treatments generally start with a thorough chart review, participation during multidisciplinary team rounding, and coordination of staff members. **Fig. 5** describes a pathway for mobility progression in stages, based on a patient's alertness and ability to follow commands. Bed activities allow assessment of a patient's ability to follow commands, functional strength, and medical responses to positional changes. Based on a patient's tolerance, they can be progressed along the continuum to transfers and upright sitting activities.

Transitions to sitting at the edge of bed can be initiated safely (**Fig. 6**), even with limited alertness, allowing further stimulation and assessment. Progression to upright sitting at this stage may require use of bedding along with at minimum a therapist anteriorly and a second posteriorly for physical support. Coordination between physical and occupational therapists can be valuable due to the extensive skill required for the management of multiple variables within a single session. From the edge of bed, core stabilization exercises can be initiated along with activities of daily living (ADLs). Use of windows, family presence, pet therapy, and other motivating factors can increase engagement and initiation of dynamic therapeutic activities.

Standing activities may require more staff or specialty equipment to assist. Manual support at the hands, upper arms, and/or blocking of the knees might be necessary, based on a patient's level of weakness. Assistive devices, can support balance and encourage use of hands for patients with upper extremity injuries. Ambulation is initiated with laterally stepping followed by pivot transfers and forward ambulation if a patient demonstrates enough strength and coordination. Before progressing away from the edge of the bed, the Egress test (originally designed for bariatric patients) can be used as a screen to determine safety.[38]

Mobilization activities should be performed with a general goal of improving a patient's strength, functional independence, and activity tolerance. However, for the burn therapist, a mindset should also be in place to perform functional movements during mobility that support goals tissue elongation for affected burn and grafted areas. Knowledge of skin biomechanics, CFUs, and common contracture patterns associated with each location of burn injury can assist with planning early mobility

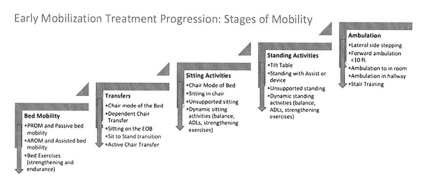

Early Mobilization Treatment Progression: Stages of Mobility

**Ambulation**
- Lateral side stepping
- Forward ambulation <10 ft.
- Ambulation to in room
- Ambulation in hallway
- Stair Training

**Standing Activities**
- Tilt Table
- Standing with Assist or device
- Unsupported standing
- Dynamic standing activities (balance, ADLs, strengthening exercises)

**Sitting Activities**
- Chair Mode of Bed
- Sitting in chair
- Unsupported sitting
- Dynamic sitting activities (balance, ADLs, strengthening exercises)

**Transfers**
- Chair mode of the Bed
- Dependent Chair Transfer
- Sitting on the EOB
- Sit to Stand transition
- Active Chair Transfer

**Bed Mobility**
- PROM and Passive bed mobility
- AROM and Assisted bed mobility
- Bed Exercises (strengthening and endurance)

**Fig. 5.** Pathway for mobility progression.

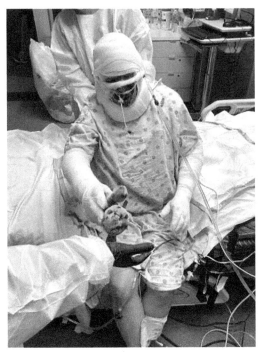

**Fig. 6.** Patient with 17% TBSA burn injuries working on upright dynamic balance, activity tolerance, and functional reaching/grasping tasks.

session, allow opportunities to incorporate active tissue stretch, and improve motor planning of injured extremities through promotion of functional ROM.[5–7,39] **Table 8** outlines opportunities to combine ROM and tissue elongation goals with functional mobility progression as scar contracture prevention continues to be the ultimate goal of burn rehabilitation.

### Mobilization Equipment

The equipment used for mobility progression can include *mechanical lifts* for supine or seated dependent transfers using specialty slings for supine or seated transfers. Some manufacturers include slings for standing and ambulation assistance. *Cardiac chairs* are essential in ICU settings, allowing upright positioning while securing with straps and lateral supports. *Tilt tables* (**Fig. 7**) can also initiate early weight-bearing activities. *Standing frames* and *sit-to-stand transition aids* permit assisted transfer training and strengthening once a patient has enough core stability to safely sit unsupported. *Ambulatory aids*, including specialty ICU walkers, are available for supported gait training while providing attachments for critical care monitors. Equipment and strapping may have to be modified based on location of a patient's open wounds and grafts. Foam padding, strap modifications, and pillows can be used to prevent increased pain and shear forces while using equipment.

### EARLY AMBULATION

The burn setting continues to lack a standardized definition or established evidence-based protocol for "early ambulation." Despite investigative efforts to shift culture,

**Table 8**
**Tissue elongation during functional mobility**

|  | Body Location | Movement |
|---|---|---|
| Rolling | Trunk | Rotation initiated with upper or lower body movements first |
|  | Upper extremity | Sidelying shoulder flexion, overhead or forward reaching |
|  | Lower extremity | Sidelying hip flexion and hip extension, knee flexion, and extension |
| Sitting | Cervical | ROM and functional tracking activities |
|  | Trunk | Composite arm and trunk movements during dynamic balance activities. Reaching outside base of support. Trunk writing and core stabilization |
|  | Upper extremities | Weight-bearing opportunity for hands. Promotion of ADLs |
|  | Lower extremities | Hip flexion, knee flexion, and ankle dorsiflexion sustained stretch |
| Standing | Upper body | Combined overhead reaching tasks for function movements and trunk elongation |
|  | Lower body | Composite trunk extension, hip extension, knee extension, and ankle dorsiflexion |
| Ambulation | Upper body | Natural arm swing and trunk mobility without assistive device. Weight-bearing and functional use of arms with assistive device |
|  | Lower body | Promotion of ankle dorsiflexion, knee and hip ROM through gait cycle |

commonly accepted practice patterns associated with lower extremity postoperative autograft management often include a conservative approach of bedrest[40] up to postoperative day (POD) 5 or later with no substantial evidence in support of this practice.[41,42] There is also a tendency to immobilize[43,44] and elevate[43,45] an extremity after autograft placement with non–weight-bearing (NWB) implemented if an involved joint is located on the lower extremity.[41] Prolonged immobilization may result in increased complications including impaired range of motion, decreased ability to perform ADLs, deconditioning, deep vein thrombosis (DVT) pulmonary embolism, prolonged hospital LOS, reduced quality of life, and reduced functional outcome.[43,44,40,47]

The concept of early ambulation dates to 1971 where ambulation occurred within 24 to 48 hours postsurgical intervention, with no compromise to skin graft adherence observed.[48] Several subsequent early ambulation studies through 2019 occurred with a variety of burn and nonburn lower extremity wounds requiring autograft placement. Within this large timeframe, inpatient care and grafting techniques have evolved, which makes generalization challenging.[47] Comparison between burn-injured patients to other injuries is also challenging due to the presence of soft tissue damage that may be significant enough to impair muscle function involved with mobility, particularly following surgical debridement of burn wounds. Subsequent autograft placement may prompt immobility of the joint to protect the grafts. Sufficient immobilization support to promote graft adherence on lower extremities during ambulation can be achieved with a posterior splint,[49] conforming cast,[41,42] or Unna boot[50] in adults. Practice patterns within the last decade have shifted toward earlier postoperative autograft ambulation[51]

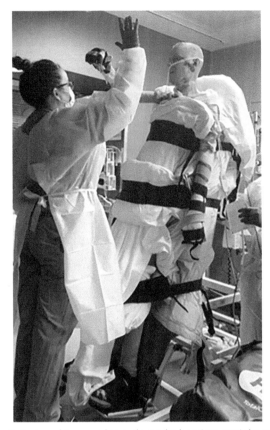

**Fig. 7.** Tilt table activity to achieve prolonged weight-bearing, upright tolerance, in combination with functional reaching tasks.

### Perceived Barriers to Early Ambulation

Postop immobilization protocols may be attributed to beliefs that skin graft loss and poor adherence occur from "shearing" forces associated with joint movement and may result in subsequent hematoma formation.[41,43,52] Other factors include tissue necrosis[43] or venous stasis and edema associated with lower extremity placed in a dependent position.[41] Early research suggests these barriers may be overcome by applying meshed autografts that allow underlying fluid to escape through the interstices.[53] Application of a firm compression dressing to the involved leg allows immediate dependent positioning and mobilization while protecting immature grafts.[53] Use of an appropriate assistive device can aid in maintaining NWB,[53] allowing mobility even in grafts that involve the foot or ankle complex.

### Graft Healing

Lower extremity skin graft adherence is not significantly impacted by timing of postoperative mobility.[41–43] Application of negative pressure wound therapy to provide stabilization and promotion of split-thickness skin graft (STSG) adherence, while allowing for movement and ambulation, may be beneficial during early ambulation but is not always associated with successful graft adherence.[40,45,52]

## Other Factors

Early ambulation may have a positive impact on pain reduction experienced at rest and with ambulation in comparison to delayed mobility,[41] which may, in turn, lead to decreased reliance on opioids for pain management.[47] Early ambulation patients guided with functionally oriented motor tasks, along with a progressive ambulation regimen without an assistive device, benefit from improved strength, endurance, decreased pain complaints, decreased return to baseline knee and/or ankle range of motion, and reduction in perceived fear and helplessness.[54] Early influence on factors that contribute to overall pain, joint mechanics, and functional use of the lower extremity during the healing phase has significant implications toward reduced risk of long-term contracture development. Early ambulation also influences a reduction in overall hospital LOS, which may result in decreased costs of care and associated decreased risk for complications such as infection or nosocomial systemic morbidities.[41,47]

## Autograft Location and Type

The propensity to initiate out of bed (OOB) activity tends to be segmented by body region. Grafts superior to the waist have the least impact on clinical decisions for imposed restrictions, which result in earlier mobility compared with grafts inferior to the waist down to the feet (waist > knees > lower legs > feet) as seen in **Fig. 8**.[55] Treatment of full-thickness skin grafts (FTSG) compared with STSG and nonmeshed (sheet) grafts has no significant influence on mobility postoperatively[51] and no difference in graft success rates between STSG and FTSG.[40]

## Proposed Practice Guidelines

Based on a systematic review of available clinical evidence and an international consensus exercise to supplement gaps in data, initiation of an early ambulation protocol after postoperative lower extremity autograft placement is recommended to commence immediately postoperatively, or within 48 hours, unless exclusion criteria are recognized (**Box 3**). Application of external compression[41,42,44,52] in a figure-of-eight pattern[55] to the involved lower extremity is recommended before ambulation to promote autograft adherence and venous return.[55] Any autograft involving a joint should be immobilized.[41,42] If the patient is initially unable to accept weight on involved lower extremity, so long as graft does not cross a joint, gradual ambulation and progressive weight-bearing can be implemented. This suggested protocol represented in

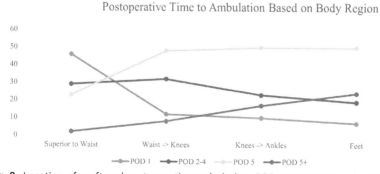

**Fig. 8.** Location of graft and postoperative ambulation. POD, postoperative day. (*Data from* Holavanahalli R, Helm P, Parry I, Dolezal C, Greenhalgh D. Select practices in management and rehabilitation of burns: a survey report. J Burn Care Res 2011;32:210-23.)

---

**Box 3**
**Guideline for early ambulation following lower extremity autograft based on burn-specific expert opinion**

Exclusion Criteria for Early Ambulation Protocol

Wound exceeding 300 cm$^2$

Autograft to the plantar aspect of the foot

Presence of a fracture

Baseline ambulation impairment

Baseline psychiatric or social conditions that affect participation

Medical status contraindicates ambulation

*Abbreviation:* cm$^2$, centimeters squared.

*Data from* Nedelec B, Serghiou M, Niszczak J, McMahon M, Healey T. Practice guidelines for early ambulation of burn survivors after lower extremity grafts. J Burn Care Res 2012;33(3):319-329

---

**Fig. 9** is intended to provide a safe and successful pathway to guide clinicians while recognizing regional and institutional differences that may influence treatment of patients in the burn population.

## Considerations

With most literature including only small uncomplicated burns and wounds[41,43,51] burn care clinicians must rely on their own evaluation of the patients' burn injury extent and location, physiologic status, cognition, preburn functional status and motor capabilities, to determine if proceeding with early ambulation efforts is in the best interest of the patient. Use of a tilt table may be necessary to support tolerance to upright if orthostatic or dependent lower extremity vascular pain limits progression.[50] The use of walking aids such as front-wheeled walkers, crutches, canes, or knee scooters may be necessary to facilitate safe progression of activity and, if indicated, offload an autografted joint.

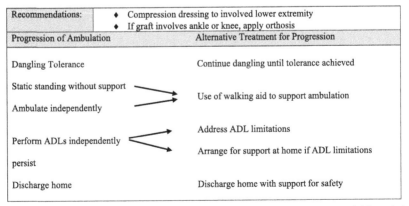

**Fig. 9.** Lower extremity autograft guideline to early ambulation. ADLs, activities of daily living. (*Data from* Nedelec B, Serghiou M, Niszczak J, McMahon M, Healey T. Practice guidelines for early ambulation of burn survivors after lower extremity grafts. J Burn Care Res 2012;33(3):319-329.)

## SUMMARY

Burn rehabilitation should commence within 24 hours of admission and be initiated with a comprehensive evaluation that addresses multiple domains of function and supportive information necessary to inform an appropriate plan of care. Burn mobility, to include progression from supine to sitting, upright, limb weight-bearing, transfers, and gait can be rendered safely for burn survivors much earlier in care than has been done historically and can be adapted to meet range of motion, strengthening, and functional independence goals efficiently and even concurrently. Contemporary, comprehensive therapy plans should not only include positioning, range of motion, edema management, strengthening, and exercise but also mobility — even while patients remain on the ICU or are in the immediate postautografting window.

## CLINICS CARE POINTS

- Whether a burn patient is an adult or child, contracture management should be the primary focus of rehabilitation throughout all phases of care.
- Increased rehabilitation times produce better outcomes in both small and large burns.
- If not managed, edema can hinder the recovery process.
- The entire care team must be well coordinated to optimize recovery and outcomes in the burn population.
- Pain control is critical to effective and humane care, and there are several adjuncts beyond opioids that can be supportive in most cases, exempting breakthrough pain.
- Burn research and evolutions in practice support early mobilization for burn survivors.
- Mobilization activities should emphasize strength, functional independence, and activity tolerance. For burns, these activities should also encourage tissue elongation of burn and graft involved areas.
- Unless exclusion criteria prohibit, early ambulation after postoperative lower extremity autograft placement is recommended to commence immediately postoperatively or, at least, within 48 hours.

## DISCLOSURE

Authors have nothing to disclose.

## REFERENCES

1. Richard RL, Hedman TL, Quick CD, et al. A clarion to recommit and reaffirm burn rehabilitation. J Burn Care Res 2008;29(3):425–32.
2. Dewey WS, Richard RL, Parry IS. Positioning, splinting, and contracture management. Phys Med Rehabil Clin N Am 2011;22(2):229–v.
3. Richard RL, Jones JA, Dewey WS, et al. Small and large burns alike benefit from lengthier rehabilitation time. J Burn Care Res 2015;36:S108.
4. Richard R, Anyan W, Kemp-Offenberg J, et al. Increased burn rehabilitation treatment time improves patient outcome. J Burn Care Res 2014;35:S100.
5. Serghiou MA, Niszczak J, Parry I, et al. Clinical practice recommendations for positioning of the burn patient. Burns 2016;42(2):267–75.
6. Richard RL, Lester ME, Miller SF, et al. Identification of cutaneous functional units related to burn scar contracture development. J Burn Care Res 2009;30(4):625–31.

7. Jacobson K, Fletchall S, Dodd H, et al. Current Concepts Burn Rehabilitation, Part I: Care During Hospitalization. Clin Plast Surg 2017;44(4):703–12.
8. Cummings GS, Crutchfield CA, Barnes MR. Orthopedic physical therapy series. Atlanta: Stokesville Publishing; 1983.
9. Zhang YT, Li-Tsang CWP, Au RKC. A Systematic Review on the Effect of Mechanical Stretch on Hypertrophic Scars after Burn Injuries. Hong Kong J Occup Ther 2017;29(1):1–9.
10. Godleski M, Oeffling A, Bruflat AK, et al. Treating burn-associated joint contracture: results of an inpatient rehabilitation stretching protocol. J Burn Care Res 2013;34(4):420–6.
11. Parry IS, Schneider JC, Yelvington M, et al. Systematic Review and Expert Consensus on the Use of Orthoses (Splints and Casts) with Adults and Children after Burn Injury to Determine Practice Guidelines. J Burn Care Res 2020;41(3):503–34.
12. Ahmadinejad M, Razban F, Jahani Y, et al. Limb edema in critically ill patients: Comparing intermittent compression and elevation. Int Wound J 2022;19(5):1085–91.
13. Li T, Yang S, Hu F, et al. Effects of ankle pump exercise frequency on venous hemodynamics of the lower limb. Clin Hemorheol Microcirc 2020;76(1):111–20.
14. Rabe E, Partsch H, Morrison N, et al. Risks and contraindications of medical compression treatment – a critical reappraisal. An international consensus statement. Phlebology:The Journal of Venous Disease 2020;35(7):447–60.
15. Cartotto R, Johnson L, Rood JM, et al. Clinical practice guideline: Early mobilization and rehabilitation of critically ill burn patients. J Burn Care Res 2022;44(1):1–15.
16. Plaza A, Adsett J, Byrnes A, et al. Physical activity levels in hospitalized adults with burn injuries. J Burn Care Res 2021;43(5):1048–54.
17. Alaparthi GK, Gatty A, Samuel SR, et al. Effectiveness, safety, and barriers to early mobilization in the Intensive Care Unit. Crit Care Res Pract 2020;2020:1–14.
18. Conceição TM, Gonzáles AI, Figueiredo FC, et al. Safety criteria to start early mobilization in Intensive Care Units. Systematic review. Rev Bras Ter Intensiva 2017;29(4).
19. Benjamin E, Roddy L, Giuliano KK. Management of patient tubes and lines during early mobility in the Intensive Care Unit. Hum Factors 2022;2:100017.
20. ONeil AM, Rush C, Griffard L, et al. 510 5-year retrospective analysis of a vented early mobility algorithm in the burn ICU. J Burn Care Res 2022;43:1129–34.
21. Romanowski KS, Carson J, Pape K, et al. American Burn Association guidelines on the management of acute pain in the adult burn patient: A review of the literature, a compilation of expert opinion, and next steps. J Burn Care Res 2020;41(6):1129–51.
22. Griggs C, Goverman J, Bittner EA, et al. Sedation and pain management in burn patients. Clin Plast Surg 2017;44(3):535–40.
23. Patterson DR, Hoflund H, Espey K, et al. Pain management. Burns 2004;30(8). https://doi.org/10.1016/j.burns.2004.08.004.
24. Sinha S, Schreiner AJ, Biernaskie J, et al. Treating pain on skin graft donor sites: Review and Clinical Recommendations. J Trauma Acute Care Surg 2017;83(5):954–64.
25. Christian LM, Graham JE, Padgett DA, et al. Stress and wound healing. Neuroimmunomodulation 2006;13(5–6):337–46.
26. Patterson DR, Carrigan L, Questad KA, et al. Post-traumatic stress disorder in hospitalized patients with burn injuries. J Burn Care Rehabil 1990;11(3):181–4.

27. Bright L, Van Der Lee L, Hince D, et al. Quantification of the negative impact of sedation and inotropic support on achieving early mobility in burn patients in ICU: A single center observational study. Burns 2021;47(8):1756–65.
28. Funk DH, Fletchall S, Velamuri SR. 72 burn rehabilitation non-invasive approach; lower extremity Burns. J Burn Care Res 2022;43.
29. Söderberg A, Karlsson V, Ahlberg BM, et al. From fear to fight: Patients experiences of early mobilization in intensive care. A qualitative interview study. Physiother Theory Pract 2020;38(6):750–8.
30. Adler J, Malone D. Early mobilization in the intensive care unit: a systematic review. Cardiopulm Phys Ther J 2012;23:5–13.
31. Bailey P, Thomsen GE, Spuhler VJ, et al. Early activity is feasible and safe in respiratory failure patients. Crit Care Med 2007;35:139–45.
32. Zhang L, Hu W, Cai Z, et al. Early mobilization of critically ill patients in the intensive care unit: a systematic review and meta-analysis. PLoS One 2019;14: e0223185.
33. Hashem MD, Parker AM, Needham DM. Early mobilization and rehabilitation of patients who are critically ill. Chest 2016;150:722–31.
34. Hodgson CL, Stiller K, Needham DM, et al. Expert consensus and recommendations on safety criteria for active mobilization of mechanically ventilated critically ill adults. Crit Care 2014;18:658.
35. Clark DE, Lowman JD, Griffin RL, et al. Effectiveness of an early mobilization protocol in a trauma and burns intensive care unit: a retrospective cohort study. Phys Ther 2013;93:186–96.
36. de Figueiredo TB, Utsunomiya KF, de Oliveira AMRR, et al. Mobilization practices for patients with burn injury in critical care. Burns 2020;46:314–21.
37. Thomsen GE, Snow GL, Rodriguez L, et al. Patients with respiratory failure increase ambulation after transfer to an intensive care unit where early activity is a priority. Crit Care Med 2008;36:1119–24.
38. Barbay K, Williams K, Berning P. The Utility of the Modified Dionne's Egress Test as a Predictor of Falls in Adult Medical and Surgical Patients. J Nurs Adm 2021; 51(12):638–44.
39. Lester ME, Hazelton J, Dewey WS, et al. Influence of upper extremity positioning on pain, paresthesia, and tolerance: advancing current practice. J Burn Care Res 2013;34(6):e342–50.
40. Reddy S, El-Haddawi F, Fancourt M, et al. The incidence and risk factors for lower limb skin graft failure. Dermatology Research and Practice 2014;2014:582080.
41. Lorello D, Peck M, Albrecht M, et al. Results of a prospective randomized controlled trial of early ambulation for patients with lower extremity autografts. J Burn Care Res 2014;35:431–6.
42. Kumar N. Effect of an early vs. late ambulation over graft take on the lower limb autograft: a comparative study. Annals of Plastic and Reconstructive Surgery 2019;3(5):1043.
43. Nedelec B, Serghiou M, Niszczak J, et al. Practice guidelines for early ambulation of burn survivors after lower extremity grafts. J Burn Care Res 2012;33(3):319–29.
44. Gawaziuk J, Peters B, Logsetty S. Early ambulation after-grafting of lower extremity burns. Burns 2018;44(1):183–7.
45. Henderson N, Fancourt M, Gilkison W, et al. Skin grafts: a rural general surgical perspective. ANZ J Surg 2009;79(5):362–6.
46. Tallon B, Lamb S, Patel D. Randomized nonblinded comparison of convalescence for 2 and 7 days after split-thickness skin grafting to the lower legs. Dermatol Surg 2009;35:634–7.

47. Lagziel T, Ramos M, Klifto K, et al. Complication with time-to-ambulation following skin grafting for burn patients: a meta-analysis and systematic review. Cureus 2021;13(8):e17214.
48. Bodenham D, Watson R. The early ambulation of patients with lower limb grafts. Br J of Plasti Surg 1971;24:20–2.
49. Richard R, Baryza M, Carr J, et al. Burn rehabilitation and research: proceedings of a consensus summit. J Burn Care Res 2009;30:543–73.
50. Dean S, Press B. Outpatient or short-stay skin grafting with early ambulation for lower-extremity burns. Ann Plast Surg 1990;25(2):150–1.
51. Parry I, Sen S, Palmieri T, et al. Current trends in practice for early mobility with the burn population. J Burn Care Res 2019;40(1):29–33.
52. Achora S, Muliira J, Thanka A. Strategies to promote healing of split thickness skin grafts: an integrative review. J Wound Ostomy Continence Nurs 2014; 41(4):335–9.
53. Sharpe D, Cardoso E, Baheti V. The immediate mobilization of patients with lower limb skin grafts: a clinical report. Br J Plast Surg 1983;36:105–8.
54. Burnsworth B, Krob M, Langer-Schnepp M. Immediate ambulation of patients with lower-extremity grafts. J Burn Care Rehabil 1992;13:89–92.
55. Holavanahalli R, Helm P, Parry I, et al. Select practices in management and rehabilitation of burns: a survey report. J Burn Care Res 2011;32:210–23.

# Inpatient Rehabilitation Following Burn Injury

Maria Twichell, MD

## KEYWORDS

• Inpatient rehabilitation • Burn • Physiatrists • Complications

## KEY POINTS

- Inpatient rehabilitation has been shown to reduce acute center length of stay (LOS) and improves functional outcomes.
- Burn survivors should meet standard InterQual criteria to be considered for IPR, including ability to tolerate and participate in greater than 3 hours of therapy daily. Per Centers for Medicare & Medicaid Services, burns are 1 of the 13 qualifying diagnoses requiring intensive rehabilitation.
- The physiatrist diagnoses and treats postburn complications including: pruritus, neuropathy, heterotopic ossification, nutrition, and dysphagia.
- The physiatrist considers interventions to address medical sequelae of injury, including pain, itch, neuropathy, psychological coping, and mood.
- The physiatrist devises and oversees an exercise program based on the survivor's functional status and goals to begin during inpatient rehabilitation that can continue in the outpatient setting.

## INTRODUCTION

As of 2012, more than 9000 burn survivors used inpatient rehabilitation (IPR) services to improve their functional outcomes after burn injury.[1] Burn injuries are 1 of the 13 diagnoses requiring intensive IPR per Centers for Medicare & Medicaid Services inclusion rule.[2] Burn survivors in IPR demonstrate outcomes similar to those admitted because of other etiologies, including stroke, acquired brain injury, spinal cord dysfunction, orthopedic conditions, and other neurologic conditions.[1] The number of burn survivors discharged to IPR can vary from 8% to 26% of patients admitted to the hospital for burn injury, depending on the state where they are located and the percentage of body surface involved.[3] It is noted that IPR for these patients helped to reduce acute center length of stay (LOS) and improves functional outcomes.[1]

LOS in IPR depends on functional limitations of the individual survivor and total body surface area (TBSA) involvement. According to the Burn Model Systems, 3.2% of burn

Department of Physical Medicine and Rehabilitation, School of Medicine, University of Pittsburgh, 3471 Fifth Avenue, Suite 910, Pittsburgh, PA 15213, USA
E-mail address: twichellmf@upmc.edu

Phys Med Rehabil Clin N Am 34 (2023) 755–765
https://doi.org/10.1016/j.pmr.2023.06.002

survivors spent 1 to 10 days in IPR, 4.6% spent 11 to 20 days in IPR, and 5.2% needed more than 21 days of IPR.[4]

Characteristics of survivors requiring comprehensive IPR services include those with more complex injuries including: large burns (>20% TBSA), especially involving the hands and feet; range of motion (ROM) restriction; inhalation injury; dysphagia; and prolonged acute course including mechanical ventilation.[1] Survivors who participated in IPR programs had a higher likelihood of returning to employment 1 year post-injury compared with those who received rehabilitation at a skilled nursing facility (SNF), long-term care hospital, or other extended care facility, despite a more severe injury.[5]

Those older than 55 years of age account for 14% of hospitalized burn survivors and are a population that require particular attention in care planning and management.[6] IPR is shown to confer a benefit to older survivors and practice models should include IPR as a discharge option for all older burn survivors. Older survivors tend to have a longer acute care hospital stay, higher likelihood of complications and death, and discharge to a nonindependent living situation, such as SNF, compared with younger survivors.[6] Discharges to an independent living location may be increased with a rehabilitation program that begins in the acute care hospitalization phase and is continued with a stay in IPR.[6]

IPR instead of SNF may provide a survivorship benefit for those greater than 60 years old. Approximately 20% of older survivors are discharged to SNF, particularly those with larger burns, inhalation injury, prolonged hospital LOS, and government-issued insurance. At follow-up (an average of 46 months postdischarge), 58.6% of those discharged to SNF were deceased compared with 24.1% of survivors discharged to home. There was no difference in comorbidities or complications between the groups to account for the difference in mortality.[7] Discharge to IPR instead of SNF allows for additional time for burn healing with onsite wound care, intensive therapies to improve functional status, and potentially less burden of care for caregivers. These benefits can increase the likelihood of home discharge, thus survivorship. In addition, caregiver support, a familiar environment, and a daily routine in a home setting may be helpful for ongoing recovery and survival of elderly burn patients.

## EVALUATION FOR INPATIENT REHABILITATION

Early physical medicine and rehabilitation consultation by a physiatrist allows involvement throughout the patient's acute care course to make appropriate rehabilitation-specific recommendations and evaluate their candidacy for IPR. Use of intensive physical and occupational therapy (PT, OT) services during the acute care phase is standard of care. It improves the functional status of the burn survivor on presentation to IPR,[8] thus affecting the likelihood of discharge to home and reducing acute care LOS.

When evaluating a burn survivor in the acute care setting, the rehabilitation team should document pertinent portions of the history and physical examination to inform the treatment plan. Essential elements of the history and physical examination include: how the burn occurred, cause, classification, and TBSA of the burn injury including the initial modified Lund-Browder chart documented by the acute care team; concomitant injuries; plans for surgical salvage versus amputation of affected limbs; weight-beating status; additional planned interventions or surgeries; pain; if clearance is granted for positioning and splinting; preinjury cognition and functional status and activity level; current activities of daily living and mobility; psychosocial components; and short- and long-term treatment goals. The examination should include measurement of edema, ROM, strength, sensation, and scar assessment.[9]

All acute surgical interventions should be completed before admission to IPR to minimize interruption of the comprehensive therapy program. However, for survivors with large burns, a planned readmission to acute care for additional surgeries after an interim of period of healing wound beds or donor sites and improving nutrition while rehabilitating in IPR is beneficial. Burn survivors in IPR that were transferred back to acute care and subsequently readmitted to IPR had a lower functional level on admission and discharge during their first IPR admission but improved at the time of their second IPR discharge to match scores of those who had only one IPR admission.[2] Although return to acute care is typically viewed as a negative outcome in the current payor system, at times it may be the best course of care.[2,9]

Burn survivors should meet standard InterQual criteria to be considered for IPR, including ability to tolerate and participate in greater than 3 hours of therapy daily, ongoing medical issues to be managed by a physiatrist with specialized rehabilitation training, and care needs that cannot be coordinated in an SNF environment.[10] Although the criteria for admission to IPR is nationally standardized, there is significant variation in use of IPR services by state. This may be attributed to differences in local physician practice habits and resources available between states. Higher age, higher TBSA (up to 70%), hospitalization at a burn center as opposed to an outlying hospital, and possession of health insurance were also identified as factors increasing the likelihood of IPR stay after acute hospitalization for burn injury.[4] It should be noted that because burn injury is included in the Medicare 60% rule (in which each IPR facility is required to document at least 60% of patients have at least 1 of 13 qualifying diagnosis)[10] it may benefit IPRs with borderline compliance to admit burn survivors.

## TREATMENT

The physiatrist managing an inpatient burn survivor needs to be adept at recognizing additional complications that may present during IPR. Symptoms may be present on admission, or not be evident until a survivor is further along in their course.

### Wound Care

Burn survivors in IPR receive daily burn wound care provided by burn-certified nurses and physicians. Wound care is scheduled to minimize interruption of therapies. Before wound care, patients are treated for anticipated procedural pain. Dressing changes and wound care of open areas are provided daily, with emollients applied to healed areas multiple times per day by nurses or occupational therapists. Emphasis is placed on patient teaching for self-management and caregiver training. Once cleared, self-management of wound care in the shower is an excellent preparation for home.

### Management of Pain

Burn survivors in IPR must have a multimodal pain medication regimen in place. An effective pain regimen should include medications that address background, breakthrough, procedural, and postoperative pain. Acutely, opiates are the foundation of pain management, but can be weaned during the rehabilitation stay. Adjuvant pain medications, such as nonsteroidal anti-inflammatory drugs and acetaminophen, can reduce the need for higher doses of opiates. Gabapentin may help to address neuropathic pain or itch.[11] A typical regimen consists of three to four doses per day of scheduled acetaminophen and gabapentin for background pain control with opiates dosed for breakthrough pain. Medications for breakthrough pain can be scheduled before anticipated therapies to maximize benefit and permit the fullest participation in rehabilitation activities.

As part of a multimodal approach to burn pain, the American Burn Association (ABA) Guidelines on the Management of Acute Pain recommends nonpharmacologic inventions, such as cognitive-behavioral therapy and virtual reality.[12] In IPR, psychologists assist with coping skills, stress and anxiety management, identifying support systems, and provide outpatient resources. Psychologists can also assist patients and caregivers in their adjustment to role changes, such as parenting or working, and changes in appearance. Education about psychological techniques including cognitive behavioral training, relaxation techniques, and cognitive restricting tasks, is helpful.[13] Providers should also treat psychological pain modifiers, such as anxiety, which may exacerbate pain. In refractory cases, benzodiazepines can reduce anxiety related to dressing changes or procedures. Psychiatry consultation can help to adjust medications to address acute stress reaction, posttraumatic stress disorder, anxiety, and insomnia.

### Pruritus

Postburn pruritus affects between 70% and 90% of adult burn survivors and reduces quality of life.[14,15] It is important to recognize and treat postburn pruritis in the IPR setting. Although no consensus has been reached, pathophysiology is postulated to include pruritogenic and neuropathic pathways involved in regeneration of tissue.[15] Neuropeptide secretion is needed to promote epidermal, connective tissue, and vascular cell proliferation. These neuropeptides also increase the sensitivity of the itch receptors, which carry itch sensation via unmyelinated C afferent fibers to the central nervous system.[16] Gabapentin or pregabalin are effective treatment options especially in chronic postburn pruritus. Topical emollients and massage also have a role in treatment. Antihistamines are generally not helpful, although hydroxyzine may be useful to decrease scratching because of its anxiolytic properties.

### Neuropathy

Please reference the article on neuropathy elsewhere in this issue for complete information; however, the rehabilitation physiatrist should be aware of the potential of neuropathy to affect the survivor in IPR. Between 10% and 37% of persons with burns are affected by peripheral neuropathies as a direct result of their injury, surgeries, positioning, and/or compression[16,17] Generalized peripheral neuropathy can also be a result of the circulating inflammatory mediators from the body's systemic response to burn injury. This manifests clinically as paresthesia and distal weakness, and affects the rehabilitative process.[14] As in the general population, neuropathies may be managed in IPR setting with PT, OT, splinting, and neuropathic pain medication.[17]

### Heterotopic Ossification

Heterotopic ossification (HO) is discussed elsewhere in this issue. However, the burn physiatrist should be aware of the potential of HO to manifest while in IPR. HO affects between 3.5% and 5.6% of persons with burns,[18,19] with the posterior elbow being the most common site.[18] In one study, the median time to clinical development of HO in burn survivors was 37 days (range, 30–40).[19] Therefore, survivors may be in acute care or in IPR at the time of initial development of HO.

A small study specific to burn injury by Crawford and colleagues[20] showed active ROM within the pain-free arc was helpful in reducing the progression of HO. Those who were engaged only in passive ROM showed progression to bone maturity and need for surgical removal.[20] Therefore, in IPR, active progressive ROM guided by therapists is recommended with gentle prolonged stretch near the end range.

*Nutrition*

Nutrition presents another challenge within inpatient burn rehabilitation. Although per os intake is preferred, supplemental enteral feeds may be used to optimize intake initially when sufficient calories cannot be taken by mouth. Once survivors can take sufficient oral intake, a nutrition consultation is important to suggest supplements for optimal nutrient and calorie balance. Total caloric needs are anywhere between 20% and 60% greater than baseline after burn injury.[21] This number can fluctuate based on the percentage of open wounds as healing occurs and activity level; supplemental feeding should decrease as healing of open burns progress to avoid overfeeding. Current recommendations to decrease muscle breakdown during the hypermetabolic state of burn recovery include a diet that is high carbohydrate (55% of calories), moderate protein (20%–25% of calories), and low fat (<20% of calories).[21]

## THERAPY CONSIDERATIONS
*Dysphagia*

Dysphagia of varying degrees was detected in 27.78% of people surviving a major burn.[22] Dysphagia after burns can complicate the provision of adequate nutrition intake, and place survivors at risk for additional complications, such as aspiration pneumonia, dehydration, or insufficient intake to meet their postburn nutritional needs. Risk factors for dysphagia after burns include larger TBSA (>18%), older age, head and face involvement, presence of inhalation injury, need for prolonged mechanical ventilation, and need for tracheostomy or escharotomy. Generalized muscle weakness and catabolism may also contribute to development.[22] All burn survivors should have an initial screening for dysphagia, especially if they have had a protracted course including ventilation, immobilization, or prolonged nonoral means of nutrition before diet initiation.

For those with identifiable dysphagia, the standard clinical protocol with visits five to seven times per week with a trained speech language pathologist (SLP) is recommended. Treatment includes standard oropharyngeal swallowing exercises, Frazier Free Water protocol,[23] and trials of advanced textures in a controlled environment before diet upgrades. Objective evaluation of swallowing function is completed by functional endoscopic evaluation of swallow or modified barium swallow. Some patients need multiple evaluations to assess progress. Rumbach and coworkers[24] demonstrated that improvement in swallowing function of those with dysphagia is the most rapid between weeks 2 and 6 after burn injury. At 6 weeks postburn, 50% of patients with initial dysphagia had complete resolution of dysphagia. That number increased to 75% by 9 weeks after injury, and 85% by the time of discharge if the hospital stay was longer than that.[24] Therefore, 15% of patients may have prolonged dysphagia after discharge from IPR. In this case, continued dysphagia treatment in the outpatient setting, including additional objective evaluations, is recommended.

*Cognition*

On admission to IPR, all burn survivors should be given a cognitive screen, and if positive, receive continued cognitive therapy by an SLP. Up to 79% of burn survivors have cognitive communication deficits on admission to IPR.[25,26] Burn survivors have lower memory scores on measures of function on admission compared with other populations in rehabilitation.[26] This holds true after accounting for confounders. Potential causes may include decreased oxygenation to the hippocampi from smoke or chemical inhalation, stress of the injury and hospital setting, delirium, and medications.[26] Delirium is a major contributor to lower cognitive scores initially. As delirium resolves with time, healing, and the rehabilitation milieu, cognitive scores improve and approximately 27% of survivors have deficits that persist past discharge (which is similar to data described in post–intensive care unit survivors).[25]

Not surprisingly, a higher cognitive score on admission is associated with a higher functional score at discharge. The burn survivors with lower cognitive scores on admission to IPR are also more likely to be discharged back to acute care within the first 72 hours of their IPR stay,[27] which may be accounted for by ongoing underlying medical complications or delirium affecting cognition.

Speech therapy to counteract cognitive changes is typically dosed 5 to 7 days per week in 30- to 60-minute sessions. The focus is on sustained attention, memory strategies, functional problem solving, and carryover of techniques and treatments from other therapy sessions. Medication management on discharge to home is also addressed to ensure adherence. The frequency of SLP sessions is decreased as cognitive status improves. Outpatient referral for SLP service is recommended for those still with deficits at the time of discharge.

### Physical and Occupational Therapy

IPR therapy is provided by PTs and OTs, preferably those who have been certified by the ABA. Burn survivors may have had comorbid conditions requiring immobility, such as prolonged ventilation caused by inhalation or other respiratory conditions, aggressive sedation for pain management, additional traumatic injuries, or mobility and ROM restrictions after recent grafting. ROM and weightbearing restrictions vary by institution and type of grafting. Therefore, early therapy focuses on elongation; stretching; maintaining ROM; contracture prevention; edema reduction; static and dynamic bracing; and more dynamic activities, such as transferring to a chair, maintaining sitting position, and supported standing. These activities, although not conferring a mortality benefit, are associated with reduced incidence of pneumonia, deep vein thrombosis, reduced number of hospital and intensive care unit days, and improved peripheral and respiratory muscle strength.[28] In addition, early mobility lays the foundation for movement and exercise in IPR.

### Hypertrophic Scarring

Burn scar massage is a key component of the IPR program to reduce or prevent more intensive treatments later in the healing process. Massage lessens the development of hypertrophic burn scar, including scar height, and improves skin vascularity and pliability and patient-described pain, pruritus, and depression.[29] Based on these data burn scar massage can be incorporated into OT treatment during IPR. It should be reiterated that scar massage is only completed over those burn and graft sites that have completely healed, not areas that are prone to shear or are receiving ongoing wound care.

### Contracture Prevention

Stretching is used to combat unopposed wound contraction and tissue shortening, asburned and grafted skin heals. It is initiated in the postoperative phase after clearance from the burn surgeons. Gentle, slow, prolonged stretching is preferred over high-velocity stretching to reduce injury to fragile tissue.[30] Despite advancements in multiple aspects of burn and rehabilitation care, some patients arrive at IPR with ROM loss. The incidence of joint contractures remains between 38% and 54%.[31]

Godleski and colleagues[32] developed a 1-hour stretching protocol incorporated into the comprehensive IPR program. In this protocol, survivors are premedicated with analgesia before therapy. They are positioned in supine and the joint of interest is stretched in one plane of motion. Once maximal stretch is reached, it is held for

3 minutes. If there is restriction in multiple planes of movement in a particular joint, the stretch is repeated in all affected planes. This is repeated for each joint of concern. It was also noted that the time spent on the stretching protocol did not adversely affect other rehabilitation outcomes, such as Functional Independence Measure score.[32] This protocol was shown to be safe and effective as part of a comprehensive inpatient rehabilitation program.

## Exercise

Exercise plays a vital role in the rehabilitation of patients with severe burns. Survivors experience several years of reduced exercise capacity and reduced pulmonary function following burn injury.[33] To counteract these changes, PTs design exercise programs individualized to each survivor and their functional needs. The physiatrist reviews the exercise plan, and daily progress toward goals to ensure optimal outcome. Disseldorp and colleagues[34] conducted a systematic review of 11 studies that showed persons with severe burns scored worse on measures of physical fitness, but survivors engaged in exercise training experienced improved lean muscle mass, strength, and reduced requirement for contracture release. The study also demonstrated improvement in physical fitness and maximal oxygen uptake.[34]

The ABA published guidelines for exercise prescription following burn injury based on 20 reports evaluating exercise prescription for adult and pediatric patients with burns. Adult patients who demonstrate less than normal strength should be prescribed a resistance and/or aerobic exercise program under supervision as early as discharge from acute care for 6 to 12 weeks.[35] These are foundational goals of exercise for burn survivors and exercise programs can commence during IPR.

## Aerobic Training

The stress response to burns includes hypermetabolic catabolism and circulating catecholamines, cortisol, and proinflammatory factors, and results in muscle wasting and cardiac dysfunction.[36] It makes sense that exercise postburn can help counteract further muscle loss attributable to these factors and prolonged immobility and strengthen cardiac function. Survivors typically have elevated heart rate and cardiac output, and many studies confirm reduced cardiorespiratory fitness in survivors compared with control subjects.[33–37] A review by Palackic and coworkers[36] outlines recommendations for a 12-week rehabilitation exercise training protocol, which could be initiated either as outpatient therapy or as part of a comprehensive IPR program. Each aerobic session should be tailored to the individual's current functional status and capabilities, while ensuring maximum safety. Typical aerobic protocol includes a heart rate of 70% to 85% of predicted maximum (220 minus age) initially for only 5 to 10 minutes, with progression to 20 to 40 minutes, three to five times per week. As patients improve, small bursts of more intense exercise (95% of predicted maximum heart rate) for a few minutes followed by a prolonged rest may be incorporated. Aerobic activity to achieve heart rate goals should be dynamic and incorporate large muscles of the legs, back, buttocks, core, and arms. Understanding that the level of deconditioning in survivors may be profound, easy walking may be enough activity initially to achieve the heart rate target. Treadmill, stationary bike, arm ergometer, and other exercise machines may be incorporated as aerobic capacity increases.

## Resistance Training

The safety of adding resistance training in burn survivors within the acute care setting has been established by Gittings and colleagues[37] in a small randomized controlled

| Table 1 | | |
| --- | --- | --- |
| Recommended progression[36] | | |
| Weeks | % of Weight | Sets/Repetitions |
| 1–3 | 50–60 | 3/10–15 |
| 4–6 | 70–75 | 3/8–10 |
| 6–11 | 75–80 | 3/8–12 |

Data from Palackic A, Suman OE, Porter C, Murton AJ, Crandall CG, Rivas E. Rehabilitative Exercise Training for Burn Injury. Sports Med. Dec 2021;51(12):2469-2482. doi:10.1007/s40279-021-01528-4.

trial. The addition of resistance training or sham resistance training in two matched and compared groups found no differences in adverse outcomes or increased LOS because of complications. There was improvement in the strength of the upper extremities in those who received resistance training compared with the standard PT group.[37] Because safety and efficacy have been established in the acute care setting, presumably when survivors are more ill, the safety and efficacy of resistance training in IPR is implied.

Resistance training programs are used to strengthen individual muscles using machines, bands, free weights, or body weight.[36,37] Therapists should provide initial instruction on form, technique, and safety, considering each individual's pain and current functional level.[37] Typical resistance exercise programs in burn survivors target large muscle groups crossing multiple joints (eg, legs, chest, back) or isolate specific movements, such as biceps curls or triceps press. Strengthening of the core should also be incorporated. Gradual progression is recommended (**Table 1**) with further increases after 12 weeks, by increasing the weight or repetitions by 5% to 10% each week.[36] This program can be initiated in the IPR setting, with instructions for continuation during outpatient PT or as a self-directed program.

## SUMMARY

IPR confers excellent benefit to those burn survivors who meet admission criteria and should always be included as a potential destination during the discharge planning. This is especially true for those who have complex injuries or are older. Physiatrists identify and manage complications within the IPR setting. Interventions can be taken to address medical sequelae of injury, including pain, itch, neuropathy, delirium, psychological coping and mood, and nutritional needs. Physiatrists also oversee and direct a rehabilitation program focusing on scar management, contracture prevention, dysphagia treatment, and evaluation and treatment of cognitive impairments. Aerobic and resistive exercise are key components of an IPR program to reduce the systemic impact of a burn injury and improve quality of life. IPR provides a steppingstone to outpatient care and long-term health for burn survivors.

## CLINICS CARE POINTS

- After completing an initial consult for a burn survivor early in their acute course, Physiatry follow up and discussion with the acute care team would ultimately occur at least once weekly. This helps provider communication, ease transition to IPR, and optimize care. It is also helpful for obtaining insurance authorization for IPR.
- Even if a burn survivor is not eligible for IPR based on current functional status, an outpatient visit with physiatry can help address unresolved pain, therapy needs and return to work evaluation.

- If the burn survivor's injuries were the result of an industrial or work-related accident, obtain consent from the survivor or their family members prior to discussing the case the the workers comp case manager.
- If the mechanism of injury included trauma or blast injury, remember to screen for concussion or brain injury.
- Any survivor who still requires opioid pain medication at the time of discharge should also receive a prescription for intranasal naloxone (also available over the counter) and have a support person trained in administration.

## DISCLOSURE

The author has nothing to disclose.

## ACKNOWLEDGMENTS

The author acknowledges Jessa Darwin who assisted with manuscript preparation.

## REFERENCES

1. Tan WH, Goldstein R, Gerrard P, et al. Outcomes and predictors in burn rehabilitation. J Burn Care Res 2012;33(1):110–7.
2. DiVita MA, Mix JM, Goldstein R, et al. Rehabilitation outcomes among burn injury patients with a second admission to an inpatient rehabilitation facility. Pharm Manag PM R 2014;6(11):999–1007.
3. Greene NH, Pham TN, Esselman PC, et al. Variation in inpatient rehabilitation utilization after hospitalization for burn injury in the United States. J Burn Care Res 2015;36(6):613–8.
4. Burn Model System, UW Rehabilitation Medicine, University of Washington, National Institute on Disability Independent Living and Rehabilitation Research, Model Systems Knowledge Translation Center. Burn Model System National Data and Statistical Center Seattle, WA: University of Washington. Available at: https://burndata.washington.edu/.
5. Espinoza LF, Simko LC, Goldstein R, et al. Postacute care setting is associated with employment after burn injury. Arch Phys Med Rehabil 2019;100(11): 2015–21.
6. Pham TN, Carrougher GJ, Martinez E, et al. Predictors of discharge disposition in older adults with burns: a study of the burn model systems. J Burn Care Res 2015;36(6):607–12.
7. Palmieri TL, Molitor F, Chan G, et al. Long-term functional outcomes in the elderly after burn injury. J Burn Care Res 2012;33(4):497–503.
8. Wright PC. Fundamentals of acute burn care and physical therapy management. Phys Ther 1984;64(8):1217–31.
9. Herndon DN. Total burn care. 5th edition. Edinburgh: Elsevier; 2018. p. 744, xix.
10. Centers for Medicare & Medicaid Services. Fact Sheet #1: Inpatient Rehabilitation Facility Classification Requirements. Available at: https://www.cms.gov/Medicare/Medicare-Fee-for-Service-Payment/InpatientRehabFacPPS/Downloads/fs1classreq.pdf. Accessed February 25, 2023.
11. Faucher L, Furukawa K. Practice guidelines for the management of pain. J Burn Care Res 2006;27(5):659–68.
12. Romanowski KS, Carson J, Pape K, et al. American Burn Association guidelines on the management of acute pain in the adult burn patient: a review of the

literature, a compilation of expert opinion, and next steps. J Burn Care Res 2020; 41(6):1129–51.

13. Cukor J, Wyka K, Leahy N, et al. The treatment of posttraumatic stress disorder and related psychosocial consequences of burn injury: a pilot study. J Burn Care Res 2015;36(1):184–92.

14. Schneider JC, Qu HD. Neurologic and musculoskeletal complications of burn injuries. Phys Med Rehabil Clin 2011;22(2):261–75, vi.

15. Carrougher GJ, Martinez EM, McMullen KS, et al. Pruritus in adult burn survivors: postburn prevalence and risk factors associated with increased intensity. J Burn Care Res 2013;34(1):94–101.

16. Chung BY, Kim HB, Jung MJ, et al. Post-burn pruritus. Int J Mol Sci 2020;21(11). https://doi.org/10.3390/ijms21113880.

17. Tu Y, Lineaweaver WC, Zheng X, et al. Burn-related peripheral neuropathy: a systematic review. Burns 2017;43(4):693–9.

18. Richards AM, Klaassen MF. Heterotopic ossification after severe burns: a report of three cases and review of the literature. Burns 1997;23(1):64–8.

19. Levi B, Jayakumar P, Giladi A, et al. Risk factors for the development of heterotopic ossification in seriously burned adults: a National Institute on Disability, Independent Living and Rehabilitation Research burn model system database analysis. J Trauma Acute Care Surg 2015;79(5):870–6.

20. Crawford CM, Varghese G, Mani MM, et al. Heterotopic ossification: are range of motion exercises contraindicated? J Burn Care Rehabil 1986;7(4):323–7.

21. Sommerhalder C, Blears E, Murton AJ, et al. Current problems in burn hypermetabolism. Curr Probl Surg 2020;57(1):100709.

22. Pavez RA, Martinez MP. Dysphagia in the burn patient: experience in a national burn reference Centre. Burns 2019;45(5):1172–81.

23. Gillman A, Winkler R, Taylor NF. Implementing the free water protocol does not result in aspiration pneumonia in carefully selected patients with dysphagia: a systematic review. Dysphagia 2017;32(3):345–61.

24. Rumbach AF, Ward EC, Cornwell PL, et al. Incidence and predictive factors for dysphagia after thermal burn injury: a prospective cohort study. J Burn Care Res 2011;32(6):608–16.

25. Hendricks CT, Camara K, Violick Boole K, et al. Burn injuries and their impact on cognitive-communication skills in the inpatient rehabilitation setting. J Burn Care Res 2017;38(1):e359–69.

26. Purohit M, Goldstein R, Nadler D, et al. Cognition in patients with burn injury in the inpatient rehabilitation population. Arch Phys Med Rehabil 2014;95(7):1342–9.

27. Bajorek AJ, Slocum C, Goldstein R, et al. Impact of cognition on burn inpatient rehabilitation outcomes. Pharm Manag PM R 2017;9(1):1–7.

28. Jacobson K, Fletchall S, Dodd H, et al. Current concepts burn rehabilitation, part I: care during hospitalization. Clin Plast Surg 2017;44(4):703–12.

29. Ault P, Plaza A, Paratz J. Scar massage for hypertrophic burns scarring: a systematic review. Burns 2018;44(1):24–38.

30. Chapman TT. Burn scar and contracture management. J Trauma Acute Care Surg 2007;62(6):S8.

31. Oosterwijk AM, Mouton LJ, Schouten H, et al. Prevalence of scar contractures after burn: a systematic review. Burns 2017;43(1):41–9.

32. Godleski M, Oeffling A, Bruflat AK, et al. Treating burn-associated joint contracture: results of an inpatient rehabilitation stretching protocol. J Burn Care Res 2013;34(4):420–6.

33. Porter C, Hardee JP, Herndon DN, et al. The role of exercise in the rehabilitation of patients with severe burns. Exerc Sport Sci Rev 2015;43(1):34–40.

34. Disseldorp LM, Nieuwenhuis MK, Van Baar ME, et al. Physical fitness in people after burn injury: a systematic review. Arch Phys Med Rehabil 2011;92(9): 1501–10.

35. Nedelec B, Parry I, Acharya H, et al. Practice guidelines for cardiovascular fitness and strengthening exercise prescription after burn injury. J Burn Care Res 2016; 37(6):e539–58.

36. Palackic A, Suman OE, Porter C, et al. Rehabilitative exercise training for burn injury. Sports Med 2021;51(12):2469–82.

37. Gittings PM, Wand BM, Hince DA, et al. The efficacy of resistance training in addition to usual care for adults with acute burn injury: a randomised controlled trial. Burns 2021;47(1):84–100.

# Rehabilitation Management of the Burned Hand

Brooke Murtaugh, OTD, OTR/L, BT-C[a],*,
Renee Warthman, MS, OTR/L, BT-C, CHT[b],
Trudy Boulter, OTR/L, CHT, BT-C[c]

## KEYWORDS

• Burns • Hand injuries • Rehabilitation

## KEY POINTS

- Hand burns result in significant disability and loss of function requiring specialized rehabilitation knowledge and expertise.
- Core clinical tenants of positioning, edema management, ROM, use of orthotics, and scar management can be applied across all phases of burn rehabilitation.
- Effective pediatric hand burn rehabilitation requires a specialized knowledge of skeletal development, burn injury, and impact of hypertrophic scars on the growth of the child.
- Multiple outcome assessments for hand burns can be implemented into clinical practice. Burn therapists must use clinical judgment in choosing the most appropriate outcome measures for the patient and their individual goals.

## INTRODUCTION

"A burn to the hand, whether it is in isolation or associated with a major systemic thermal injury, continues to pose one of the greatest challenges to the surgeon and the rehabilitation team."[1] Burns of the hand account for small total body surface area (TBSA) burn injury, approximately 3%, but can have significant functional consequences. Additionally, hands are the most frequently affected in burn injury.[2] Outside of larger TBSA involvement, partial and full thickness burns to the hand are classified as a major burn injury and require specialized burn intervention.[3] Intricate anatomy of the hand includes multiple bones, joints, muscles, tendons, ligaments and connective tissue that coalesce in a precise biomechanical and kinematic interplay to allow humans to engage in daily activities that require various grasp and pinch patterns.[4]

[a] Department of Rehabilitation Programs, Madonna Rehabilitation Hospitals, 5401 South Street, Lincoln, NE 68506, USA; [b] Arizona Burn Center, Valleywise Health Medical Center, 2601 East Roosevelt Street, Phoenix, AZ 85008, USA; [c] Children's Hospital Colorado Burn Center, 13123 East 16th Avenue, Aurora, CO 80045, USA
* Corresponding author.
*E-mail address:* bmurtaugh@madonna.org

Phys Med Rehabil Clin N Am 34 (2023) 767–782
https://doi.org/10.1016/j.pmr.2023.05.001
1047-9651/23/© 2023 Elsevier Inc. All rights reserved.

Burns to the hand and upper extremity can occur through multiple mechanisms including flame, scald, contact, electrical or chemical exposure.[5] In adult burn injury, the most likely hand pattern involvement includes the dorsal aspects of the hand. In pediatrics, the volar aspects of the hands are more typically involved due to children exploring objects or falling on a hot surface.[6,7] Partial and full thickness burns to the dorsal and or volar aspects of the hand and wrist can result in significant disability by limiting joint and skin range of motion (ROM), functional grasp and pinch patterns required to complete basic daily functions such as dressing, bathing, toileting, home management and work-related tasks.[8] Furthermore, studies have reported that individuals with hand burns were 73% less likely to return to work 2 years post injury.[9,10] Multiple joint contractures can lead to deformities of digit(s) and in the most severe cases, digit amputation.[11] This results in cosmetic changes and visible scars that can negatively impact the individual's psychological and psychosocial wellbeing and quality of life.[2,12,13]

Rehabilitation must begin as soon as possible following burn injury and continue throughout long-term phases of recovery.[6] Multidisciplinary rehabilitation is essential for the recovery of function after burn injury to the hands and upper extremity in the acute and post-acute phases.[14] Rehabilitation team members across the continuum should include: burn surgeon, advanced practice provider, Physical Medicine and Rehabilitation physician, physical therapy (PT), occupational therapy (OT), nursing, pharmacy, psychology, child life specialist for pediatrics, the patient and family.[15]

## ANATOMY OF THE HAND AND IMPACT OF BURN INJURY

Knowledge of the anatomy of the hand is the foundation for successful treatment. Understanding the delicate balance of the skeletal and ligamentous structure, joint range of motion, intrinsic and extrinsic musculature, anatomical differences in the skin and underlying tissue on the volar and dorsal aspect provides valuable information during assessment. The dermis on the palmar aspect of the hand is one of the thickest in the body, making it less mobile while also providing protection. In contrast, the skin and subcutaneous tissue on the dorsal aspect of the hand is much thinner, allowing for more mobility. Therefore, burn injuries to the dorsal hand and digits can more easily affect the deeper structures and result in deformities including true boutonnière, pseudo boutonnière, and swan neck of the digits which can be less amenable to reconstruction in the burn-injured hand. Care must be taken to protect and preserve the integrity of the extensor hood when burns to the dorsal aspect of the digit are present.[3,16] Knowledge of these structures will provide key information of risk factors and guide therapeutic interventions. Following a burn injury to the hand, risk factors that may impact the long-term structures are dictated by the initial depth of injury as well as interventions, both surgical and therapeutic, that were provided from the time of injury through the rehabilitative phase.

Key anatomical constructs of the hand that support function.

- Carpus has an intricate balance of stability and mobility. The stability of the central portion contrasts the mobility of the ulnar aspect of the hand and the arthrokinematics of the thumb.
- The arthrokinematics of the thumb, the unique characteristics of the CMC joint, the thumb ray, and the power and precision of the thenar musculature support its intricate function.
- The cam-shaped structure of the MCP joint of the digits and their associated collateral ligaments warrant prolonged positioning of the MP joint of the adult hand at 60 to 90° to avoid a claw hand.

- PIP joints, collateral ligaments, and extensor mechanism support joint alignment at rest and during extension.
- Complex vasculature and peripheral nerves support blood flow and sensation of the hand.
- Arches of the hand promote grasp.

Rehabilitation of the burned hand must consider cutaneokinematics, how the skin moves in response to joint ROM, and how that will impact the function of the hand and wrist as the burn injury and subsequent scar formation evolves[17,18] Cutaneous functional units (CFUs) are fields of skin that functionally contribute to the range of motion. These fields extend beyond the area of skin that approximates the joint.[19,20] The concept of CFUs is an evolving theory around which an understanding of cutaneokinematics can be based. This concept has led to several principles that are beneficial when managing the burned hand; adjacent joint positions impact the amount of skin recruitment necessary to permit full ROM,[21] and greater degrees of joint ROM require serial recruitment of greater percentages of the associated CFUs well beyond the joint itself.[17–19] The CFU paradigm provides a context for evaluating how a burn may affect the movement and function of a hand and help guide the clinician anticipate and proactively address these potential issues. Understanding CFUs should also guide a therapist's approach to treatment strategies, including the range of motion, positioning, and orthotic management.

## PHASES OF BURN REHABILITATION

Burn rehabilitation is conceptualized into phases that help guide interventions. Literature stratifies these phases as acute, intermediate, and long-term.[16,22] Phases of rehabilitation and wound healing often overlap and can occur simultaneously within the same hand. The acute phase of rehabilitation is the time from injury to 50% wound closure or skin grafting has been initiated. Early excision and grafting are ideal in the management of deep partial and full thickness hand burns to the dorsal surface as this expedites wound closure, decreases edema, and allows the earlier return of function.[6,11,14] The intermediate phase is from 50% wound closure extending to complete closure. The long-term phase of rehabilitation is wound closure or discharge from the acute burn setting until the patient has received maximum benefit from rehabilitation.[16] Interventions within the long-term phase are built upon care and treatment provided in the acute and intermediate phases.[23] Long-term phase of rehabilitation can last months, years or even a lifetime. Therapeutic interventions are required during each phase to maximize outcomes and mitigate the risk of disability. Many clinical concepts and treatment modalities for the burned hand can be applied across all phases of burn rehabilitation dependent upon the patient's presentation, continued needs, and therapeutic goals.

## EVALUATION OF THE BURNED HAND

Evaluation of a hand burn should occur as soon as possible following injury.[24] The emphasis of the burn evaluation varies based on the stage of wound healing and phase of rehabilitation. The patient's ability to participate provides critical information when evaluating hand burns. A thorough burn evaluation should include the assessment of multiple domains focused on patient characteristics and a comprehensive wound assessment (including location, depth of injury, and exposed structures) to allow the therapist to anticipate areas of potential dysfunction.[16](**Fig. 1**). The evaluation will assist in identifying areas of "risk" to the hand that have the potential to

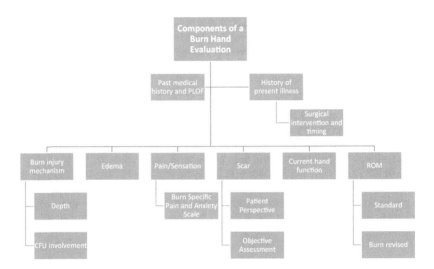

**Fig. 1.** Components of hand burn evaluation.

complicate and impede recovery of function. **Table 1** highlights additional areas of risk to consider during evaluation (see **Table 1**). Discerning the cause of limitations is imperative to direct the plan of care, therapeutic interventions, and dosing.

ROM should be assessed with a standard and revised goniometric methodology to determine the underlying cause of ROM restrictions. When restrictions are present, differential diagnosis to identify the root cause of movement limitation is imperative to guide effective treatment. that is, skin or scar contracture, soft tissue, musculotendinous, joint, and skeletal malalignment. A recently revised goniometric approach includes the consideration of CFUs, cutaneokinematics and scar on the range of motion.[18] This updated approach, published by Richard and colleagues (2017), utilizes the measurement of composite movement patterns which are a more reliable indication of the available ROM for functional hand use. These measurement methods appreciate the unique characteristics of the skin, involved CFUs and resulting impairment from burn injury. Furthermore, this evidence-based paradigm integrates the impact of functional positions for objective assessment of progress and accurate clinical documentation.[18,25] Goal development should focus on maintaining current ROM and functional abilities, protecting new autografts and exposed anatomical structures.[16] Therapeutic goals and care plan are fluid and continually modified as progress is made and the patient transitions through the phases of rehabilitation. Goals should be person-centered, measurable, functional, and promote engagement in life roles.[26]

## PAIN AND SENSITIVITY WITH HAND BURNS

Burn injury has been described as one of the most painful traumas an individual can experience.[27] A paucity of evidence exists specifically addressing post-burn hand pain and management. However, evidence suggests increased complaints of pain with burns to the upper extremity.[28] Pain can vary in intensity and be instigated by multiple sources such as wounds, dressing changes, surgical procedures, neuropathic pain, movement and psychological factors[29] Experience of pain can be a significant factor in patient resistance or non-compliance within rehabilitation programs. Pain can be an ongoing challenge throughout all phases of burn rehabilitation and can

**Table 1**
**Areas of risk and functional implications for hand burns**

| Complications of the Burned Hand | Functional Implications | Orthoses to Mitigate Complications |
|---|---|---|
| Edema | • Compromise of extensor and flexion mechanisms<br>• Risk for clawed hand deformity | Resting Hand<br>• MCP joints 60–90°<br>• Wrist 0–20° extension |
| 1st Webspace | • Narrowing of webspace<br>• Shortening/collapse of webspace<br>• Loss of grasp, opposition | C-bar<br>• Radial or palmar<br>Static Opponens |
| Loss of thumb | • Loss of 45%–50% of hand function | • Thermoplastic prosthetic<br>• Consider surgical consultation for reconstruction |
| Deep Partial/ Full Thickness Dorsal Hand Burn | • Loss of extensor mechanism integrity<br>• Terminal slip of extensor tendon<br>• Boutonniere & Mallet deformities | Resting hand splint<br>• Wrist in extension<br>• PIP and DIP extension<br>• MCP flexion over 60° |
| Partial Thickness Doral Hand Burns | • Loss of composite flexion | Resting hand splint<br>• Wrist neutral<br>• MCP 60° flexion<br>• PIP and DIP slight flexion |
| Palmar Hand Burn | • Palmar Cupping deformity<br>• Loss of digit extension and abduction<br>• Loss of thumb radial abduction<br>• Loss of wrist extension<br>• Loss of weight bearing ability | Palmar expansion<br>• Palmar expansion with digit extension splint<br>• Palmar expansion cast (must incorporate the forearm) |
| Exposed Tendons | • Tendon desiccation<br>• Loss of function<br>• Boutonnière deformity | Immobilization orthoses as needed<br>• Avoid overstretch<br>• Keep tendon moist |
| Wrist Flexion Contracture | • Impacts hand function<br>• Loss of grip strength | Wrist cockup splint<br>• 10–30° wrist extension |

become chronic lasting for months and years.[22,30] Past evidence confirms individuals experiencing chronic pain are at a higher risk for depression, PTSD, suicidal ideation, and anxiety.[24,27,29] Furthermore, sensory deficits can result after burn injury to the dermis of the hand thus exacerbating the patient's experience of pain and discomfort. Numbness, paresthesia, or hypersensitivity can occur from injury to sensory structures in the skin and peripheral nerve injury from deep burns or compartment syndromes. Pain and loss of sensation can significantly impact hand function.[31]

## NEUROPATHY IN HAND BURNS

Post-burn neuropathy has been widely documented with localized neuropathies reported at an incidence of 15% to 37%.[32] Neuropathy can result from the depth of burn injury, compression or injury to the peripheral nerves secondary to edema, eschar and scar formation in both thermal and electrical injuries.[33] Polyneuropathies can occur as a result of critical illness and prolonged ICU stay.[3,32,34] Additionally, positioning of the burned upper extremity can place mechanical strain on peripheral nerves contributing to neuropathy.[35] Lester and colleagues (2013) conducted a study that demonstrated positioning the axilla above 90° increased symptoms of numbness and tingling. The findings of this study also supported positioning across multiple joints influences tension throughout the peripheral nerve increasing parasthesias.[35]

The hand is susceptible to the development of mononeuropathies as ulnar, median, and radial nerves are compromised in deep burns, positioning protocols, and compression due to edema and compression dressings.[32,36] Risk factors for neuropathy of the hand include positioning of the wrist in hyperextension and positioning the elbow in flexion and pronation. Additional risk factors to consider are upper extremity positioning along or over bedrails, use of wrist restraints, and interventional procedures.[32] Therapists must use caution when implementing positioning protocols, splints, and compression therapy to monitor for signs and symptoms of neuropathy. Evidence does support the regeneration and healing of peripheral nerves over time after burn injury for some patients.[36] Positioning and range of motion should be used to prevent neuropathy-related contractures during the recovery period.

## EDEMA MANAGEMENT

Edema is a common sequela of burn injury that can be problematic in the hand and should be addressed early and throughout the rehabilitation process. Edema can impede wound healing, result in deeper burn conversion, lead to compartment syndrome, impact function, and contribute to increased scar formation. As edema persists it becomes fibrotic, overtime leading to brawny edema and thus more difficult to manage resulting in long-term functional impairment.[37] Elevation of the hand in the first 48 to 72 hours post burn injury is critical to decrease the impact of edema on wound conversion and the development of compartment syndrome.[38] Elevation can be achieved by placing the hand above heart level. This is effective in reducing or preventing worsening edema and aids in supporting circulation.[16,23,38] Even in isolated hand burns, elbow positioning should be considered as supporting the elbow in extension will improve lymphatic drainage from the hand.[37]

Compression is an evidence-supported intervention to manage and decrease edema, improve ROM and function.[39,40] Introducing wrapping techniques, including self-adhesive and cotton wraps has been shown to be effective in managing hand edema. Care should be taken when incorporating ROM with compression wrapping as this can lead to shear and tissue breakdown. Compression wrapping hands should be completed by a skilled therapist to avoid complications. Interim garments provide early pressure for scar management when a custom glove may not yet be feasible. Off-the-shelf compression options should be used with care as they do not provide the custom-graded compression that wrapping techniques impart. If an off-the-shelf product is utilized and compression is not consistently graded from distal to proximal, this could lead to an increase in edema in certain areas. The use of chip bags (foam pieces of varying size and density incased in material) is a strategy used in conjunction with elevation, compression and is beneficial as edema becomes more fibrotic. Chip bags are placed with netting or light wrap and can be placed on the volar and dorsal aspects of the hand (**Fig. 2**). When possible, active range of motion (AROM) of the hand should be encouraged and will aid in decreasing edema by increasing lymphatic flow.[37,41]

## ORTHOTIC USE IN HAND BURNS

Orthoses and casting are valuable tools for managing the burned hand. These are positional aides to prevent contractures, support wound healing, and enhance function across all stages of rehabilitation.[24,42,43] Published clinical practice guidelines endorse

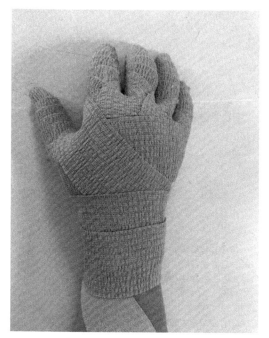

**Fig. 2.** Compression wrapping for edema management.

the use of orthoses and casts after burn injury.[44] However, evidence suggests significant heterogeneity within splinting practices by therapists.[43] Orthoses can have multiple clinical objectives focused on counteracting contractile forces, protecting delicate structures from further injury, increasing or preserving range of motion and facilitating function.[11,16,17,43] **(Table 2)**

Design and fabrication should be goal driven and follow biomechanical principles. The use of an orthosis should be balanced with the phases of healing and rehabilitation goals to support optimal outcomes. Clinical experience suggests that orthotic positioning with hand CFUs at maximal length before and after autograft may lead to more rapid gains in ROM and function (**Fig. 3**).

Various materials are utilized for the fabrication of orthoses including fiberglass, polyester cast tape, soft cast, plaster, and a variety of thermoplastics. For the purpose of this article, casting will be discussed as another material choice with its own unique characteristics. It is important to be familiar with the different properties of each material and how they can be used together to accomplish treatment goals. Casting is an

| Table 2 | |
|---|---|
| **Clinical objectives for orthoses implementation** | |
| Protective | • Edema management<br>• Wound healing<br>• Immobilization of new skin grafts |
| Preventative | • Counteracting contractile forces of burn scar |
| Restorative | • Improving loss of range of motion<br>• Promoting function |

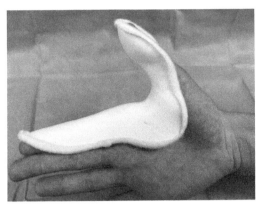

**Fig. 3.** 1st webspace thermoplast orthotic.

effective intervention for focused prolonged positioning and scar management.[42,44] When casting is identified as an appropriate intervention, understanding the properties of different casting tape will guide clinical decision making, including material, timing, and precautions with use. For example, fiberglass or circumferential plaster casting materials may not be ideal when close monitoring of an inpatient setting is not available. Soft cast material or a removable orthosis, may be more appropriate as it can be removed easily at home if significant discomfort or edema arise.[45] (**Fig. 4**)

The following should be addressed with orthotic implementation.

- Ongoing fit assessment (especially when used with bulky dressings and fluctuating edema)[46]
- Acknowledge the risk of orthotic migration and negative sequelae of sheer and friction
- Assess for areas of potential pressure and monitor wear time appropriately
- Determine dosage or wear time to achieve optimal outcome
- Assess functional impact of orthosis wear.

The art of fabrication and use of orthoses requires a strong knowledge of contractile forces that will impact long-term function and then design a program that includes balanced sustained stretch of structures and fields of skin which are "at risk" for

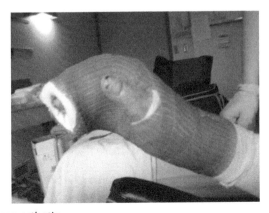

**Fig. 4.** Soft cast tape orthotic.

contracture while providing a wear schedule with adequate dosage to meet treatment goals. More than one orthosis is typically required to address complex positioning needs of the hand based on the burn pattern and structures impacted to support hand function. For example, in a circumferential hand burn, a positioning program that alternates between flexion and extension is beneficial. Incorporating a palmar extension orthosis at night and then emphasizing flexion during the day balances the positioning needs and promotes function. Although the burn resting hand orthosis is a standard positioning device for a dorsal burn, adjustments should be made based on patient-specific factors.[24] The use of a hand-based thumb opponens orthosis can assist in increasing hand function by placing the thumb in a more functional position to facilitate a functional grasp. See **Fig. 5**.

**Table 3** outlines different types of orthoses and clinical considerations for use.

## RANGE OF MOTION

ROM is an integral part of rehabilitation to counteract the contractile forces of burn wound healing that can lead to loss of motion.[47,48] Achieving or preserving full ROM is paramount for recovery of hand function.[3,14,49] An understanding of the involved CFUs will help guide the motions that should be emphasized and that are prone to contracture based on the pattern of injury. Accurate assessment of planes of motion prone to contracture allows the clinician to pro-actively address and anticipate potential problems. This is critical when managing the burned hand due to the intricate movements and the delicate structures that are easily impacted by the forces of burn scar formation.

Patients at highest risk for loss of ROM are those with autografts, larger number of CFU involvement, and prolonged bed rest.[47] AROM exercises should be encouraged early and often post burn injury to decrease edema, improve available ROM, increase strength, and decrease the risk of tendon adhesions.[50] Early post-operative AROM

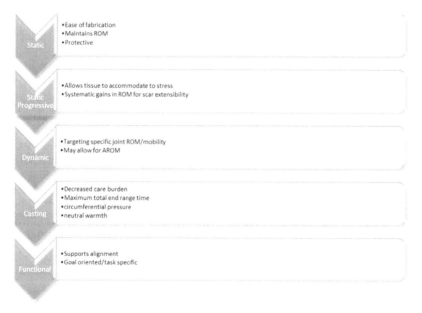

**Fig. 5.** Types of orthoses and considerations for use.

| Table 3 | |
|---|---|
| **Types of orthoses and considerations for use** | |
| Static | • Ease of fabrication<br>• Maintains ROM<br>• Protective |
| Static Progressive | • Allows tissue to accommodate to stress<br>• Systematic gains in ROM for scar extensibility |
| Dynamic | • Targeting specific joint ROM/mobility<br>• May allow for AROM |
| Casting | • Decreased care burden<br>• Maximum total end range time<br>• Circumferential pressure<br>• Neutral warmth |
| Functional | • Supports alignment<br>• Goal oriented/task specific |

has been shown to be safe for hand grafts beginning post-operative day #1 when directed by a therapist and performed with the dressings removed.[50] If AROM is not feasible, passive range of motion (PROM) should be implemented. Specificity of hand placement and support of joint and soft tissue structures during ROM is important to obtain desired motion, protect healing structures, and maintain appropriate arthrokinematic movement.

AROM and functional hand activities take priority when there is no longer a need to protect the deeper anatomical structures or recent skin grafts. As AROM continues to improve, integrating strengthening activities to recover grip and pinch within the various hand patterns facilitates movement against forces of hypertrophic scar and progression toward improved function[40] Strength is achieved through focused resistive hand and upper extremity exercises as well as functional tasks that the patient engages in throughout their day. It is recommended to prescribe resistive training of 8 to 12 repetitions per exercise, 2 to 3 times per week to build strength and endurance.[16] Patients and families should be educated and trained on a home exercise program focused on PROM, AROM and strengthening[24,51]

## SCAR MANAGEMENT

Scar contracture can have a devastating impact on the multi-planar joints and intricacies of hand function. Scar formation and contracture is a result of multiple factors.[47] Various hand and digit deformities can result from unmitigated hypertrophic scar formation and maturation.[22] These include intrinsic minus deformity with hyperextension of the MCPs and hyper-flexion of the PIPs, as well as swan neck and pseudo-boutonniere deformities.[3,16] Scar management for the hand is most successful through early multi-modal interventions that include positioning, orthotics, compression therapy and use of silicone products.[11,24,48] Concave surfaces, such as webspaces between digits, are particularly important to provide early and consistent compression to counteract scar webspace creep. This is a common complication of hand burns, limiting the hand's ability to abduct digits for functional grasp and release.[11]

## PEDIATRIC HAND BURNS

Children are curious by nature and learn about their world through tactile exploration. This places toddlers at high risk for sustaining burn injuries to the hand. Nearly 250,000 pediatric burns occur every year with 50% of those burns involving the upper extremity and hand.[52] Common injuries include spill scald burns, electrical injuries, friction burns, and heat contact burns. Armed with the awareness of normal development, the clinician is better equipped to discern accidental and non-accidental injury. Non-accidental trauma is an important consideration in situations when there is a delay in care, inconsistent report of the injury mechanism, there are clear lines of demarcation, or when the size, shape, or depth of the injury does not match the history provided. These burn injuries warrant additional investigation and support from child abuse specialists and pertinent authorities.[53]

Care of the pediatric hand burn requires an experienced practitioner to facilitate optimal outcomes. The early months of treatment are critical for the pediatric patient. A study by Omar (2022) demonstrated children make significant functional improvement in the first 6 months after discharge from the burn center.[54] Therapist(s) treating hand burns must have a comprehensive knowledge of hands, burns, and pediatrics to promote optimal recovery. The pediatric patient differs from the adult in skeletal growth and the development of the musculoskeletal structures that support the developing hand. The pediatric hand is comprised of both cartilaginous structure, developing long bones, and ligamentous laxity. Normal development of hand function, sensory-motor system and skeleton mature simultaneously. Developmental sequence lays the foundation for the hand to develop the strength and integrity used for locomotion, exploration, and fine manipulation. Children develop functional strength through weight-bearing, weight shifting, reaching, and tactile exploration. The development of thick, fibrous, inextensible scar tissue has devastating functional consequences for the developing pediatric patient due to the strength of the contractile forces of the wound bed in combination with the developmental growth of the hand. The inability of scar tissue to accommodate growth will result in contracture and loss of hand function over time.[55] Clinical tenants of positioning and orthotic use are key features of rehabilitation of the pediatric hand burn. Often, the growth of the burned extremity exceeds the rate of scar stretch necessitating many pediatric hand burns to be followed by burn specialists into adulthood.[56] Ongoing assessment throughout the growing years can provide timely interventions to restore function and enhance the developmental and reintegration needs of the child.

Burn-specific positioning guidelines, based on the mature musculoskeletal structures of the adult, do not always apply to the pediatric patient. Ligamentous laxity associated with the MP joint in the pediatric hand allows for prolonged positioning in MP extension. This allows sustained positioning of palmar expansion following a palmar burn. Additionally, the developing carpus is cartilaginous in nature which allows for positioning of the wrist in more extreme positions of extension without median nerve palsy symptoms that may be present adult population when placed in a similar position.[57] It is a natural phenomenon for the child to use the wrist in greater than 30° of wrist extension. Benefits of the malleability of the upper extremity have corresponding drawbacks when ideal positioning is not achieved. The MP joint of the thumb is typically hyper-mobile in the pediatric hand making effective positioning of the first ray challenging. Optimal positioning of the thumb is realized when the emphasis on alignment occurs at the level of the CMC joint. Deep burn injury and subsequent scarring increase the risk of the finger pulling into flexion and rotating on its axis causing a rotary deformity of the digit.[57,58]

Burn injuries and hypertrophic scars encompassing multiple CFUs of the upper extremity affects the delicate balance of reach and grasp for the child. The pull of a scar across the forearm and wrist can alter the stability of the carpus on the distal radio-ulnar joint impacting hand position relative to the forearm.[58] Palmar burns can be especially difficult to manage in the pediatric patient. Properties of wound contracture, characteristics of palmar skin, the mobile pediatric skeleton, and the imbalance of grip strength versus extensor strength create specific challenges.[54,58] Attention must be paid to palmar expansion, the palmar arches of the hand, and the position of the thumb in relation to the function of the hand. Maintaining palmar expansion is preferred compared to restoring this position after contracture.

The use of orthoses or intermittent casting may be indicated to help the child sustain tissue length. Sustained stretch improves elasticity and length of contracted tissue.[42] Dosage needed to maintain tissue length is individualized based on the child's injury and their unique biology. Orthoses may be designed to prevent contractures, correct an existing problem, position for function, or protect the injured or repaired structure.[45,55] A single orthosis rarely achieves all the rehabilitative goals for the pediatric hand. Fabrication of an orthosis for a child requires clinical decision that are not applicable to the adult hand burn. These include:

- Avoid using a small orthosis that may be a choking hazard such as a finger-based orthosis
- Child's ability to remove the orthosis
- Complications of donning and doffing the orthosis by the caregiver
- Wearing time or dosage and impact on the parents and child's schedule.

Pediatric burn rehabilitation is most successful with a multidisciplinary team approach. The therapeutic approach should incorporate play and enjoyable activities versus rote exercise. Omar and colleagues (2012) found children who engaged in play activities as part of their hand burn rehabilitation improved function and reported less pain than those who performed rote ROM activities.[59] When a pediatric burn injury occurs, the whole family is impacted and it is necessary to meet the needs of the child and family.[56] It is essential the child's caregivers be incorporated into treatment decisions from the time of the initial injury and subsequent care to promote long-term recovery. Building rapport with the child and family is important as relationships established during the rehabilitation often continue until the child reaches skeletal maturity or no longer requires skilled intervention.

## OUTCOME ASSESSMENT FOR HAND BURNS

A battery of outcome assessments are required to evaluate the efficacy of hand burn rehabilitation interventions to demonstrate value-based healthcare for reimbursement purposes and provide feedback on progress to the patient and clinician.[15,60] Outcome assessments focus on multiple domains including: patient-reported outcomes, component outcome measures such as ROM or Vancouver Scar Scale, and performance-based measures including the Jebsen-Taylor Hand Function Test or the Sollerman Hand Function Test.[8,22,60–62] (**Table 4**). A recent systematic review by Kittrick (2021) identified 25 outcome measures that captured properties of the International classification of functioning, disability, and health (ICF) and evaluated the validity and reliability of the assessments. The results of the systematic review identified only one outcome measure, the Michigan Hand Function Questionnaire, assessed all components of ICF including body structure, function, activity, and participation.[63] However, this study found ROM and grip strength were the outcome measures most frequently used with reported validity and reliability. The burn therapist must be familiar with the outcome measures applicable to measuring outcomes for hand burns and utilize clinical judgment in deciding which outcome assessments are most appropriate to provide meaningful results to guide continued care decisions.

**Table 4**
**Burn-specific outcome assessment measures**

| Patient Reported Outcome Measures | • Burn Specific Health Scale<br>• Burn Specific Health Scale-Brief<br>• Young Adults Burns Outcomes Questionnaire<br>• Pediatric Quality of Life Inventory (PedsQL)<br>• Burn Specific Pain Anxiety Scale<br>• Disabilities of the Arm, Shoulder, and Hand (DASH)<br>• Michigan Hand Questionnaire<br>• Patient Observer Scar Assessment (POSAS) |
|---|---|
| Component Outcome Measures | • Figure 8-edema<br>• Vancouver Scar Scale<br>• PROM/AROM<br>• Grip Strength<br>• Sensation<br>• 9-hole Peg Test |
| Performance-Based Outcome Measures | • Sollerman Hand Function Test<br>• Jebsen-Taylor Hand Function Test<br>• Functional Independence Measure (FIM |

## SUMMARY

Burns of hand can result in significant disability and loss of function. Recovery of hand burns is complex and requires focused, specialized rehabilitation within all phases of recovery for adult and pediatric patient. Effective management requires intensive focus starting in the early hours and days of the acute phase of rehabilitation through the months and years post-injury. Key interventions applied to the hand at all phases of rehabilitation include: edema management, positioning, orthotics, ROM, scar management, and use of reliable outcome assessment. Therapeutic goals for the burned hand focus on the achievement of optimal ROM, strength, function, and independence. Return of hand function after burn injury improves the quality of life and probability of return to school, work and meaningful life roles.

## CLINICS CARE POINTS

- Partial and full thickness burns to the hands are classified as major burn injury and require specialized burn intervention.

- The concepts of cutaneoukinematics and cutaneous functional units (CFUs) of the hand and adjacent fields of skin must be applied to promote successful rehabilitation.

- Evaluation and identification of areas of "risk" to the hand is imperative to development of an effective plan of care.

- Pediatric hand burns requires an experienced practitioner to facilitate optimal outcomes.

- Valid and reliable outcome measures should be used to assess progress of the burned hand to demonstrate value-based rehabilitation.

## DISCLOSURE

Authors do not have any commercial, financial, or non-financial conflicts of interest or disclosures related to the content included within this article.

## REFERENCES

1. Cartotto R. The burned hand: optimizing long-term outcomes with a standardized approach to acute and subacute care. Clin Plast Surg 2005;32(4):515–27, vi.
2. Dunpath T, Chetty V, Van Der Reyden D. Acute burns of the hands – physiotherapy perspective. Afr H Sci 2016;16(1):266.
3. Kowalske KJ. Hand Burns. Phys Med Rehabil Clin 2011;22(2):249–59.
4. Jones LA, Lederman SJ. Human hand function. New York: Oxford University Press; 2006.
5. Dargan D, Himmi G, Anwar U, et al. A comparison of the epidemiology of isolated and non-isolated hand burns. Burns 2022. https://doi.org/10.1016/j.burns.2022.05.018. S0305-4179(22)00125-5.
6. Kamolz LP, Kitzinger HB, Karle B, et al. The treatment of hand burns. Burns 2009; 35(3):327–37.
7. McBride JM, Romanowski KS, Sen S, et al. Contact Hand Burns in Children: Still a Major Prevention Need. J Burn Care Res 2020;41(5):1000–3.
8. Sizoo SJM, van Baar ME, Jelsma N, et al. Outcome measures to evaluate the function of the hand after burns; a clinical initiative. Burns Open 2021;5(3):162–7.
9. Quinn T, Wasiak J, Cleland H. An examination of factors that affect return to work following burns: A systematic review of the literature. Burns 2010;36(7):1021–6.
10. Mason ST, Esselman P, Fraser R, et al. Return to work after burn injury: a systematic review. J Burn Care Res 2012;33(1):101–9.
11. Sorkin M, Cholok D, Levi B. Scar Management of the Burned Hand. Hand Clin 2017;33(2):305–15.
12. Mc Kittrick A, Gustafsson L, Hodson T, et al. Exploration of individuals perspectives of recovery following severe hand burn injuries. Burns 2022. https://doi.org/10.1016/j.burns.2022.04.026. S0305-S4179(22)00102-00104.
13. Martin L, Byrnes M, McGarry S, et al. Social challenges of visible scarring after severe burn: A qualitative analysis. Burns 2017;43(1):76–83.
14. Pan BS, Vu AT, Yakuboff KP. Management of the Acutely Burned Hand. J Hand Surg Am 2015;40(7):1477–84 [quiz: 1485].
15. Allorto N, Atieh B, Bolgiani A, et al. ISBI Practice Guidelines for Burn Care, Part 2. Burns 2018;44(7):1617–706.
16. Serghiou MA, Ott S, Whitehead C, et al. Comprehensive rehabilitation of the burn patient. In: Herndon D, editor. Total burn care. 4th edition. Philadelphia: Elsevier; 2012. p. 517–49.
17. Jacobson K, Fletchall S, Dodd H, et al. Current Concepts Burn Rehabilitation, Part I. Clin Plast Surg 2017;44(4):703–12.
18. Parry I, Richard R, Aden JK, et al. Goniometric Measurement of Burn Scar Contracture: A Paradigm Shift Challenging the Standard. J Burn Care Res 2019;40(4):377–85.
19. Richard RL, Lester ME, Miller SF, et al. Identification of Cutaneous Functional Units Related to Burn Scar Contracture Development. J Burn Care Res 2009; 30(4):625–31.
20. Yelvington ML, Parry I. Integration of Cutaneous Functional Units Principles in Burn Rehabilitation: A Diffusion of Innovations Assessment. J Burn Care Res 2023. https://doi.org/10.1093/jbcr/irad007. irad007.
21. Richard R, Steinlag R, Staley M, et al. Mathmatic model to estimate change in burn scar length required for joint range of motion. J Burn Care Rehabil 1996;17:436–43.
22. Cowan AC, Stegink-Jansen CW. Rehabilitation of hand burn injuries: Current updates. Injury 2013;44(3):391–6.

23. Abu-Sittah GS, El Khatib AM, Dibo SA. Thermal injury to the hand: review of the literature. Ann Burns Fire Disasters 2011;24(4):175–85.

24. Dodd H, Fletchall S, Starnes C, et al. Current Concepts Burn Rehabilitation, Part II. Clin Plast Surg 2017;44(4):713–28.

25. Richard R, Parry IS, Santos A, et al. Burn Hand or Finger Goniometric Measurements: Sum of the Isolated Parts and the Composite Whole. J Burn Care Res 2017;38(6):e960–5.

26. Yoshida A, Yamamoto M, Li-Tsang CWP, et al. A systematic review assessing the effectiveness of hand therapy programmes in adults with burns using the International Classification of Functioning, Disability and Health framework. Nagoya J Med Sci 2022. https://doi.org/10.18999/nagjms.84.4.689.

27. Kim DE, Pruskowski KA, Ainsworth CR, et al. A Review of Adjunctive Therapies for Burn Injury Pain During the Opioid Crisis. J Burn Care Res 2019;40(6):983–95.

28. Dunpath T, Chetty V, Van Der Reyden D. The experience of acute burns of the hand - patients perspectives. Disabil Rehabil 2015;37(10):892–8.

29. Browne AL, Andrews R, Schug SA, et al. Persistent Pain Outcomes and Patient Satisfaction With Pain Management After Burn Injury. Clin J Pain 2011;27(2): 136–45.

30. Wiechman SA. Psychosocial recovery, pain, and itch after burn injuries. Phys Med Rehabil Clin N Am 2011;22(2):327–45, vii.

31. Moore ML, Dewey WS, Richard RL. Rehabilitation of the Burned Hand. Hand Clin 2009;25(4):529–41.

32. Schneider JC, Qu HD. Neurologic and musculoskeletal complications of burn injuries. Phys Med Rehabil Clin N Am 2011;22(2):261–75, vi.

33. Ferguson JS, Franco J, Pollack J, et al. Compression Neuropathy: A Late Finding in the Postburn Population: A Four-Year Institutional Review. J Burn Care Res 2010;31(3):458–61.

34. Kowalske K, Holavanahalli R, Helm P. Neuropathy After Burn Injury. J Burn Care Rehabil 2001;22(5):353–7.

35. Lester ME, Hazelton J, Dewey WS, et al. Influence of Upper Extremity Positioning on Pain, Paresthesia, and Tolerance: Advancing Current Practice. J Burn Care Res 2013;34(6):e342–50.

36. Gabriel V, Kowalske KJ, Holavanahalli RK. Assessment of Recovery From Burn-Related Neuropathy by Electrodiagnostic Testing. J Burn Care Res 2009;30(4): 668–74.

37. Mortimer PS. Therapy approaches for lymphedema. Angiology 1997;48(1): 87–91.

38. Smith MA, Munster AM, Spence RJ. Burns of the hand and upper limb–a review. Burns 1998;24(6):493–505.

39. Edwick DO, Hince DA, Rawlins JM, et al. Randomized Controlled Trial of Compression Interventions for Managing Hand Burn Edema, as Measured by Bioimpedance Spectroscopy. J Burn Care Res 2020;41(5):992–9.

40. Edger-Lacoursière Z, Deziel E, Nedelec B. Rehabilitation interventions after hand burn injury in adults: A systematic review. Burns 2022. https://doi.org/10.1016/j.burns.2022.05.005. S0305-4179(22)00114-0.

41. Schuind F, Burny F. Can algodystrophy be prevented after hand surgery? Hand Clin 1997;13(3):455–76.

42. Dewey WS, Richard RL, Parry IS. Positioning, splinting, and contracture management. Phys Med Rehabil Clin N Am 2011;22(2):229–47, v.

43. Khor D, Liao J, Fleishhacker Z, et al. Update on the Practice of Splinting During Acute Burn Admission From the ACT Study. J Burn Care Res 2022;43(3):640–5.

44. Parry IS, Schneider JC, Yelvington M, et al. Systematic Review and Expert Consensus on the Use of Orthoses (Splints and Casts) with Adults and Children after Burn Injury to Determine Practice Guidelines. J Burn Care Res 2020;41(3): 503–34.

45. Choi YM, Nederveld C, Campbell K, et al. A Soft Casting Technique for Managing Pediatric Hand and Foot Burns. J Burn Care Res 2018;39(5):760–5.

46. Richard R, Ward RS. Splinting Strategies and Controversies. J Burn Care Rehabil 2005;26(5):392–6.

47. Lensing J, Wibbenmeyer L, Liao J, et al. Demographic and Burn Injury-Specific Variables Associated with Limited Joint Mobility at Discharge in a Multicenter Study. J Burn Care Res 2020;41(2):363–70.

48. Finnerty CC, Jeschke MG, Branski LK, et al. Hypertrophic scarring: the greatest unmet challenge after burn injury. Lancet 2016;388(10052):1427–36.

49. Williams T, Berenz T. Postburn Upper Extremity Occupational Therapy. Hand Clin 2017;33(2):293–304.

50. Dewey WS, Cunningham KB, Shingleton SK, et al. Safety of Early Postoperative Range of Motion in Burn Patients With Newly Placed Hand Autografts: A Pilot Study. J Burn Care Res 2020;41(4):809–13.

51. Ardebili FM, Manzari ZS, Bozorgnejad M. Effect of Educational Program Based On Exercise Therapy on Burned Hand Function. World J Plast Surg 2014;3(1): 39–46.

52. Dodd AR, Nelson-Mooney K, Greenhalgh DG, et al. The effect of hand burns on quality of life in children. J Burn Care Res 2010;31(3):414–22.

53. Pawlik MC, Kemp A, Maguire S, et al. Children with burns referred for child abuse evaluation: Burn characteristics and co-existent injuries. Child Abuse Negl 2016; 55:52–61.

54. Omar MT, Ibrahim ZM, Salama AB. Patterns and predictors of hand functional recovery following pediatric burn injuries: Prospective cohort study. Burns 2022; 48(8):1863–73.

55. Thomas R, Wicks S, Dale M, et al. Outcomes of Early and Intensive Use of a Palm and Digit Extension Orthosis in Young Children After Burn Injury. J Burn Care Res 2021;42(2):245–57.

56. Feldmann ME, Evans J, O SJ. Early Management of the Burned Pediatric Hand. J Craniofac Surg 2008;19(4):942–50.

57. Norbury WB, Herndon DN. Management of Acute Pediatric Hand Burns. Hand Clin 2017;33(2):237–42.

58. Birchenough SA, Gampper TJ, Morgan RF. Special considerations in the management of pediatric upper extremity and hand burns. J Craniofac Surg 2008; 19(4):933–41.

59. Omar MTA, Hegazy FA, Mokashi SP. Influences of purposeful activity versus rote exercise on improving pain and hand function in pediatric burn. Burns 2012; 38(2):261–8.

60. Johnson SP, Chung KC. Outcomes Assessment After Hand Burns. Hand Clin 2017;33(2):389–97.

61. Weng LY, Hsieh CL, Tung KY, et al. Excellent reliability of the Sollerman hand function test for patients with burned hands. J Burn Care Res 2010;31(6):904–10.

62. Kowalske K. Outcome Assessment After Hand Burns. Hand Clin 2009;25(4): 557–61.

63. Mc Kittrick A, Gustafsson L, Marshall K. A systematic review to investigate outcome tools currently in use for those with hand burns, and mapping psychometric properties of outcome measures. Burns 2021;47(2):295–314.

# Hypertrophic Scar

Shyla Kajal Bharadia[a], Lindsay Burnett, RN, BScN, MN, NP[b],
Vincent Gabriel, MD, MSc, FRCPC[c,d,e],*

## KEYWORDS

- Burn scar • Hypertrophic scar • Scar evolution • Scar measurement

## KEY POINTS

- Wound healing post-burn frequently results in the formation of hypertrophic scar, with non-trivial impact on patient quality of life.
- The natural history of scar includes the peaking, then regression of troublesome scar features such as pain, pruritus, discolouration, contractility, and raised volume, though without return to a pre-injury state.
- Objective quantification of the natural history of burn scar characteristics is important in both research and clinically, regarding the assessment of wound progression and treatment effect
- Scar characteristics can be modulated by various conservative treatments, with different treatments targeting different characteristics, suggesting the use of combination therapies to manage hypertrophic burn scar.

## INTRODUCTION

Burns are traumatic tissue injuries accompanied by various physiological and psychological morbidities.[1-3] Scar is the most apparent pathognomonic characteristic of burn injury and can be classed as normotrophic or pathologic which includes hypertrophic and keloid scars, each of which differs in their clinical presentation and cellular and molecular characterisation.[4,5] Where normotrophic scarring represents ideal wound healing, undesired hypertrophic scarring following burn injury is common.[6] Owing to abnormalities in wound healing, hypertrophic scars are functionally and visually

[a] Cumming School of Medicine, University of Calgary, Foothills Medical Centre, 1403-29 Street Northwest, Calgary, Alberta T2N 2T9, Canada; [b] Alberta Health Services, University of Calgary, Foothills Medical Centre, 1403-29 Street Northwest, Calgary, Alberta T2N 2T9, Canada; [c] Department of Clinical Neurosciences, University of Calgary, Foothills Medical Centre, 1403-29 Street Northwest, Calgary, Alberta T2N 2T9, Canada; [d] Department of Surgery, University of Calgary, Foothills Medical Centre, 1403-29 Street Northwest, Calgary, Alberta T2N 2T9, Canada; [e] Medical Director, Calgary Firefighters Burn Treatment Centre, Foothills Medical Centre, 1403-29 Street Northwest, Calgary, Alberta T2N 2T9, Canada
* Corresponding author. Foothills Medical Centre, 1403-29 Street Northwest, Calgary, Alberta T2N 2T9, Canada
E-mail address: vince.gabriel@albertahealthservices.ca

Phys Med Rehabil Clin N Am 34 (2023) 783–798
https://doi.org/10.1016/j.pmr.2023.05.002
1047-9651/23/© 2023 Elsevier Inc. All rights reserved.
pmr.theclinics.com

distinct from uninjured skin. These fibrotic scars cause significant patient burden socially (due to appearance), functionally (due to contractures), and economically (due to the cost of scar treatment).[3,7,8] Herein, we describe the formation, evolution, management, and measurement modalities of the hypertrophic burn scar over time. This review should be instructive to burn patients, orienting them along their burn recovery journey, as well as burn care practitioners for the corroboration of temporal change in the clinical phenotypes of hypertrophic scar.

### Anatomy of the Skin and Burn Classification

Human skin is stratified into the epidermis, dermis, and hypodermis (or subcutaneous tissue); each of these 3 layers is uniquely characterized and contributes to the skin's many functions.

The epidermis is the most superficial layer of the skin forming a protective, robust outer barrier. It is segregated into different strata as characterized by keratinocyte (the principal epidermal cell) status.[9] Conferring this skin layer its functions are the structure and organization of keratinocytes throughout each epidermal layer, as well as 3 additional cell types: melanocytes, Merkel cells, and Langerhans cells.[9] Keratinocytes originate in the basal layer of the epidermis and progressively differentiate as they migrate toward the surface of the skin.[9] The water-insoluble intermediate filament protein keratin is produced by keratinocytes and accumulates during keratinocyte maturation through the epidermal strata.[9] Linking of keratinocytes via desmosomes facilitates the skin's ability to accommodate mechanical strain.[9] Nearing the surface of the skin, keratinocytes are terminally differentiated and termed corneocytes.[9] Here, anucleate and organelle-less corneocytes participate in protection against extrinsic assault, pathogen invasion, and water loss.[9] Renewal of the epidermis is achieved by desquamation and basal cell proliferation.[9] Other cellular components that encompass epidermal function and properties are melanocytes which produce pigment and defend against ultraviolet radiation, Merkel cells which account for tactile reception, and specialized immune cells, Langerhans cells.[9,10] The epidermis plays an essential role in re-epithelialization during wound healing.

Inferior to the epidermis is the dermis. Comprised of 2 differentially organized layers of connective tissue, the dermis is responsible for the skin's mechanical properties.[9,11] Papillary dermis lies underneath the epidermis and consists of loose connective tissue whereas the deeper reticular dermis consists of dense connective tissue.[11] Residing in the dermis are the dermal appendages (hair follicles, glands), sensory nerves, and vasculature.[9,11] The mechanical role of the dermis is supplemented by the thermoregulatory, secretory, and sensory functions that are imparted by these structures. Extracellular proteins, namely collagen, characterize the dermal matrix and are produced by the primary cell of the dermis: the fibroblast.[9] Depending on their localization within this skin layer, the phenotype and morphology of dermal fibroblasts varies.[12,13] Not only is the inflammation of the dermis associated with scar formation, but the dermal structures affected by burn injuries disrupting this skin layer mediate burn complications such as sensory dysfunction.[4]

A loose connective tissue punctuated with vasculature, nerves, and fat cells, the hypodermis is the inmost layer of the skin overlaying fascia, muscle, and bone.[9] The hypodermis participates in endocrine functions, insulates the body, acts as an energy reservoir, and absorbs shock.[9–11]

Burns violate, to varying extents, these layers of the skin–burn injury classification is therefore dependent on wound depth. Colloquially referred to as first, second, and third degree, burns may be described on a continuum of superficial, partial-, or full-thickness depths respectively. Superficial burn wounds disrupt the epidermis only, whereas superficial and deep partial-thickness burn wounds obliterate the epidermis and penetrate to some extent into the dermis. The most severe, full-thickness burns damage the epidermis and dermis completely. Symptomology of burn injury corresponds to the affected skin composition and adnexa which in turn is related to burn depth.

## Resolution of the Burn Wound and Pathology of the Hypertrophic Scar

Ideal wound healing following cutaneous injury such as burns would involve complete regeneration of the damaged tissue, as observed in fetal and oral mucosa wounds.[5] However, post-natal wound healing tends toward fibrosis rather than regeneration. Wound healing follows 4 dynamic, integrated processes: hemostasis, inflammation, proliferation, and remodeling.

### Typical wound healing

The hemostatic phase of wound healing mediates blood clot development, forms a provisional matrix within the clot, and assembles cytokines and growth factors required for downstream healing processes.[14] Hemostasis is promoted by platelet aggregation and vasoconstriction; platelet degranulation also releases growth factors and cytokines into the wound bed that advance the wound healing response.[14,15] Among the mediators released by platelets are transforming growth factor-$\beta$ (TGF-$\beta$), platelet-derived growth factor (PDGF), vascular endothelial growth factor (VEGF), and chemokine ligand 5 (CCL5).[15]

The accruement of pro-inflammatory mediators during the hemostatic stage begins the transition to inflammation. In essence, the wound inflammatory response functions to clear the injury of pathogenic substances, cell debris, and found a wound environment capable of the tissue repair process. Neutrophils, the earliest immune cells present in the injury site, perform wound debridement and are responsible for the secretion of a myriad of growth factors and cytokines that elicit immune and healing responses.[14,16] Further, neutrophils recruit macrophages.[16] Differentiated from circulating monocytes, or derived from skin-resident macrophages, macrophages appear in the wound bed a few days after injury.[14–16] Positioned as antigen presenting and phagocytic cells, macrophages ensure protection and cleaning of the inflamed wound while also mitigating the immune response via phagocytic eradication of neutrophils.[14–16] Macrophages are crucial to maintaining wound healing processes by their production of growth factors related to extracellular matrix (ECM) production and cell proliferation; these growth factors include TGF-$\beta$.[14] Phenotypic alterations in wound macrophage populations supports the progression from the inflammatory to proliferative phase.[15,16] Other immune cells, including T-cells and mast cells, fulfill additional healing activities (for example, promoting endothelial permeability) and augment the pool of cytokines and growth factors already secreted by macrophages and neutrophils.[16]

The proliferative phase of wound healing may be described in 3 components concerning reepithelialization, filling of the wound with granulation tissue, and angiogenesis. A ubiquitous mechanism of reepithelialization in both partial- and full-thickness burn wounds, the progression and fusion of stimulated keratinocytes across the wound's blood clot facilitates the formation of the new epidermal layer.[14,16] In partial-thickness burns, closure by keratinocyte migration from the wound periphery is accompanied by epithelial cells derived from stem cells in the bulge of hair follicles and sweat glands.[16] Angiogenesis is critical to re-establishing tissue perfusion and the provision of nutrients and oxygen. A complement of growth factors (such as VEGF, PDGF, and basic fibroblast growth factor bFGF) commence blood vessel development by stimulating sprouting of endothelial cells into the injury site wherein continued proliferation and maturation of these sprouts develops a new network of vasculature.[14] Vascular, highly cellular granulation tissue substitutes the provisional matrix created by the blood clot in the initial stages of wound healing, preceding scar tissue formation.[14] Fibroblasts are activated by various factors and enter the wound site where they function to deposit ECM components such as collagen, fibronectin, and proteoglycans.[14,16]

As the final and lengthiest phase in wound healing, remodeling serves to replace granulation tissue with scar tissue that intends to resemble uninjured skin composition and structure when mature. Overall, restructuring of the tissue, slowing of synthetic and proliferative processes, and removal of cells characterize the remodeling phase.[14,15] Type III collagen is converted into type I; the scar contracts; scar tissue becomes less perfused and vascular.[14,15] Over time, this remodeling of connective tissue enables the scar to naturally regress up until the point of maturation, when its features stagnate. A study elucidating the length of hypertrophic scar maturation found that hypertrophic burn scars develop around 6 months post-injury and on average mature in around 2.5 years.[17] Although temporary spontaneous regression improves scar quality, the scar still may not resemble adjacent uninjured skin when it is mature and further improvements in scar characteristics are accommodated only by therapeutic intervention.

### Healing disruptions in a wound closed by hypertrophic scar

Hypertrophic scars are the product of an aberrant wound healing process and show discordant architecture and composition compared to normally healed tissue. The inflammatory phase of wound healing may be robust in the healing burn wound, accentuating ECM deposition and promoting fibrosis through irregular cytokine and growth factor expression. ECM components in hypertrophic scar are either grossly overproduced or are decreased in amount. Contributing to matrix abundance, collagen expression is increased in hypertrophic scar.[18] Not only is collagen synthesis greater in hypertrophic scars, but the ratio of type I to III collagen is altered as well.[16] The proteoglycans versican and biglycan are also matrix molecules that are plentiful in hypertrophic scar, whereas the proteoglycan decorin is diminished.[19–21] Importantly, decorin suppresses the production and activity of TGF-$\beta$1.[22,23] TGF-$\beta$ is recognized as a potent mediator of fibrosis, participating in a range of events that establish scar; its pro-fibrotic isoform (TGF-$\beta$1) is increased in hypertrophic scar whereas the anti-fibrotic isoform (TGF-$\beta$3) is reduced.[18,20] TGF-$\beta$ is among the many molecules dysregulated to enable hypertrophic scar development (**Table 1**). Mature post-burn scars retain the molecular abnormalities of the more severe early post-burn hypertrophic scar to an extent.[19]

### Temporal Characterization and Evaluation of the Hypertrophic Burn Scar

Cellular and molecular abnormalities associated with hypertrophic scarring are manifest in the scar's clinical features. The hypertrophic burn scar is elevated, erythematous, inelastic, contractile, pruritic, and painful, causing patients significant, long-term functional and cosmetic concern. As such, burn scar assessment and therapeutic management constitute much of the post-injury burn patient burden after acute treatment of the wound. Scar treatments aiming to address complexities of the post-burn scar, such as discolouration, itch, or contracture, can relieve burn survivors of poor scar quality and function if effective. However, treatment regimens are not guaranteed, nor is scar so easily manipulated after it matures. So, a comprehensive understanding of burn scar characteristics and their anticipated evolution is important

**Table 1**
**Non-exhaustive summary of common molecular markers of hypertrophic scar**

| Molecular Marker | Marker Test(s) | Released by | Contribution to Hypertrophic Scar Phenotype | Hypertrophic Scar Expression |
|---|---|---|---|---|
| TGF-β | In situ hybridization, immunohistochemistry, Western blot (for TGF-β receptor), serum analysis | Macrophages, keratinocytes, fibroblasts, platelets | Pro-fibrotic | Increased TGF-β1, Reduced TGF-β3 |
| IGF-1 | Immunohistochemical staining, reverse transcriptase-polymerase chain reaction, Northern analysis, in situ hybridization | Sweat and sebaceous glands | Pro-fibrotic | Increased |
| Collagen | In situ hybridization, immunohistochemistry | Fibroblasts | Pro-fibrotic | Increased |
| Decorin | Immunohistochemistry | Fibroblasts | Anti-fibrotic | Reduced |
| Versican | Immunohistochemistry | Fibroblasts | Pro-fibrotic | Increased |
| Biglycan | Immunohistochemistry | Fibroblasts | Pro-fibrotic | Increased |

Abbreviations: IGF-1, insulin-like growth factor-1; TGF-β, transforming growth factor-β.

given their value as clinical indicators of firstly, the state and natural progression of scar and secondly, scar therapy impact. At 6 to 12 months post-burn, hypertrophy is documented to be at its greatest; at 18 to 24 months post-burn, hypertrophy declines.[24] While experienced burn clinicians rely on anecdotal knowledge to inform their understanding of scar quality and progression over time, instrumented and objective scar assessment may be employed as a standardized method to capture clinically relevant scar variables over time for the longitudinal evaluation of the burn scar.

Considering the utility of documenting burn scar features longitudinally, later in discussion we describe the mechanisms of commonly measured burn scar characteristics, their change over time, and methodologies for the assessment of these characteristics. **Table 2** summarizes longitudinal or long-term burn scar studies reviewed in this article. Visualization of temporal change in burn scar features is shown in **Fig. 1**.

### Hypertrophic scars are thick and raised

Hypertrophic scars exhibit increased epidermal thickness as well as the upregulation of particular proteoglycans.[19–21,25,26] While not all proteoglycans are increased in concentration in hypertrophic scar, such as the anti-fibrotic proteoglycan decorin, these molecules contribute to positive scar volume by overhydrating the scar.[20,21,25] Numerous descriptive clinical scales including the assessment of burn scar thickness have been implemented in clinical practice, in addition to objective approaches aiming to capture scar thickness or volume. The Vancouver Scar Scale (VSS) and Patient and Observer Scar Assessment Scale (POSAS) are widely used in burn scar evaluation and consider subjectively rated scar thickness on a numerical scale.[27] VSS burn scar estimations are completed only by clinicians, whereas POSAS estimations are completed by both patients and clinicians. In terms of the objective quantification of burn scar thickness or volume, imaging techniques such as high-frequency ultrasound and stereophotogrammetry have shown utility, though ultrasonic descriptions of skin thickness are limited and stereophotogrammetry is relatively new as a burn care modality.[28–31] Non-instrumented and invasive, biopsy (and histological assessment) provides an alternative objective approach to scar thickness assessment.[24,28]

Raised scars are characteristic following burns of sufficient depth and scar thickness is assessed as greater in more severe burn injuries.[32,33] As with all burn scar characteristics progressing along a normal healing trajectory, scar thickness will peak in elevation after the formation of the scar, then diminish as time post-burn increases. Scars of the upper extremity, lower extremity, and trunk differ in the development of their relative thickness.[34] Upper extremity burn scars display the longest increase in thickness up to 4 months post-burn and the smallest reduction in thickness 7 months post-burn compared to trunk (intermediate duration of increase, intermediate reduction in thickness), and lower extremity (shortest duration of increase, greatest reduction in thickness) scars over the same 7 month period.[34] Considering variability within subjective as well as between objective versus subjective estimation of burn scar thickness, thickness of the scar shows an overall decrease 1 year post-burn or remains unchanged from 6-months post-burn.[35,36] However, hypertrophic scar thickness still exceeds that of normal skin thickness at 1 year and elevated scars are a concern for the majority of burn patients decades after their injury.[2,35]

### Hypertrophic scars are inelastic and contractile

Poor biomechanical properties of the hypertrophic burn scar are manifestations of the altered molecular and cellular composition of ECM. The inelasticity of scar is attributed to reduced elastic fibers in the scar tissue and scar contracture–a major impediment to

**Table 2**
Summary of selected longitudinal or long-term burn scar quality studies

| Author(s) | Method(s) of Scar Assessment | Primary Scar Feature(s) Measured | Assessment Time Points Post-Burn |
|---|---|---|---|
| Holavanahalli et al,[1] 2016; Holavanahalli et al,[2] 2010 | Patient report, physical examination | General issues related to the skin post-burn, including scar | Once, ≥3 y |
| Spronk et al,[32] 2019 | Patient scale of the POSAS | Pain, pruritus, color, thickness, relief, pliability | Once, ≥5 y |
| Nedelec et al,[31] 2008; Nedelec et al,[35] 2014; Nedelec et al,[70] 2019; Nedelec et al,[78] 2015 | DermaScan C (Cortex Technology, Handsund, Denmark), Cutometer (Courage + Khazaka Electronic, Cologne, Germany), Mexameter (Courage + Khazaka Electronic, Cologne, Germany) | Thickness, pliability, erythema, and pigmentation | 3, 6, 12 mo |
| van der Wal et al,[36] 2012; van der Wal et al,[46] 2013 | DermaSpectrometer (Cortex Technology, Hadshund, Denmark), POSAS | Color, pliability, thickness, relief, pain, pruritus, vascularization, pigmentation | 3, 6, 12 mo |
| Goei et al,[43] 2017 | POSAS, DermaSpect- rometer (Cortex Technology, Hadshund, Denmark), Cutometer (Courage + Khazaka Electronic, Cologne, Germany) | Color, vascularization, pigmentation, elasticity/pliability, pain, pruritus, thickness, relief, surface area | 3, >18 mo |
| Muller et al,[44] 2021 | Nimble, Cutometer (Courage + Khazaka Electronic, Cologne, Germany), POSAS | Stiffness/pliability | 3, 6, 9, 12 mo |
| Edger-Lacoursière et al,[34] 2021 | DermaScan C (Cortex Technology, Handsund, Denmark), Cutometer (Courage + Khazaka Electronic, Cologne, Germany), Mexameter (Courage + Khazaka Electronic, Cologne, Germany), VAS | Thickness, pliability, erythema, pigmentation, pain, itch | 2, 3, 4, 5, 6, and 7 mo |

*Abbreviations:* POSAS, patient and observer scar assessment scale; VAS, visual analogue scale.

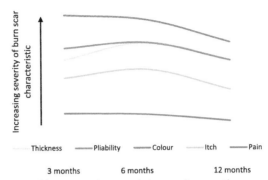

Fig. 1. Broad trajectory of burn scar characteristic severity over the course of 1 year according to averaged patient POSAS scores at 3, 6, and 12 months post-burn. POSAS, patient and observer scar assessment scale.

mobility–is largely attributed to myofibroblast contractility as imparted by the cell's expression of α-smooth muscle actin.[12,26,37] Myofibroblast differentiation is, notably, evoked by TGF-β1.[38] Burn scar elasticity and stiffness are measured during clinical interactions, with options for subjective and objective assessment. Again, the POSAS and VSS offer subjective evaluation of scar elasticity and stiffness through the pliability scale for clinicians (POSAS and VSS) and the stiffness scale for patients (POSAS). Instrumented measurement of burn scar elasticity involves an assortment of techniques by which applied forces are used to elucidate the biomechanical properties of scar. The Cutometer (Courage + Khazaka Electronic, Cologne, Germany), which utilizes negative pressure deformation to measure the skin's viscoelastic properties, and the Dermal Torque Meter (Dia-Stron Limited, Broomall, PA), which implements a torsion-based deformation technique, have been used in burn scar assessment.[31,39–41] Another device that objectively evaluates burn scar pliability based on deformation is the tissue tonometer.[42]

The nascent burn scar exhibits reduced pliability; generally, as time since burn increases so does the pliability of the scar.[35,36,43] When stratified by burned region, scars of the trunk do not show a significant change in pliability up to 7 months post-burn while upper and lower extremity scars become more pliable over this time.[34] Interestingly, despite the common increase in pliability 1 year post-burn, the trajectory of scar pliability is variant in the months preceding this progress. Where a large cohort study reported observer POSAS scores of pliability to worsen 6 months after burn, reports of burn scar stiffness have either increased then diminished at 12 months or have shown consistent improvement in stiffness.[36,44] Burn scar pliability does not return to normal even 1 year post-burn.[35]

### Hypertrophic scars are discolored
Burn scars are dyschromic due to disrupted melanin content and a change in vascularity following the injury.[45] Melanin content corresponds to scar pigmentation, which can be either hyper or hypopigmented, and vascularity to scar redness. Clinical burn care captures scar color via subjective color scoring, standard clinical photography, and through objective modalities. The POSAS asks patients to rate scar color on the whole, whereas both the POSAS and VSS ask observers to rate the independent contributors to scar color: vascularity and pigmentation. Reflectance spectroscopy is one method by which objective color assessment can be accomplished-tristimulus colorimeters and narrowband simple reflectance meters utilize reflectance spectroscopy

to output vascularity and pigmentation values. The Mexameter (Courage + Khazaka Electronic, Cologne, Germany), a narrowband simple reflectance meter, is a device commonly cited in the evaluation of burn scar color; the Colorimeter (Courage + Khazaka Electronic, Cologne, Germany), which is based on tristimulus colorimetry, is also used in scar assessment.[31,39,46] Laser-based techniques may be used as a measure of perfusion, but not pigmentation.[24,47]

Early on, burn scars are more erythematous than pigmented.[43] While erythema at 3 months post-burn is significantly greater than in uninjured skin, objective scar assessment showed pigmentation to be marginally less than that of normal skin.[35] Region-specific increasing patterns in pigmentation may be observed in upper and lower extremity burn scars and scars of the trunk, at least from 2 to 7 months after burn.[34] Regarding erythema, trunk, upper extremity, and lower extremity scar redness all decrease 7 months post-burn, although upper extremity scars show the longest increase in redness at 4 months post-burn prior to the aforementioned decrease.[34] Burn scar color improves 1 year after injury, credited to a reduction in erythema and vascularity, and enhancement in the pigmentation of the tissue.[35,36] Nonetheless, scar color is perhaps one of the most disparate features of the post-burn scar, long-term.[32]

### Hypertrophic scars are pruritic

Normally, unmyelinated nerve fibers in the skin moderate the perception of itch, as stimulated by cell-secreted substances for example,[48] Itch can also be neuropathic in origin, resulting from injury that damages and alters nervous reception and relay of pruritic sensation.[48] Post-burn pruritus consists of both normal and neuropathic mechanisms of itch.[48] Keratinocytes and immune cells, such as mast cells, secrete itch-promoting substances; hypertrophic scars have increased mast cell populations and neuropeptides related to itch.[48,49] As a subjective sensation, no instrumented measure of pruritus exists. However, several scar scales include itch as a patient-reported outcome in their evaluation of scar features, such as the POSAS, or are solely purposed for the measurement of pruritus. The latter category of assessment tools captures a more comprehensive view of post-burn pruritus. For example, the recently described pruritus severity scale considers items such as the duration, severity, and frequency of itch.[50] The 5D itch scale collects similar ratings of duration and itch intensity, but has also been validated for change over time and incorporates an important component related to the impact of itch on daily activities.[51]

One year after burn, itch subsides though pruritus is a predominant and chronic concern for patients as they recover from their burn injury,[2,36] Individuals suffering from more severe burns have higher perceptions of itch, in contrast to those with less severe burn, at or greater than 5 years following their injury.[32]

### Hypertrophic scars are painful

Though the mechanism of burn scar pain is largely unsettled, neuropathic pain appears to play a role in the chronic sensory aberrancies of burn scar.[52] Recent evidence also suggests hyperalgesia may be triggered through events leading to excessive collagen deposition that aggravates mechanical stimulation at the scar site.[53] Similar to the evaluation of burn scar pruritus, objective, clinical measures of scar pain are non-existent–subjective pain scales are utilized. Commonly employed pain scales include the Visual Analog Scale, POSAS, Burn Specific Pain Anxiety Scale, Numeric Rating Scale, Brief Pain Inventory, and McGill Pain Questionnaire.[34,53–55] The POSAS is the only scale intended for scar pain specifically, and asks of patients ratings of the scar pain and sensations they experience in the past week.

Regarding the development of pain, pain often peaks within the first 6 months post-burn, then decreases.[36] Scar pain persists long-term, though to a lesser degree than pruritus.[2]

### Risk Factors for Hypertrophic Scar

Risk factors for hypertrophic scar can be considered modifiable or non-modifiable. Non-modifiable risk factors are those where no action can be taken to reduce the possibility of hypertrophic scar development, such as age (with reduced propensity for scar in the elderly), race, and genetics.[56–58] Modifiable risk factors for hypertrophic scar are those where preventative actions may reduce the possibility of hypertrophic scar development. In both pediatric and adult burns, wounds that heal within 21 days have a lesser (although not zero) risk of developing hypertrophic scar.[58,59] As well, hypertrophic scarring is associated with bacterial colonization.[60] Accordingly, burn injury management should aim to promote rapid wound healing while also reducing infection rates in order to achieve the most desirable scar outcomes. Acute wound management including wound excision and selectivity in wound dressings have shown utility in reducing bacterial colonization and accelerating the rate of wound healing.[61–63] Compared to time to healing and bacterial colonization, mechanical stretch has less conclusively been implicated as a modifiable risk factor for hypertrophic scarring. Quatresooz and colleagues reported hypertrophic scars to show increased tension as compared to atrophic scars.[64] Mechanical tension may be involved in wound healing further suggesting stretch to play a role in hypertrophic scar development, for example, by promoting the fibroblast to myofibroblast transition.[65] At the same time, mechanical stretch (such as massage) has been employed as treatment for the post-burn hypertrophic scar.[66] Common clinical practice where burned regions are kept mobile to maintain functional movement against contractile forces also obscures the relationship between hypertrophic scar development and mechanical stretch.

### Non-operative Scar Management Therapeutics

Non-operative manipulation of hypertrophic scar includes both physical, pharmacologic, and device-based modalities.

Several types of lasers have been employed in the management of scar, including fractional ablative $CO_2$ (fCO2), intense pulsed light (IPL), and pulsed dye light (PDL) lasers. Attenuation of scar volume using fCO2 lasers (10,600 nm) is achieved via ablation-the laser forms microscopic holes in the tissue by targeting water in abnormal collagen, facilitating scar remodeling.[67] The PDL (585 or 595 nm) diminishes scar erythema through photothermolysis of hemoglobin.[67] Although not well described, IPL (515–1200 nm) likely limits vascular proliferation thus reducing scar dyschromia.[67]

Silicone gel sheeting, the use of pressure garments, and massage are among physical treatments that attempt to modulate scar. Ubiquitously used to both treat established burn scar and prevent the progression of incipient wounds to scar, pressure garments limit perfusion to scar tissue and modify collagen synthesis.[68] Additionally, the physical barrier of a pressure garment may alleviate the desire to excoriate and provide aesthetic appeal given a covering of the scarred area. Silicone gel sheets provide a soft, flexible wound covering impacting scar through the provision of local hydration, increased temperature, and regulation of growth factors that may increase collagenase production.[69] Massage may exert its effect through mechanical adjustment of scar tissue arrangement and edema.[70]

Pharmacologic modalities addressing scar symptomatology include intralesional steroid injections and a gamut of other medications. Intralesional steroid injections work to mitigate scar by eliciting vasoconstriction and anti-inflammatory effects.[71] Further, needle infiltration mechanically degrades fibrotic tissue and may promote more appropriate wound healing.

Lastly, transcutaneous electrical nerve stimulation (TENS) and extracorporeal shock wave therapy (ESWT) utilize electrical impulses and sound waves, respectively, to lessen troublesome scar characteristics.[72] Where impulses delivered through TENS block afferent nerves responsible for pain and pruritus signaling, ESWT dismantles collagenous scar tissue.[72]

While a variety of therapeutic avenues exist to promote scar regression, there is no one treatment that addresses all aspects of scar. As such, combinational and individualized approaches are superior to isolated treatment regimens for hypertrophic scar. Pressure garments, silicone gel sheeting, fCO2 laser and intralesional steroid injections have been shown to depress scar and improve scar contractility.[67–69,73–79] While no intervention exists to enhance scar hypopigmentation, IPL and PDL minimize hypertrophic scar hyperpigmentation and erythema, respectively.[79] Topical agents commonly applied for hyperpigmentation include immune-modulating agents, such as hydroquinone. Pharmacologic treatment for pain and pruritus overlaps in the use of gabapentin and ESWT, for example,[72] Additional pharmacologic treatment for pruritus includes but is not limited to antihistamines and serotonin receptor antagonists.[72] Burn scar massage may potentiate redress in burn scar characteristics, though with low and variable evidence.[70,77]

## DISCUSSION

Hypertrophic scarring is a pathological outcome of wound healing common in survivors of burn injury, and the post-burn hypertrophic scar is not benign.[6] While the experienced burn care practitioner may provide a suggestive timeline of wound healing and attenuation of hypertrophic scar characteristics, reference to the quantification of the burn scar over time is important in both clinical and research environments. A database consolidating temporal change in the burn scar is useful for informing patients of an expected and realistic scar trajectory, monitoring scar treatment, and as a control for clinical trials assessing scar characteristics in response to novel treatment—overall, accurate and standardized reference for the evolution of the post-burn scar may assist in providing care and therapies that objectively yield better scar outcomes. The reliability and accuracy of objective measurement tools make them attractive for the creation of such a database, though it is important to note that some symptoms of the burn scar (such as pain and itch) are not appropriately measured using objective tools. Our lab is undertaking a long-term cohort study utilizing instrumented measures of scar to develop a longitudinal human scar database for the advancement of burn scar care and research.

## SUMMARY

Hypertrophic burn scars present as pruritic, red, raised, inelastic, contractile, and painful due to a discordant healing process. As a result, hypertrophic scars cause patients long-term burden, impacting their participation in daily activities due to social and functional concerns. Through a lengthy remodeling process, scar symptoms may be reduced in severity; however, the scar may never return to its pre-injury skin state. So, patients' individual burn scar trajectories may vary, but those with normal wound healing can expect natural improvements in the quality of their scar over time which may be enhanced or expedited by the implementation of a scar therapy program. Although a number of subjective and objective modalities are available for the measurement of burn scar features, changes in these features over time is not well-documented in the literature. Evolution of the burn scar, via objective assessment, is warranted and offers clinical and research utility.

## CLINICS CARE POINTS

- Burn clinicians should relay the natural evolution of hypertrophic scar characteristics over time, including the initial worsening of scar, to provide patients with a prognostic course for their scar
- The natural trajectory of scar should be considered when determining the use and timing of scar interventions to elicit the most benefit
- The evolution of burn scar characteristics may be best measured using objective clinical instruments, where appropriate. Such objective measurements may be used for individual patient assessment to track wound healing progression, treatment impact, and in patient education

## DISCLOSURE

The authors have nothing to disclose.

## FUNDING

SB received funding from an Alberta Innovates Summer Research Studentship (AI SRS).

## REFERENCES

1. Holavanahalli RK, Helm PA, Kowalske KJ. Long-term outcomes in patients surviving large burns: the musculoskeletal system. J Burn Care Res 2016;37(4): 243–54.
2. Holavanahalli RK, Helm PA, Kowalske KJ. Long-term outcomes in patients surviving large burns: the skin. J Burn Care Res 2010;31(4):631–9.
3. Thombs BD, Notes LD, Lawrence JW, et al. From survival to socialization: a longitudinal study of body image in survivors of severe burn injury. J Psychosom Res 2008;64(2):205–12.
4. Ogawa R. Keloid and hypertrophic scars are the result of chronic inflammation in the reticular dermis. Int J Mol Sci 2017;18(3):606.
5. Karppinen S.M., Heljasvaara R., Gullberg D., et al., Toward understanding scarless skin wound healing and pathological scarring. F1000Res. 2019;8:F1000 Faculty Rev-787. https://doi.org/10.12688/f1000research.18293.1.
6. Bombaro KM, Engrav LH, Carrougher GJ, et al. What is the prevalence of hypertrophic scarring following burns? Burns 2003;29(4):299–302.
7. Mirastschijski U, Sander JT, Zier U, et al. The cost of post-burn scarring. Ann Burns Fire Disasters 2015;28(3):215–22.
8. Leblebici B, Adam M, Bağiş S, et al. Quality of life after burn injury: the impact of joint contracture. J Burn Care Res 2006;27(6):864–8.
9. Kolarsick PAJ, Kolarsick MA, Goodwin C. Anatomy and Physiology of the Skin. Journal of the Dermatology Nurses' Association 2011;3:203–13.
10. Baroni A, Buommino E, De Gregorio V, et al. Structure and function of the epidermis related to barrier properties. Clin Dermatol 2012;30(3):257–62.

11. Nguyen AV, Soulika AM. The dynamics of the skin's immune system. Int J Mol Sci 2019;20(8):1811.
12. Kwan PO, Tredget EE. Biological principles of scar and contracture. Hand Clin 2017;33(2):277–92.
13. Sorrell JM, Baber MA, Caplan AI. Site-matched papillary and reticular human dermal fibroblasts differ in their release of specific growth factors/cytokines and in their interaction with keratinocytes. J Cell Physiol 2004;200(1):134–45.
14. Reinke JM, Sorg H. Wound repair and regeneration. Eur Surg Res 2012;49(1): 35–43.
15. Mahdavian Delavary B, van der Veer WM, van Egmond M, et al. Macrophages in skin injury and repair. Immunobiology 2011;216(7):753–62.
16. Čoma M, Fröhlichová L, Urban L, et al. Molecular changes underlying hypertrophic scarring following burns involve specific deregulations at all wound healing stages (inflammation, proliferation and maturation). Int J Mol Sci 2021;22(2):897.
17. Kant S, van den Kerckhove E, Colla C, et al. Duration of scar maturation: retrospective analyses of 361 hypertrophic scars over 5 years. Adv Skin Wound Care 2019;32(1):26–34.
18. Zhang K, Garner W, Cohen L, et al. Increased types I and III collagen and transforming growth factor-beta 1 mRNA and protein in hypertrophic burn scar. J Invest Dermatol 1995;104(5):750–4.
19. Scott PG, Dodd CM, Tredget EE, et al. Immunohistochemical localization of the proteoglycans decorin, biglycan and versican and transforming growth factor-beta in human post-burn hypertrophic and mature scars. Histopathology 1995; 26(5):423–31.
20. Honardoust D, Varkey M, Marcoux Y, et al. Reduced decorin, fibromodulin, and transforming growth factor-β3 in deep dermis leads to hypertrophic scarring. J Burn Care Res 2012;33(2):218–27.
21. Kwan P, Desmouliere A, Tredget EE. Molecular and cellular basis of hypertrophic scarring. In: Herndon, DN. Total burn care. 5th Edition. Amsterdam: Elsevier; 2018. p. 455–65.
22. Zhang Z, Li XJ, Liu Y, et al. Recombinant human decorin inhibits cell proliferation and downregulates TGF-beta1 production in hypertrophic scar fibroblasts. Burns 2007;33(5):634–41.
23. Zhang Z, Garron TM, Li XJ, et al. Recombinant human decorin inhibits TGF-beta1-induced contraction of collagen lattice by hypertrophic scar fibroblasts. Burns 2009;35(4):527–37.
24. Oliveira GV, Chinkes D, Mitchell C, et al. Objective assessment of burn scar vascularity, erythema, pliability, thickness, and planimetry. Dermatol Surg 2005; 31(1):48–58.
25. Scott PG, Ghahary A, Tredget EE. Molecular and cellular aspects of fibrosis following thermal injury. Hand Clin 2000;16(2):271–87.
26. Choi YH, Kim KM, Kim HO, et al. Clinical and histological correlation in post-burn hypertrophic scar for pain and itching sensation. Ann Dermatol 2013;25(4): 428–33.
27. Bae SH, Bae YC. Analysis of frequency of use of different scar assessment scales based on the scar condition and treatment method. Arch Plast Surg 2014;41(2): 111–5.
28. Agabalyan NA, Su S, Sinha S, et al. Comparison between high-frequency ultrasonography and histological assessment reveals weak correlation for measurements of scar tissue thickness. Burns 2017;43(3):531–8.

29. Su S, Sinha S, Gabriel V. Evaluating accuracy and reliability of active stereophotogrammetry using MAVIS III Wound Camera for three-dimensional assessment of hypertrophic scars. Burns 2017;43(6):1263–70.

30. Peake M, Pan K, Rotatori RM, et al. Incorporation of 3D stereophotogrammetry as a reliable method for assessing scar volume in standard clinical practice. Burns 2019;45(7):1614–20.

31. Nedelec B, Correa JA, Rachelska G, et al. Quantitative measurement of hypertrophic scar: interrater reliability and concurrent validity. J Burn Care Res 2008; 29(3):501–11.

32. Spronk I, Polinder S, Haagsma JA, et al. Patient-reported scar quality of adults after burn injuries: a five-year multicenter follow-up study. Wound Repair Regen 2019;27(4):406–14.

33. Wallace HJ, Fear MW, Crowe MM, et al. Identification of factors predicting scar outcome after burn in adults: a prospective case-control study. Burns 2017; 43(6):1271–83.

34. Edger-Lacoursière Z, Nedelec B, Marois-Pagé E, et al. Systematic quantification of hypertrophic scar in adult burn survivors. European Burn Journal 2021;2: 88–105.

35. Nedelec B, Correa JA, de Oliveira A, et al. Longitudinal burn scar quantification. Burns 2014;40(8):1504–12.

36. van der Wal MB, Vloemans JF, Tuinebreijer WE, et al. Outcome after burns: an observational study on burn scar maturation and predictors for severe scarring. Wound Repair Regen 2012;20(5):676–87.

37. Shin D, Minn KW. The effect of myofibroblast on contracture of hypertrophic scar. Plast Reconstr Surg 2004;113(2):633–40.

38. Desmoulière A, Geinoz A, Gabbiani F, et al. Transforming growth factor-beta 1 induces alpha-smooth muscle actin expression in granulation tissue myofibroblasts and in quiescent and growing cultured fibroblasts. J Cell Biol 1993;122(1): 103–11.

39. Baumann ME, DeBruler DM, Blackstone BN, et al. Direct comparison of reproducibility and reliability in quantitative assessments of burn scar properties. Burns 2021;47(2):466–78.

40. Boyce ST, Supp AP, Wickett RR, et al. Assessment with the dermal torque meter of skin pliability after treatment of burns with cultured skin substitutes. J Burn Care Rehabil 2000;21(1 Pt 1):55–63.

41. Busche MN, Thraen AJ, Gohritz A, et al. Burn scar evaluation using the Cutometer® MPA 580 in comparison to "Patient and Observer Scar Assessment Scale" and "Vancouver Scar Scale". J Burn Care Res 2018;39(4):516–26.

42. Lye I, Edgar DW, Wood FM, et al. Tissue tonometry is a simple, objective measure for pliability of burn scar: is it reliable? J Burn Care Res 2006;27(1):82–5.

43. Goei H, van der Vlies CH, Tuinebreijer WE, et al. Predictive validity of short term scar quality on final burn scar outcome using the Patient and Observer Scar Assessment Scale in patients with minor to moderate burn severity. Burns 2017;43(4):715–23.

44. Müller B, Mazza E, Schiestl C, et al. Longitudinal monitoring and prediction of long-term outcome of scar stiffness on pediatric patients. Burns Trauma 2021; 9:tkab028.

45. Tyack ZF, Pegg S, Ziviani J. Postburn dyspigmentation: its assessment, management, and relationship to scarring–a review of the literature. J Burn Care Rehabil 1997;18(5):435–40.

46. van der Wal M, Bloemen M, Verhaegen P, et al. Objective color measurements: clinimetric performance of three devices on normal skin and scar tissue. J Burn Care Res 2013;34(3):e187–94.
47. Brusselaers N, Pirayesh A, Hoeksema H, et al. Burn scar assessment: a systematic review of objective scar assessment tools. Burns 2010;36(8):1157–64.
48. Chung BY, Kim HB, Jung MJ, et al. Post-burn pruritus. Int J Mol Sci 2020;21(11).
49. Kwak IS, Choi YH, Jang YC, et al. Immunohistochemical analysis of neuropeptides (protein gene product 9.5, substance P and calcitonin gene-related peptide) in hypertrophic burn scar with pain and itching. Burns 2014;40(8):1661–7.
50. Beecher SM, Hill R, Kearney L, et al. The pruritus severity scale-a novel tool to assess itch in burns patients. Int J Burns Trauma 2021;11(3):156–62.
51. Elman S, Hynan LS, Gabriel V, et al. The 5-D itch scale: a new measure of pruritus. Br J Dermatol 2010;162(3):587–93.
52. Mewa Kinoo S, Singh B. Complex regional pain syndrome in burn pathological scarring: a case report and review of the literature. Burns 2017;43(3):e47–52.
53. Shu F, Liu H, Lou X, et al. Analysis of the predictors of hypertrophic scarring pain and neuropathic pain after burn. Burns 2022;48(6):1425–34.
54. Meyer WJ III, Martyn JAJ, Wiechman S, et al. Management of pain and other discomforts in burned patients. In: Herndon DN, editor. Total burn care. 5th edition. Amsterdam: Elsevier; 2018. p. 679–99.
55. Finnerty CC, Jeschke MG, Branski LK, et al. Hypertrophic scarring: the greatest unmet challenge after burn injury. Lancet 2016;388(10052):1427–36.
56. Bond JS, Duncan JAL, Sattar A, et al. Maturation of the human scar: an observational study. Plast Reconstr Surg 2008;121(5):1650–8.
57. Sood RF, Hocking AM, Muffley LA, et al. Genome-wide association study of post-burn scarring identifies a novel protective variant. Ann Surg 2015;262(4):563–9.
58. Deitch EA, Wheelahan TM, Rose MP, et al. Hypertrophic burn scars: analysis of variables. J Trauma 1983;23(10):895–8.
59. Chipp E, Charles L, Thomas C, et al. A prospective study of time to healing and hypertrophic scarring in paediatric burns: every day counts. Burns Trauma 2017; 5:3.
60. Baker RH, Townley WA, McKeon S, et al. Retrospective study of the association between hypertrophic burn scarring and bacterial colonization. J Burn Care Res 2007;28(1):152–6.
61. Barret JP, Herndon DN. Effects of burn wound excision on bacterial colonization and invasion. Plast Reconstr Surg 2003;111(2):744–50, discussion 51–2.
62. Daryabeigi R, Heidari M, Hosseini SA, et al. Comparison of healing time of the 2 degree burn wounds with two dressing methods of fundermol herbal ointment and 1% silver sulfadiazine cream. Iran J Nurs Midwifery Res 2010;15(3):97–101.
63. Beheshti A, Shafigh Y, Zangivand AA, et al. Comparison of topical sucralfate and silver sulfadiazine cream in second degree burns in rats. Adv Clin Exp Med 2013; 22(4):481–7.
64. Quatresooz P, Hermanns JF, Paquet P, et al. Mechanobiology and force transduction in scars developed in darker skin types. Skin Res Technol 2006;12(4):279–82.
65. Junker JP, Kratz C, Tollbäck A, et al. Mechanical tension stimulates the transdifferentiation of fibroblasts into myofibroblasts in human burn scars. Burns 2008; 34(7):942–6.
66. Cho YS, Jeon JH, Hong A, et al. The effect of burn rehabilitation massage therapy on hypertrophic scar after burn: a randomized controlled trial. Burns 2014;40(8): 1513–20.

67. McLaughlin J, Branski LK, Norbury WB, et al. Laser for burn scar treatment. In: Herndon DN, editor. Total burn care. 5th edition. Amsterdam: Elsevier; 2018. p. 648–54.
68. Kim JY, Willard JJ, Supp DM, et al. Burn scar biomechanics after pressure garment therapy. Plast Reconstr Surg. Sep 2015;136(3):572–81.
69. Bleasdale B, Finnegan S, Murray K, et al. The use of silicone adhesives for scar reduction. Adv Wound Care 2015;4(7):422–30.
70. Nedelec B, Couture MA, Calva V, et al. Randomized controlled trial of the immediate and long-term effect of massage on adult postburn scar. Burns 2019;45(1): 128–39.
71. Mony MP, Harmon KA, Hess R, et al. An updated review of hypertrophic scarring. Cells 2023;12(5):678.
72. Sinha S, Gabriel VA, Arora RK, et al. Interventions for postburn pruritus. Manuscript submitted for publication.
73. Khalid FA, Mehrose MY, Saleem M, et al. Comparison of efficacy and safety of intralesional triamcinolone and combination of triamcinolone with 5-fluorouracil in the treatment of keloids and hypertrophic scars: randomised control trial. Burns. Feb 2019;45(1):69–75.
74. Zhuang Z, Li Y, Wei X. The safety and efficacy of intralesional triamcinolone acetonide for keloids and hypertrophic scars: a systematic review and meta-analysis. Burns. Aug 2021;47(5):987–98.
75. Abedini R, Sasani P, Mahmoudi HR, et al. Comparison of intralesional verapamil versus intralesional corticosteroids in treatment of keloids and hypertrophic scars: A randomized controlled trial. Burns. Sep 2018;44(6):1482–8.
76. Engrav LH, Heimbach DM, Rivara FP, et al. 12-Year within-wound study of the effectiveness of custom pressure garment therapy. Burns. Nov 2010;36(7): 975–83.
77. Anthonissen M, Daly D, Janssens T, et al. The effects of conservative treatments on burn scars: a systematic review. Burns. May 2016;42(3):508–18.
78. Nedelec B, Carter A, Forbes L, et al. Practice guidelines for the application of nonsilicone or silicone gels and gel sheets after burn injury. J Burn Care Res 2015;36(3):345–74.
79. Seago M, Shumaker PR, Spring LK, et al. Laser treatment of traumatic scars and contractures: 2020 international consensus recommendations. Lasers Surg Med. Feb 2020;52(2):96–116.

# Burn Injury Complications Impacting Rehabilitation

Matthew Godleski, MD[a],*, Miranda Yelvington, MS, OTR/L, BT-C[b],
Stephanie Jean, MD, MSc, FRCPC[c]

## KEYWORDS

- Burns • Rehabilitation • Therapy • Contracture • Peripheral nerve injury
- Heterotopic ossification • Amputation • Dysphagia

## KEY POINTS

- Successful post-burn rehabilitation requires an understanding of a wide range of complications to maximize functional recovery.
- Contracture is one of the most common complications requiring multi-modal prevention and treatment as well as a clear understanding of the physiological role of skin in joint movement and the impact of post-burn contracture upon that function.
- Burn injury causes complications beyond the skin, including peripheral nerve injury, heterotopic ossification, and dysphagia.
- Post-burn amputation can be a significant challenge following burn injury and local soft tissue injury can complicate prosthesis use and prescription.
- Many survivors of burn injury will experience symptoms from altered skin physiology, pain, and pruritis, each of which requires education and management.

## INTRODUCTION

Burn injuries can cause a host of functional complications both directly within the injured skin as well as in a number of other organ systems.[1–3] Understanding these potential complications–their prevention, early detection, and treatment–is a core foundation of post-burn injury care and rehabilitation. It is also important to recognize that many of these complications can be delayed by weeks or months following the initial trauma, emphasizing the importance of sustained rehabilitation care and screening during all phases of care, including the community.[4]

---

[a] Department of Physical Medicine and Rehabilitation, Sunnybrook Health Sciences Centre, University of Toronto, St. John's Rehab, 285 Cummer Avenue, Toronto, Ontario M2M 2G1, Canada; [b] Department of Rehabilitation, Arkansas Children's Hospital, 1 Children's Way, Slot 104, Little Rock, AR 72202, USA; [c] Department of Physical Medicine and Rehabilitation, Institut de Réadaptation Gingras-Lindsay de Montréal (Darlington), Université de Montréal, 6300 Avenue Darlington, Montréal, Québec H3S 2J4, Canada
* Corresponding author.
*E-mail address:* matthew.godleski@sunnybrook.ca

Phys Med Rehabil Clin N Am 34 (2023) 799–809
https://doi.org/10.1016/j.pmr.2023.06.020

The review presented here is by no means exhaustive. Some common complications such as hypertrophic scarring and the psychological impact of burn–including acute and posttraumatic stress disorders and fear avoidance–will be addressed separately but should also be considered key areas of rehabilitation critical to long-term functional recovery and quality of life. Complications specific to the mechanism of injury–such as polytrauma or electrical injury–must also be considered in terms of their complications but are outside the scope of this work.

## CONTRACTURE

Contracture is defined as a loss of range of motion (ROM) or malalignment of anatomic structures. In the setting of burn injury, it frequently occurs as a result of the development of scar tissue and wound contraction. Contractures are present in 18-50% of all burn survivors and have been associated with delayed wound healing, decreased mobility, decreased ability to complete daily activities, and suboptimal restoration of quality of life.[5–11] Larger burn size and longer length of stays have been correlated with greater risk of adult and pediatric burn scar contractures.[5,12,13] Hypertrophic scars have decreased pliability compared to nonburned skin, resulting in less available skin excursion to allow joint articulation.[14] Loss of ROM directly contributes to loss of function for burn survivors.[11,15] Prevention and treatment remain some of the hallmark goals of post-burn therapy.[1]

Burn rehabilitation, focusing on cutaneous functional units (CFUs), provides a cutaneokinematic approach to addressing these rapidly forming burn scar contractures. This approach considers the impact on skin and scar extensibility on ROM and provides principles to guide scar prevention interventions. The first of these principles recognizes the change in length of body segments as joint ROM occurs, resulting in the need for tissue elasticity to allow this excursion.[16] For this excursion to occur, skin is recruited well beyond the area of the joint being mobilized. Additionally, the position of the adjacent joints, which also recruit from the same skin pools, directly impacts the amount of skin available for recruitment and ROM.[16]

The size of the burn and location within a specific CFU has been found to negatively correlate with the available ROM of the joint.[17] Greater demands for joint ROM require greater recruitment from the impacted CFU.[16] A cutaneokinematic goniometric approach based on CFU concepts has been suggested.[10] This revised goniometric method can be used to complete objective measurements of burn scar contractures to provide an assessment of the impact of a patient's scar on their joint movements.

There are multiple techniques for contracture prevention, including positioning, orthoses, and stretching.[18–20] The therapy approach will need to be adjusted throughout the course of recovery, both to reflect the changing needs of the patient as well as their general medical status, level of consciousness, pain control, and functional capacity. Contracture prevention programs should be a key foundation of burn therapy knowledge and programs.[4]

Treatment programs also need to consider the numerous locations of potential contracture and their varying care needs and complications. Beyond the joints of the limbs, soft tissue contracture can impact multiple other anatomical locations. The formation of facial scars can be functionally limiting as well as cosmetically undesirable. Scars impacting the perioral areas and oral commissures can lead to microstomia (restricted mouth opening). The decreased oral aperature resulting from microstomia can lead to difficulty with oral intake, difficulty with oral hygiene, and can cause limitations in communication that should be monitored in a comprehensive fashion.[21] Multiple treatment approaches exist for microstomia prevention, though there is currently no standard of care.[19] Ocular involvement can include direct lid injury and complications of contracture such as ectropion and lagopthalmos and can lead to lasting ocular damage without appropriate management.[22] The genitalia can also be impacted by burn contracture, and this can contribute to a host of challenges that may impact sexual function following injury.[23]

## PERIPHERAL NERVE INJURY

The incidence of reported burn-related peripheral nerve injury varies widely.[24,25] It may appear in the acute phase or develop at any time during recovery.[26] Peripheral nerve injury by be the result of direct causes such as thermal or electrical injury or as a complication of escharotomies or fasciotomies or may be indirect as a result of edema formation, inflammatory response, heterotopic ossification or as a result of prolonged immobilization and positioning.[26]

The incidence of reported peripheral nerve injuries following burn injury varies depending on the methodology of the study, with cited ranges of 2-29% or more, and a suggested mean incidence of 6.4% based on a review of available literature. Nerve injury is usually associated with larger burns, more days on mechanical ventilation, increased surgical requirements, longer periods of hospitalization, and electrical current mechanisms of injury.[24,26] High voltage electrical injury particularly stands out as a high-risk etiology, with an odds ratio of over four times that of others with major burn injury.[24]

Focal peripheral nerve injury typically occurs local to the burn injury, but can also arise as a consequence of other features of burn injury such as critical illness, edema, or compartment syndrome. Particularly during periods of reduced level of consciousness, pressure or stretch from ICU or surgical positioning as well as potentially bulky dressings, need to be considered as potential causes of neuropathy.[18] Axonotmesis is often noted over demyelination in cases of larger and deeper burn injuries.[27] Focal injury incidence typically follows that of entrapment neuropathies, with the median, ulnar, and fibular nerves most often at-risk and the upper extremity a more common site than the lower.[24–26,28] The prognosis for peripheral nerve injury can often be favorable.[28] It is also important to note that non-burn specific neuropathies such as critical illness polyneuropathy and myopathy can also co-exist with burn associated nerve injuries.[29]

Nerve injury is not limited to the primary peripheral nerves, as the dermal damage associated with deeper burns will also directly injury distal nerve endings, leading to an increased threshold for detecting light touch, cold, and heat and a subsequent loss of perceived skin sensation.[2,30] The prognosis for skin-level injuries to nerve endings is more guarded.[30]

## HETEROTOPIC OSSIFICATION

Heterotopic ossification (HO) is a rare but potentially debilitating complication of burn injury. Reports show between a 0.15-5.6 percent incidence of this complication in people with burn injuries.[31] Associated risk factors have been identified, including, larger burn size, requiring mechanical ventilation, prolonged periods of immobilization and the need for grafting procedures.[32] These are all factors that relate to more severe injuries and there is no clear causative factor for the development of HO.

The elbow is the most common site for post-burn HO formation, followed by the shoulder, hip, and knee.[3] Loss of movement at these joints can directly impact the patient's independence with the performance of activities of daily living, often taking away the patient's ability to perform tasks such as dressing themselves, eating independently, or participating in self-care activities and can cause mobility limitations and increased pain. The most significant correlation between loss of range of motion and HO presence has been found in patients with 20% total body surface area burned or greater.[31]

When present, HO can lead to increased pain, decreased movement, and can worsen the formation of burn scars by preventing skin stretching and ROM. There should be a low threshold for screening, particularly if noted at the elbow joint. As HO worsens, the patient may experience muscle weakness and nerve impairment. HO is often identified clinically by a rapid loss of motion of a joint and reports of pain with movement and is confirmed by imaging.[33] While the early literature notes theoretical concerns about mobilization having a role in triggering HO, more recent literature has endorsed the use of ongoing ROM exercises, especially in cases of worsening ROM and functional limitations.[34,35] Nonburn injury literature has inconsistently noted a potential role for radiation therapy, nonsteroidal anti-inflammatory medications, and bisphosphonates for HO, but there is limited literature in burn injury. Given its negative impact on recovery, many patients may require surgical intervention to regain movement and function of the impacted extremity. The timing of surgery must be carefully considered in the context of post-burn recovery and skin healing, but recurrence rates are typically low.[36,37]

## AMPUTATION

Amputation in the context of burn injuries remains rare,[38–42] but when present causes significant quality of life and functional changes. Across many studies, the incidence of amputation has been estimated to be in between 1% and 6%, irrespective of burn etiologies,[38–41] with the exception of electrical injuries which will be addressed later in discussion.

Burn injuries sometimes results in deep thermal burn which leads to extensive soft-tissue necrosis, and therefore makes the limb unsalvageable.[43,44] Soft-tissue necrosis can also be complicated by local infection, and this can lead to systemic infection such as sepsis.[43] Amputation has been clearly shown to improve survival[38,39,44,45] when necessary to manage nonviable or recalcitrantly infected tissue.[44,46] However, there is a bimodal distribution of time to amputation that has been described in the literature: early amputation which has been described in the first two to three days after the burn injury compared to delayed amputation.[39] Early amputation from unsalvageable limbs has been shown to decrease more efficiently infection rate,[43,45] and mortality by 27%.[43] Delays in amputation can increase the incidence of infection.[43]

Burn-related amputations regarding the upper extremities are more frequent than the one regarding the lower extremities.[38,39,41,44,47] Overall, there is more minor amputation than major amputation in this population.[38,48] Minor amputation includes finger and toe amputations.[38] Major amputation typically includes transhumeral and transradial amputation for the upper extremity and transfemoral, transtibial and partial foot for the lower extremity.[38] In the minor amputation groups, there is usually a ratio of two fingers amputation for one toe amputation.[38,40]

Amputations are most often performed on older males with flame burn injury.[40,41,48] However, risk factors to have an amputation in the setting of a burn injury when controlled for confounding variables includes electrical injuries, burn size and depth, presence of comorbidities, nonwhite race, inhalation injury, and a greater degree of impaired consciousness.[38–42,44,46–48] In many studies, there is more amputation resulting from flame burn injuries since electrical burn injuries are rarer.[39] Yet, between 76% and 83% of burn-related amputations are attributable to electrical burn injuries[38] and it may be particularly accountable for upper extremity amputations.[44] Even more, the likelihood of amputation is increased from 13 to 14 times when there is an electrical injury.[38–40] Most often, the electrical injury victim that needs amputation are in majority working males.[38,39,41]

With amputation resulting from burns, rehabilitation difficulty significantly increases.[45] In fact, amputations related to burn are not as characteristic as when they are performed in the context of orthopedic trauma or following a vascular or diabetic pathology. In order to maintain bone and soft tissue, skin grafts, and muscle flaps are widely used after a burn injury.[45,49] Those factors can complicate the prosthetic fitting given they will need more adaptation of the prosthetic components, and the socket will often be from an odd shape.[45] Also, there are more complications arising from the decrease skin quality and lack of skin elasticity, as grafts are more likely to create skin adhesions and are more prone to tissue breakdown.[38,41,45,50] Furthermore, skin adhesion as well as hypertrophic scarring can result in skin and joint contracture,[38,41,45] which can limit the use of a prosthesis, even more when there is a short functional range.[45] Another factor limiting prosthetic fitting is altered skin sensation whether it is secondary to hypo- or hypersensitivity. Hyposensitivity can translate in lack of protection from increase pressure over nonweightbearing areas and increase friction, which will lead to more skin breakdown.[45,50,51] On the other hand, hypersensitivity which can arise from thinner skin and soft tissues as well as hypertrophic scarring also limits the prosthetic fitting whether during the donning and doffing or when it comes to tolerating the liner or socket pressure.[45] Burn-related heterotopic ossification will also change the shape of the residual limb, the available range of motion, the pressure a stump can tolerate and will impact the use of a prosthesis given the pain it can be associated to.[52] Finally, burns are often the result of polytraumatic injuries, which will impact the prosthetic fitting as much as the prosthetic rehabilitation.[45]

As mentioned earlier, electrical injuries more frequently result in amputation, as there is more deep tissue destruction, ischemia, and nerve damage.[39,43,45] Peripheral neuropathy, commonly seen after an electrical injury will further impact the amputation as it can lead to more limb weakness, decrease range of motion, and even decrease the electromyogram signals needed to control a myoelectric prosthesis.[45] Besides, cognitive impairments related to electrical injuries can impact the prosthetic candidacy and the use of a prosthesis.[45]

## ALTERED SKIN PHYSIOLOGY

The skin is the largest organ in the human body and it plays a range of physiological roles including the sense of touch, temperature regulation, and moisturization of the skin. Many of these functions are disrupted by injury to the dermis and typically remain impaired after autografting. Long-term physiological skin changes should be considered in recovery and patient education as they frequently persist and can have lasting functional consequences.[2]

Temperature regulation is a key function of the skin, with many of the effectors residing in skin function, such as vascular redistribution of blood via vasodilation and vasoconstriction as well as local mechanisms such as sweating and piloerection. Post-injury, these processes remain impaired with consequent decreased heat and cold tolerance relative to the size of skin injured, though heat acclimation exercises may improve heat tolerance over time.[30,53,54] Heat intolerance remains one of the most common long-term complaints of burn survivors, including the risk of heat stroke particularly in those with larger TBSA injuries.[2,55] Despite this, patients with burn injury can exercise safely with appropriate education and symptom monitoring, even without medical supervision.[55]

The loss of sebaceous glands and oil production can cause problems with pruritis, dry skin, and need for artificial moisturization both during the acute phase, when it is likely further exacerbated by the healing process, and remains one of the most common long-term complaints following major burn injury.[2] Beyond the need for early education and establishment of treatment plans, alterations in skin oil may need to be considered for activities and employment that are accompanied by exposure to chemical irritants, dry heat, or cleaning materials.

## PAIN AND PRURITIS

Burn injury-associated pain can be a significant barrier to recovery and rehabilitation and often results in the use of high doses of both narcotic and nonnarcotic pain medication. Pain is associated with burns of all sizes, and all degrees, and can affect the survivor's performance of all activities of daily living, including sleep, work, mood, and quality of life. Procedures such as dressing changes, debridement, and therapy interventions typically result in more pain than resting positions; however, these procedures are necessary for recovery and return to optimal quality of life for the burn survivor.[56] Patients with extensive burns may undergo hours of therapy daily, including prolonged stretching and range of motion, to limit the development of contractures. Burn injury-associated pain can be a significant barrier to recovery and rehabilitation. For burn survivors, procedural pain that occurs with predictable events such as therapy is often short lasting but high-intensity.[57]

From a pharmacological perspective, the management of pain during the rehabilitation phase of care will often require a foundation of neuropathic pain medications and over-the-counter analgesics.[58] Opiates may be necessary particularly for procedural and breakthrough pain associated with wound care and intensive therapy, but should be first-line for weaning in favor of nonopiate medications prior to discharge to the community. Of the neuropathic pain medication options, gabapentin and pregabalin have received particular study and have been shown to benefit patients with burn injury.[59–61]

The Model Systems Knowledge Translation Center (MSKTC) reports no correlation between the size and degree of burn and the severity of pain experienced but endorses the need for nonmedication adjuncts for pain management for all burn survivors.[62] Alternative pain management strategies have been investigated with burn survivors, including massage, guided imagery, hypnosis, aromatherapy, music therapy, vibration, and virtual reality.[63–66] The American Burn Association (ABA) recommends nonpharmacological techniques for every patient as an adjunct to pharmacological measures.[56] Screening fear-avoidance and fostering resilience are also key areas for ensuring best management of pain and tolerance of therapy.[67,68]

Pruritis is another common negative sensation for patients recovering from burn injury, both in the short- and long-term phases of recovery.[2,69] The pathophysiology of itch is complicated in burn injury and can be the outcome of a host of factors including histamine release, the inflammatory stages of healing, edema, nerve injury, skin dryness, and central sensitization.[69] Management strategies include neuropathic pain agents, topical treatments, and laser therapy.[59,61,69–72] Anti-histamines have also been studied in post-burn pruritus, but with mixed results.[71,73,74]

## DYSPHAGIA

Dysphagia is defined as a difficulty safely and effectively swallowing.[75,76] Dysphagia after a burn injury was for a long time assumed to be a secondary side effect of the following combination: burn to the head and neck, increased TBSA burned ($\geq$18%

TBSA), prolonged intubation and mechanical ventilation, prolonged critical illness, severe deconditioning, and associated muscle atrophy.[76–78] The incidence of dysphagia in the global burn population has been estimated to be 6 to 11%, but the incidence in the above-mentioned context has been estimated to be 73%.[77,78]

Inhalation injury was more recently described as a causative agent of dysphagia.[79] Inhalation injury is described by the inhalation of fire elements such as smoke when in an enclose space.[76,78] The incidence of dysphagia in a burn population with inhalation injury regardless of its severity has been estimated to be 87 to 90%.[77,78] Interestingly, there is no correlation between incidence of dysphagia and inhalation injury severity.[79] Usually, dysphagia secondary to inhalation injury will be more severe at presentation compared to dysphagia from general burn patient.[78] Dysphagia after an inhalation injury will also take more time to resolve (mean: 30 vs. 2 days), and even if not clinically detectable, will leave more persistent laryngeal pathology in the long term.[78,79] However, the grade of inhalation injury (grade 1 vs. 2) does not impact the duration of dysphagia nor if the patients are discharged with dysphagia.[79]

## SUMMARY

Burn injury can cause a wide range of complications that can impact patient recovery far beyond the immediate needs of wound care and skin grafting. Rehabilitation programs need to be poised to identify these issues across all phases of care as well as have effective education and treatment modalities.

## CLINICS CARE POINTS

- Burn injuries can cause a host of functional complications both directly within the injured skin as well as in a number of other organ systems.

- Contracture should be considered through the lens of cutaneokinematics. Prevention and treatment often employ a multi-modal approach that evolves through the phases of care.

- Peripheral nerve injury can occur in both discrete peripheral nerves in the upper and lower extremities as well as in distal nerve endings within the injured skin.

- Heterotopic ossification is a relatively rare but very functionally challenging complication often requiring both difficult therapy as well as potential consideration of surgical resection.

- Amputation can be required in more severe burn injuries and can complicate the use and prescription of protheses due to the likelihood of injured soft tissue in the residual limb.

- Altered skin physiology, pain, and pruritis can cause patient discomfort in a variety of ways and require a comprehensive approach in terms of patient education, monitoring, and treatment.

- Dysphagia can occur with burn injury and inhalational injury, supporting the need for interdisciplinary teams that include speech and language pathology.

## DISCLOSURE

The authors have nothing to disclose.

## REFERENCES

1. Esselman PC, Thombs BD, Magyar-Russell G, et al. Burn rehabilitation: state of the science. [Review] [353 refs]. Am J Phys Med Rehabil 2006;85:383 413.

2. Holavanahalli RK, Helm PA, Kowalske KJ. Long-term outcomes in patients surviving large burns: the skin. J Burn Care Res 2010;31:631–9.

3. Holavanahalli RK, Helm PA, Kowalske KJ. Long-term outcomes in patients surviving large burns: the musculoskeletal system. J Burn Care Res 2016;37(4): 243–54.

4. Parry I, Forbes L, Lorello D, et al. Burn rehabilitation therapists competency tool-version 2: an expansion to include long-term rehabilitation and outpatient care. J Burn Care Res 2017;38(1):e261–8.

5. Godleski M, Lee AF, Goverman J, et al. Quantifying contracture severity at hospital discharge in adults: a burn model system national database study. J Burn Care Res 2018;39(4):604–11.

6. Goverman J, Mathews K, Goldstein R, et al. Adult contractures in burn injury: a burn model system national database study. J Burn Care Res 2016. https://doi.org/10.1097/BCR.0000000000000380.

7. Goverman J, Mathews K, Goldstein R, et al. Pediatric contractures in burn injury: a burn model system national database study. J Burn Care Res 2016. https://doi.org/10.1097/BCR.0000000000000341.

8. Leblebici B, Adam M, Bağiş S, et al. Quality of life after burn injury: the impact of joint contracture. J Burn Care Res 2006;27(6):864–8.

9. Dobbs ER, Curreri PW. Burns: analysis of results of physical therapy in 681 patients. J Trauma 1972;12(3):242–8.

10. Parry I, Richard R, Aden JK, et al. Goniometric measurement of burn scar contracture: a paradigm shift challenging the standard. J Burn Care Res 2019; 40(4):377–85.

11. Schneider JC, Holavanahalli R, Helm P, et al. Contractures in burn injury: defining the problem. J Burn Care Res 2006;27(4):508–14.

12. Yelvington M, Godleski M, Lee AF, et al. Contracture severity at hospital discharge in children: a burn model system database study. J Burn Care Res 2021;42(3):425–33.

13. Spronk I, Legemate CM, Dokter J, et al. Predictors of health-related quality of life after burn injuries: a systematic review. Crit Care 2018;22(1):160.

14. Arno AI, Gauglitz GG, Barret JP, et al. Up-to-date approach to manage keloids and hypertrophic scars: a useful guide. Burns 2014;40(7):1255–66.

15. Korp K, Richard R, Hawkins D, et al. Refining "functional" in burn recovery outcomes. J Burn Care Res 2011;32:S160.

16. Richard RL, Lester ME, Miller SF, et al. Identification of cutaneous functional units related to burn scar contracture development. J Burn Care Res 2009;30:625–31.

17. Parry I, Sen S, Sattler-Petrocchi K, et al. Cutaneous functional units predict shoulder range of motion recovery in children receiving rehabilitation. J Burn Care Res 2017;38(2):106–11.

18. Serghiou MA, Niszczak J, Parry I, et al. Clinical practice recommendations for positioning of the burn patient. Burns 2016;42(2):267–75.

19. Parry IS, Schneider JC, Yelvington M, et al. Systematic review and expert consensus on the use of orthoses (splints and casts) with adults and children after burn injury to determine practice guidelines. J Burn Care Res 2020;41(3): 503–34.

20. Godleski M, Oeffling A, Bruflat AK, et al. Treating burn-associated joint contracture: results of an inpatient rehabilitation stretching protocol. J Burn Care Res 2013;34(4):420–6.

21. Couture MA, Calva V, de Oliveira A, et al. Development and clinimetric evaluation of the mouth impairment and disability assessment (MIDA). Burns 2018;44(4): 980–94.
22. Cabalag MS, Wasiak J, Syed Q, et al. Early and late complications of ocular burn injuries. J Plast Reconstr Aesthetic Surg 2015;68(3):356–61.
23. Pandya AA, Corkill HA, Goutos I. Sexual function following burn injuries: literature review. J Burn Care Res 2015;36(6):e283–93.
24. Kowalske K, Holavanahalli R, Helm P. Neuropathy after burn injury. J Burn Care Rehabil 2001;22(5):353–7 [discussion: 352].
25. Khedr EM, Khedr T, el-Oteify MA, et al. Peripheral neuropathy in burn patients. Burns 1997;23:579–83.
26. Tu Y, Lineaweaver WC, Zheng X, et al. Burn-related peripheral neuropathy: a systematic review. Burns 2017;43(4):693–9.
27. Coert JH. Pathophysiology of nerve regeneration and nerve reconstruction in burned patients. Burns 2010;36(5):593–8.
28. Gabriel V, Kowalske KJ, Holavanahalli RK. Assessment of recovery from burn-related neuropathy by electrodiagnostic testing. J Burn Care Res 2009;30(4): 668–74.
29. Mc Kittrick A, Kornhaber R, Harats M, et al. Critical care polyneuropathy in burn injuries: an integrative review. Burns 2017;43(8):1613–23.
30. Nedelec B, Quanzhi H, Ismahen S, et al. Sensory perception and neuroanatomical structures in normal and grafted skin of burn survivors. Burns 2005;31: 817–30.
31. Yelvington M, Godleski M, Lee AF, et al. A comparison of contracture severity at acute discharge in patients with and without heterotopic ossification: a Burn Model System National Database Study. J Burn Care Res 2019. https://doi.org/10.1093/jbcr/irz031.
32. Hu X, Sun Z, Li F, et al. Burn-induced heterotopic ossification from incidence to therapy: key signaling pathways underlying ectopic bone formation. Cell Mol Biol Lett 2021;26(1):34.
33. Foster N, Kornhaber R, McGarry S, et al. Heterotopic Ossification in adults following a burn: a phenomenological analysis. Burns 2017;43(6):1250–62.
34. Coons D, Godleski M. Range of motion exercises in the setting of burn-associated heterotopic ossification at the elbow: case series and discussion. Burns 2013;39(1):e34–8.
35. Ranganathan K, Loder S, Agarwal S, et al. Heterotopic ossification: basic-science principles and clinical correlates. J Bone Joint Surg Am 2015;97(13): 1101–11.
36. Pontell ME, Sparber LS, Chamberlain RS. Corrective and reconstructive surgery in patients with postburn heterotopic ossification and bony ankylosis: an evidence-based approach. J Burn Care Res 2015;36(1):57–69.
37. Hunt JL, Arnoldo BD, Kowalske K, et al. Heterotopic ossification revisited: a 21-year surgical experience. J Burn Care Res 2006;27(4):535–40.
38. Bartley CN, Atwell K, Purcell L, et al. Amputation following burn injury. J Burn Care Res 2019;40(4):430–6.
39. Soto CA, Albornoz CR, Peña V, et al. Prognostic factors for amputation in severe burn patients. Burns 2013;39(1):126–9.
40. Gurbuz K, Demir M, Basaran A, et al. Most prominent factors contributing to burn injury-related amputations: an analysis of a referral burn center. J Burn Care Res 2022;43(4):921–5.

41. Li Q, Wang LF, Chen Q, et al. Amputations in the burn unit: a retrospective analysis of 82 patients across 12 years. Burns 2017;43(7):1449–54.
42. Carrougher GJ, McMullen K, Mandell SP, et al. Impact of burn-related amputations on return to work: findings from the burn injury model system national database. J Burn Care Res 2019;40(1):21–8.
43. Yowler CJ, Mozingo DW, Ryan JB, et al. Factors contributing to delayed extremity amputation in burn patients. J Trauma 1998;45(3):522–6.
44. Tarim A, Ezer A. Electrical burn is still a major risk factor for amputations. Burns 2013;39(2):354–7.
45. Fergason JR, Blanck R. Prosthetic management of the burn amputation. Phys Med Rehabil Clin N Am 2011;22(2):277–99, vi.
46. Viscardi PJ, Polk HC Jr. Outcome of amputations in patients with major burns. Burns 1995;21(7):526–9.
47. Pedrazzi N, Klein H, Gentzsch T, et al. Predictors for limb amputation and reconstructive management in electrical injuries. Burns 2022. https://doi.org/10.1016/j.burns.2022.08.007.
48. Liu M, Zhu H, Yan R, et al. Epidemiology and outcome analysis of 470 patients with hand burns: a five-year retrospective study in a major burn center in Southwest China. Med Sci Mon Int Med J Exp Clin Res 2020;26:e918881.
49. Parry IS, Mooney KN, Chau C, et al. Effects of skin grafting on successful prosthetic use in children with lower extremity amputation. J Burn Care Res 2008;29(6):949–54.
50. Anderson WD, Stewart KJ, Wilson Y, et al. Skin grafts for the salvage of degloved below-knee amputation stumps. Br J Plast Surg 2002;55(4):320–3.
51. Ward RS, Hayes-Lundy C, Schnebly WA, et al. Prosthetic use in patients with burns and associated limb amputations. J Burn Care Rehabil 1990;11(4):361–4.
52. Edwards DS, Clasper JC. Heterotopic ossification: a systematic review. J R Army Med Corps 2015;161(4):315–21.
53. Davis SL, Shibasaki M, Low DA, et al. Sustained impairments in cutaneous vasodilation and sweating in grafted skin following long-term recovery. J Burn Care Res 2009;30(4):675–85.
54. Schlader ZJ, Ganio MS, Pearson J, et al. Heat acclimation improves heat exercise tolerance and heat dissipation in individuals with extensive skin grafts. J Appl Phys 2015;119(1):69–76.
55. Palackic A, Suman OE, Porter C, et al. Rehabilitative exercise training for burn injury. Sports Med 2021;51(12):2469–82.
56. Romanowski KS, Carson J, Pape K, et al. American burn association guidelines on the management of acute pain in the adult burn patient: a review of the literature, a compilation of expert opinion and next steps. J Burn Care Res 2020;41(6):1152–64.
57. James DL, Jowza M. Principles of burn pain management. Clin Plast Surg 2017;44(4):737–47.
58. Summer GJ, Puntillo KA, Miaskowski C, et al. Burn injury pain: the continuing challenge. J Pain 2007;8(7):533–48.
59. Gray P, Kirby J, Smith MT, et al. Pregabalin in severe burn injury pain: a double-blind, randomised placebo-controlled trial. Pain 2011;152(6):1279–88.
60. Kaul I, Amin A, Rosenberg M, et al. Use of gabapentin and pregabalin for pruritus and neuropathic pain associated with major burn injury: A retrospective chart review. Burns 2018;44(2):414–22.
61. Kneib CJ, Sibbett SH, Carrougher GJ, et al. The effects of early neuropathic pain control with gabapentin on long-term chronic pain and itch in burn patients. J Burn Care Res 2019;40(4):457–63.

62. Duchin ER, Moore M, Carrougher GJ, et al. Burn patients' pain experiences and perceptions. Burns 2021;47(7):1627–34.

63. de Jesus Catalã CA, Pan R, Rossetto Kron-Rodrigues M, et al. Virtual Reality therapy to control burn pain: systematic review of randomized controlled trials. J Burn Care Res 2022;43(4):880–8.

64. Coffey R, Buchert J, Ruiz A, et al. 620 the effectiveness of aromatherapy in an urban-based, safety-net hospital on pain and anxiety. J Burn Care Res 2022;43(Supplement_1):S151–2.

65. Fratianne RB, Prensner JD, Huston MJ, et al. The effect of music-based imagery and musical alternate engagement on the burn debridement process. J Burn Care Rehabil 2001;22(1):47–53.

66. Gillum M, Huang S, Kuromaru Y, et al. Nonpharmacologic management of procedural pain in pediatric burn patients: a systematic review of randomized controlled trials. J Burn Care Res 2022;43(2):368–73.

67. Langlois J, Vincent-Toskin S, Duchesne P, et al. Fear avoidance beliefs and behaviors of burn survivors: a mixed methods approach. Burns 2021;47(1):175–89.

68. Kornhaber R, Bridgman H, McLean L, et al. The role of resilience in the recovery of the burn-injured patient: an integrative review. Chron Wound Care Manag Res 2016;3(Issue 1):41–50.

69. Zachariah JR, Rao AL, Prabha R, et al. Post burn pruritus–a review of current treatment options. Burns 2012;38(5):621–9.

70. Nedelec B, Rachelska G, Parnell LK, et al. Double-blind, randomized, pilot study assessing the resolution of postburn pruritus. J Burn Care Res 2012;33(3):398–406.

71. Bell PL, Gabriel V. Evidence based review for the treatment of post-burn pruritus. J Burn Care Res 2009;30(1):55–61.

72. Ebid AA, Ibrahim AR, Omar MT, et al. Long-term effects of pulsed high-intensity laser therapy in the treatment of post-burn pruritus: a double-blind, placebo-controlled, randomized study. Lasers Med Sci 2017;32(3):693–701.

73. Ahuja RB, Gupta R, Gupta G, et al. A comparative analysis of cetirizine, gabapentin and their combination in the relief of post-burn pruritus. Burns 2011;37(2):203–7.

74. Baker RA, Zeller RA, Klein RL, et al. Burn wound itch control using H1 and H2 antagonists. J Burn Care Rehabil 2001;22(4):263–8.

75. Merriam-Webster. (n.d.). Dysphagia. In Merriam-Webster.com dictionary. Available at: https://www.morriam-webster.com/dictionary/dysphagia. Accessed March 20, 2023.

76. Vo E, Kurmis R, Campbell J, et al. Risk factors for and characteristics of dysphagia development in thermal burn injury and/or inhalation injury patients: a systematic review protocol. JBI Database System Rev Implement Rep 2016;14(1):31–43.

77. Rumbach AF, Ward EC, Cornwell PL, et al. Incidence and predictive factors for dysphagia after thermal burn injury: a prospective cohort study. J Burn Care Res 2011;32(6):608–16.

78. Clayton NA, Ward EC, Rumbach AF, et al. Influence of inhalation injury on incidence, clinical profile and recovery pattern of dysphagia following burn injury. Dysphagia 2020;35(6):968–77.

79. Weiner B, Halfacre H, Lee J, et al. 525 dysphagia in thermal injury: the impact of inhalation injury on incidence and recovery. J Burn Care Res 2022;43(Supplement_1):S97–8.

# Key Exercise Concepts in the Rehabilitation from Severe Burns

Eric Rivas, PhD[a], Josh Foster, PhD[b], Craig G. Crandall, PhD[c],
Celeste C. Finnerty, PhD[d], Oscar E. Suman-Vejas, PhD[d,*]

## KEYWORDS

• Burns • Exercise • Aerobic • Resistance • Thermoregulation • Heat • Scar
• Contracture

## KEY POINTS

- An exercise training program for whole-body rehabilitation can be beneficial during the inpatient and outpatient stage of burn care. These benefits are physical, as well as psychosocial.
- Related to thermoregulation, burn survivors can have severely impaired thermoregulation which is related to the size of the burn injury.
- If the environmental conditions are temperate, and the workload is mild to moderate, a burn survivor can safely perform physical activity. In hot climates if the duration of activity is longer than ~30 minutes or less. If the environmental conditions are warm/hot and/or the workload is hard, physical activity for longer than ~30 min can cause excessive elevations in core temperature.
- Some studies have reported that exercise programs can reduce scar severity and the need for subsequent surgical interventions.

## ESSENTIALS OF EXERCISE REHABILITATION TRAINING DURING THE IN-PATIENT STAGE

Numerous studies have demonstrated the benefits of exercise in counteracting the detrimental effects of bed rest, and post-discharge exercise is crucial for maintaining physical function, lean body mass, and metabolic recovery after major burn injuries.[1–3]

---

[a] Microgravity Research, In-Space Solutions, Axiom Space Headquarters, 1290 Hercules Avenue, Houston, TX 77058, USA; [b] Department of Internal Medicine, University of Texas Southwestern Medical Center, Institute for Exercise and Environmental Medicine (IEEM), Texas Health Presbyterian Hospital Dallas, 5323 Harry Hines Boulevard, Dallas, TX 75390, USA; [c] Division of Cardiology, Department of Internal Medicine, University of Texas Southwestern Medical Center, Institute for Exercise and Environmental Medicine (IEEM), Texas Health Presbyterian Hospital Dallas, 7232 Greenville Avenue, Suite 435, Dallas, TX 75231, USA; [d] Department of Surgery, Division of Surgical Sciences, University of Texas Medical Branch, 301 University Boulevard, Galveston, TX 77555-1220, USA
* Corresponding author.
*E-mail address:* oesuman@utmb.edu

Phys Med Rehabil Clin N Am 34 (2023) 811–824
https://doi.org/10.1016/j.pmr.2023.05.003
1047-9651/23/© 2023 Elsevier Inc. All rights reserved.

Bed rest is known to have negative effects on a patient's well-being,[4] cardiorespiratory capacity,[5] lean body mass (LBM),[6] and bone and whole-body metabolism.[6,7] A recent study showed that sedated adults on mechanical ventilation who received exercise and mobilization had better outcomes than those who received only sedation.[8] The managing physician must consider the patient's current medical condition, medical comorbidities, premorbid functional level, and cardiovascular and respiratory reserves. External factors, such as timing after a skin graft, the presence of lines, and staffing, must also be considered. While the issue of staffing is critical, future studies should investigate how mobilization can decrease complications and justify the necessary staffing for physical and occupational therapists.

Exercise during the in-patient stage may offer important benefits that may improve recovery and prevent long-term complications. The patient should have clearance by the attending medical doctor for exercising. Factors such as respiratory reserve, oxygen saturation, hemoglobin level, platelet count, a stable white blood cell count, infection status, and blood glucose levels, febrile status, mental alertness and neurologic status, as well as orthopedic limitations such as unstable spine or fracture, severe osteoporosis, or unstable bone metastasis should all be also considered.[9] Another factor to consider is the timing for getting up and exercising after a skin graft. Although numerous studies have shown that ambulation is safe on the day of grafting for lower leg burns in otherwise healthy patients with smaller burns, the risk of losing precious skin graft in a patient with a large burn should be considered against the potential trade-off of additional ventilator days and a poorer outcome at hospital discharge. This area of research is not well developed and requires more understanding.

### Essentials of Rehabilitation Exercise Training During Outpatient Stage

With advancements in acute burn care in recent decades, survival rates for patients with severe burns (up to 90% of total body surface area) have greatly increased. However, the accompanying metabolic and cardiovascular complications may persist for up to 3 years post-injury.[10] As a result, there is now a growing recognition of the importance of implementing strategies to promote faster recovery and decrease long-term morbidity following a severe burn. Rehabilitation exercise training (RET) has been shown to effectively restore lean body mass, glucose and protein metabolism, cardiorespiratory fitness, and muscle strength in burn survivors.[1,11–14] RET has been reported to control for edema, decreases tendon adherence, joint stiffness, capsular shortening and muscle atrophy, burn scar contractures and improves physical conditioning in burned patients[13] .[15,16] Despite its proven safety and efficacy, RET is not commonly incorporated into rehabilitation programs for outpatients with severe burns. It is highly recommended is that all patients with severe burns should receive a long-term progressive resistance exercise training (PRET) prescription plan, as metabolic, endocrine, and cardiovascular complications persist.[17–21] Therefore, we recommend that a long-term exercise prescription plan be considered for all patients with severe burns as a means of restoring function and reducing post-burn morbidity.

Pediatric burn patients experience elevated muscle breakdown for up to 1 year after discharge.[22] The importance of RET such as resistance exercise is highlighted by work from Chang and colleagues[23] that reported a 10% loss of lean body mass (LBM) can negatively impact immune function, while a 20% loss can impair wound healing, and a 30% loss of LBM is associated with increased mortality. In addition, a 30% loss of LBM increases the likelihood of developing pneumonia and pressure sores, which further increases the risk of mortality by 50%. Burn survivors often face challenges when attempting to resume normal activities and reintegrate into society due to the loss of lean body mass (LBM), resulting in muscle weakness and other related health issues. However, progressive resistance exercise training (PRET) can help enhance LBM and strength, ultimately reversing the negative effects of burn injury on body composition and metabolism. It is worth noting that in all cases studied, a 40% loss of LBM resulted in death.[23] Other studies that utilized RET have reported positive results. For example, the use of resistance exercise training (RET), including concurrent aerobic and resistance exercise, can increase lean body mass (LBM) in burned children by approximately 5% over a period of 6 to 12 weeks.[2,3,12,24–29] Long-term effects of RET were also evaluated by Wurzer and colleagues[26] in children who started the program at the time of hospital discharge and continued for approximately 2 years post-burn. Results indicated that RET improved muscle strength and cardiopulmonary fitness compared to standard of care at discharge, and these benefits persisted at 12 to 24 months post-injury. Similar results were observed in adult patients following a 6-week RET program that included both aerobic and resistance exercise.[30] Both boys and men showed similar increases in lean and fat mass by approximately 4% and 7%, respectively, after a 6 to 12-week RET program performed after hospital discharge.[31] RET has also been shown to improve skeletal muscle strength and increase total LBM in children with large burns (>50% TBSA) compared to SoC, without worsening hypermetabolism.[3] Furthermore, other studies have reported that 6 to 12 weeks of RET does not exacerbate hypermetabolism post-burn.[25,32]

Cardiovascular complications are reported after severe burn trauma. The cardiovascular system responds acutely to burn trauma by elevating resting cardiac output and heart rate, which is associated with myocardial degeneration and ventricular hypertrophy.[17,18,33] Chronic hyper-sympathetic innervation can cause cardiac deficiency and local myocardial hypoxia.[17,18] Pulmonary function is also affected by major burn trauma, with impaired spirometry function lasting several months post-burn, leading to reduced cardiorespiratory fitness. Cardiorespiratory fitness (CRF), a standard health measure, reflects the integrative capacity of cardiac, pulmonary, circulatory, and skeletal muscle systems. Studies have demonstrated that CRF remains lower than normative values for years post-injury, highlighting the need for long-term rehabilitation exercise training.[18] Notably, the decrease in burn-injured children and adults' CRF-the measure of the body's ability to supply and use oxygen during maximal exercise.[34] Lower CRF values were reported by Willis and colleagues, Ganio and colleagues,[35] and Cambiaso-Daniel and co-workers[36] reported in burned patients, both adults and children, up to several years after their injury.

In summary, immediately following hospital discharge, RET can restore LBM and exercise capacity, while also improving quality of life.[2,3,12,37] Notably, 6- to 12-week RET programs that include concurrent aerobic and resistance training have been shown to improve CRF (+19%), strength (+37%), and LBM (+11%) in patients post-discharge.[13,38–40] Similar concepts have been applied in several studies of adult burn survivors, with a 12-week rehabilitative exercise program resulting in improvements in aerobic capacity, occupational performance,[41] muscle strength, LBM,[38,42] and quality of life.[43] This highlights the need for long-term rehabilitation exercise training.

Prior to an RET program, patients should be evaluated from baseline fitness levels utilizing standards in exercise prescription. The patient's physical and mental abilities are also assessed by the appropriate qualified ehabilitation provider, who then uses the results of this evaluation to tailor the training program in terms of frequency, intensity, time, type, volume, and progression. Muscle strength can be evaluated through isokinetic dynamometry testing, and the Three Repetition Maximum Test or 10 to 12

Repetition Maximal Test can determine a safe and effective weight load for resistance training. For a complete description of these standard tests refer to.[44] The measured maximal heart rate during the progressive exercise test and the maximal value for the three-repetition maximum can then be used to prescribe exercise as a percentage of cardiovascular and resistive exercise shown in **Table 1**.

Severely burned children and adults can benefit from RET that positively impacts their cardiorespiratory system, musculoskeletal system, and body composition. Several studies have shown the benefits of a 6 to 12-week combined aerobic and resistance training program. See Table 1 for general prescriptive guidelines that have been used successfully in population with severe burn injuries. For a complete description of the previous Shiners Hospitals for Children-Galveston RET program see reference.[44]

### Burn Injuries and Long-Term Cardiovascular Health

While research aimed at improving immediate outcomes after severe burn injuries is essential, the long-term consequences are often overlooked, resulting in a lack of clarity regarding the health-related effects years after the injury. Studies utilizing epidemiological analyses sought to address this gap by examining all-cause mortality and various measures of morbidity burden in burn survivors years after the injury. These studies indicate that burn survivors have mortality rates 1.3 to 1.8 times higher than non-burned groups.[21,45,46] Consistent with this observation, individuals who previously sustained severe burn injuries have 1.5-fold more hospital admissions and 2.9-fold more hospitalization days for "circulatory diseases" years after the burn injury.[21] From that same set of studies, the burned cohort had higher admission rates for ischemic heart disease, heart failure, cerebrovascular disease, as well as a greater

| Table 1<br>Exercise rehabilitation training prescription guidelines | | |
|---|---|---|
| **RET Program Prescription** | **Cardiovascular Fitness** | **Resistive Fitness** |
| Frequency | 3–5 sessions/wk | At least 2 times/wk |
| Intensity | Moderate intensity between 70% and 85% HR peak or $Vo_2$ peak. High-intensity exercise can be prescribed at >90% $Vo_2$ peak | 20% of total body mass for the upper body and 40% of total body mass for the lower body, with 3 sets and 8–15 repetitions per set. |
| Time | Continuous moderate intensity 20–40 min; High-intensity intervals, lasting 1–2 min, with 3–4 min recovery and 4–5 repetitions. | No time limit |
| Volume | Time volume is 150 min/wk, physical activity ambulation >5000–12000 steps/d | No established volume |
| Progression | Should start with what they can accomplish and an individualize progressive increase over time. | |
| Major considerations | Safety is the highest priority, so progress should be slow, techniques should be taught properly, and exercise prescription should be individualized based on the severity of burns and physical limitations. | |

incidence of stroke. Furthermore, burn survivors have a higher risk of developing diabetes, hypertension, coronary artery disease, and heart failure for up to 8 years after the injury.[47] Although the underlying mechanisms responsible for these adverse outcomes in burn survivors remain unclear, similar negative effects are observed in sedentary non-burned individuals.

Long-term consequences of severe burn injuries include challenges associated with impaired temperature regulation, hypertrophic scars, hyperpigmentation, psychosocial barriers, decreased cutaneous sensation, and a lower quality of life.[48–53] Fatigue and muscle weakness are also prevalent, affecting over 50% of individuals a decade or more after the injury, with fatigue being a major barrier to returning to work and performing daily activities.[54] Importantly, burn survivors have profoundly reduced aerobic capacity many years after the injury. Specifically, one study found that ~75% of subjects who sustained major burn injuries at least 2 years prior had a peak oxygen uptake (VO2peak; a measure of aerobic fitness) in the lowest 20th percentile rankings, relative to sex and age adjusted non-burned individuals.[35] Similar observations are found when the obtained data were compared with normative VO2peak values from the American Heart Association, with 88% of the burned cohort being below age-adjusted normative VO2peak values[55] and the Aspenes and colleagues dataset, with 80% of the burned cohort have a VO2peak in the lowest quartile.[56] It is important to emphasize that in non-burned individuals, such low VO2peak values are associated with increased cardiovascular-specific and all cause morbidity and mortality.[35,56–60] Moreover, drawing from data relating percentile rankings of VO2peak with mortality,[57] ~75% of severely burned individuals have a 3 to 5 fold greater mortality risk, values consistent with the aforementioned epidemiological findings.

A lower aerobic capacity is associated with elevated cardiovascular risk factors, reduced quality of life, reduced ability to perform functions of daily living, and a greater reliance on dependent care as they age. Importantly, well-healed burn survivors can improve their aerobic capacity through an aggressive exercise training regimen.[30,43] For example, it was recently demonstrated that well-healed burn survivors can appropriately improve their aerobic capacity through an aggressive 6-month community-based exercise training regimen,[30] or after a supervised 12-week exercise training regimen.[43] Such a training regimen also improves blood pressure and ventilatory responses to exercise.[61,62] These findings strongly suggest that the primary etiology for a low VO2peak in well-healed burn survivors is likely related to reduced physical activity in this population, while bed rest associated with length of ICU stay in the acute phase of the injury may also contribute.[63] In summary, severe burn injuries can have a host of long-term consequences that impact a survivor's quality of life. Fatigue and muscle weakness are prevalent issues, while reduced aerobic capacity can lead to an increased risk of several health conditions and a greater reliance on dependent care. However, through an aggressive exercise training regimen, well-healed burn survivors can improve their aerobic capacity, potentially reducing their risk of developing further health complications.

### *Burn Injuries and Thermoregulation*

Proper regulation of body temperature during physical activity is an important factor that can influence exercise tolerance. High body temperatures place an additional demand on the cardiovascular system that culminates in an elevated cardiovascular strain and an accompanying increased perception of effort.[64] Furthermore, high internal/core or skin temperatures can decrease thermal comfort, which likely decreases one's willingness to engage in physical activity. Body temperature homeostasis is maintained via a balance between heat accumulation (from internal and/or external sources) and heat dissipation.[65] Consequently, core body temperature will increase if the rate of heat accumulation is greater than that of heat dissipation. Typically, heat stroke is associated with a core temperature of greater than 40 °C, yet core temperatures of only 38 °C (ie, a 1 °C elevation from rest) can induce a significant increase in heart rate and sweat loss, even in resting subjects.[66–68] Sweating and elevations in skin blood flow are the primary mechanisms by which humans dissipate heat. For example, for each 1 g of sweat that evaporates from the skin surface, ~2400 J of heat energy is removed from the body.[69] The physical process of evaporative cooling also reduces blood temperature at the skin surface, such that cooler blood returns to the body core from the skin. However, if these heat-dissipating responses are insufficient relative to heat gain from metabolism and the environment, core body temperature will continually rise during physical activity, reducing one's desire to perform that physical activity, and potentially culminating in heat stroke.

The capacity for grafted skin to increase skin blood flow and sweating during heat stress is effectively absent, with these limitations persisting throughout the individual's life.[70] Such responses result in excessive elevations in core body and skin temperatures during physical activity, the extent of which is dictated by the size of the area of burned versus non-injured skin.[63,71,72] Furthermore, a heightened perception of heat stress that accompanies these elevated core body and skin temperatures has been documented in burn survivors.[71] Consistent with these laboratory observations, 72% of burn survivors report "problems in hot temperature" ~17 years post-injury. It is important to note that the risk of overheating in burn survivors may be specific to activity in hot ambient environments. A previous study examined the core body temperature responses in burn survivors to 1-h moderate-intensity exercise in a hot (40 °C) and neutral (25 °C) environment and observed differing responses.[73] During exercise at 40 °C, the magnitude of the increase in core temperature was proportional with the size of the burn injury, and heart rate was ~25 b/min greater in those with burns greater than 40% body surface area. However, there were no differences in core temperature during exercise in the 25 °C environment between non-burned individuals and burn survivors, regardless of the size of their injuries. These findings demonstrate that it is safe for burn survivors to perform moderate-intensity exercise if the air temperature is ≤ 25 °C. It is also worth noting that the extent to which burn injuries increase core temperature during activity in the heat is dependent on the activity level/intensity.[74] At a low activity level of ~ 4 METS, there were no differences in core temperature at 60 min of exercise in the heat between control and high burn surface areas of 60%. However, at a moderate intensity of ~ 6 METS in the same heated condition, a burn size of 40% and 60% resulted in greater core temperatures compared with non-burned control individuals.

### Cooling Methods for Burn Survivors

Investigations have pursued several methods to help curtail excessive core temperature rises in burn survivors during physical activity in the heat. In non-burned subjects, physiological adaptation (acclimatization) to the heat occurs after 1 to 3 weeks of daily exposure to a hot environment.[75] The primary adaptation to heat acclimation is an increase in the sweating responses; that is, in heat acclimated subjects, sweating is activated at a lower core temperature threshold, sweat output is elevated for a given core temperature, maximum sweat output per gland is elevated, and the sweat becomes more dilute, such that less electrolytes are lost.[75–79] Interestingly, 7 days of heat acclimation induced favorable sweating adaptations in the non-injured skin of burn survivors (burn surface area ranging from 17% to 75%), such that core temperature and heart rate were significantly reduced during exercise in the heat after acclimation.[72] Importantly, sweating from grafted skin remained almost completely absent regardless of heat acclimation status, such that those with very high surface area burns (ie, approximately > 60%) may not realize the full benefits heat acclimation.

An effective and practical method to mitigate rises in core temperature in burn survivors may be to intermittently spritz the grafted skin with water using a spray bottle. Such water spray applied to grafted skin will replicate the effect of sweating, in that the water will evaporate from the skin surface and provide a cooling effect. In lab studies, water spray is typically applied every 5 minutes, or when the grafted skin is no longer wet. It is also beneficial to apply warm, instead of cold, water since warm water is generally better tolerated from a subjective perspective, and warm water will evaporate more efficiently from the skin surface compared with cold water. In environments at or below 33 °C air temperature, increasing the air speed with an electric fan can also have profound heat loss effects, especially if humidity is high.[80] Increasing the air speed increases convective heat loss while also improving the rate of sweat evaporation. In air temperatures above 33 °C, electric fans will have, at-best, a negligible effect on core temperature responses. However, in a similar manner to a convective oven, fans are likely to increase the core temperature if used in a hot environment (ie, $\geq$ 40 °C). Finally, wetted clothing also decreases physiological strain during heat exposure, though this observation has not be verified in burn survivors.[81]

### Application to Exercise Rehabilitation

The data presented above have important implications for rehabilitation practices post-burn injury. Overall, the greater incidence of mortality in burn survivors up to 30 years post-injury is largely due to low aerobic capacity secondary to a sedentary lifestyle, given that low aerobic capacity is linked to greater morbidity and mortality. Therefore, improving aerobic capacity with exercise training, as previously discussed, should improve health-related quality of life in burn survivors years after the injury. Importantly, similar benefits of a community based (ie, outpatient) exercise training program were reported in the pediatric population.[3,82] Finally, a combined aerobic and resistance exercise training program increased psychological domains on the burn-specific health scale, but only after 12-weeks training.[83] Overall, physical activity appears to be an important and beneficial aspect of rehabilitation in burn survivors.

### Knowledge Gaps in Thermoregulation

Currently, there is an absence of research investigating the impact of burn injury on core temperature in outdoor environments. The main difference outdoors is the potential for substantial additional heat gain from solar radiation.[84] While activity at low to moderate intensities is safe for burn survivors at 25 °C indoors, it is likely these thresholds will be reduced with direct sun exposure (ie, higher solar radiation). Moreover, further studies are required to determine how the interaction between different air temperatures and humidity may alter core temperature responses, that is, is exercise at 25 °C safe in burn survivors only at low to moderate humidity levels. If activity is undertaken outdoors in the sun, wearing white, loose-fitting clothing is the most effective method to reduce the effect of solar radiation on the thermal and cardiovascular strain. However, exercising indoors (ie, in a gym environment) should be initially recommended to avoid potential complications with high humidity and/or solar radiation. With regard to exercise training programs, more work is needed to determine to psychological benefits of training, since these responses are typically underreported in comparison to the physiological/functional benefits. Finally, studies are needed to determine if regular physical activity negates the epidemiological reports of increased morbidity and mortality in burn survivors decades following the initial injury. To date, no studies have evaluated the potential benefit of consistent physical activity on morbidity and/or mortality risks in burn survivors.

## The Role of Exercise Movement in Scarring and Contractures

Following a burn, scars and contractures can limit motion, be a source of pain and itch, create dissatisfaction with appearance, and negatively impact quality of life.[85,86] Scarring is one of the most problematic sequelae for burn survivors, with 55% of survivors more than 10 years post injury reporting continued difficulty.[87,88] Conservative, non-invasive strategies for managing burn scars include massage, splinting and positioning, stretching, and exercise/mobilization.[39,40,89] Although rehabilitation regimens may include movement (passive and active), strength training, and aerobic workouts to build endurance, improve lean body mass, and improve range of motion,[40] the influence of exercise on scar-related outcomes is rarely evaluated.[39,90–94] The few studies reporting scarring-related outcomes, however, suggest that exercise programs can reduce scar severity and the need for subsequent surgical interventions.[13,95,96] The need for scar release surgeries was reduced in pediatric burn survivors participating in a 12- week supervised, in-hospital exercise program with concurrent physical and occupational therapy compared to a cohort that did not exercise.[96] Similarly, comparison of pediatric burn survivors participating in an intensive physical exercise program to those who did not revealed that although the severity of initial injuries were comparable, exercise was associated with an approximate 60% reduction in contracture releasing surgeries.[96] In a study comparing conventional scar management to exercise and physiotherapy in adult burn survivors, range of motion improved and severity of post burn hypertrophic scarring was reduced with exercise.[95]

## Knowledge Gaps in Exercise-Induced Effects on Contractures

Scar development and maturation are modulated by myriad factors, including mechano-physiological conditions, the presence of contractile myofibroblasts, and the influence of inflammatory cells and molecules.[97] Throughout the rehabilitative period, a combination of reconstructive surgeries, laser resurfacing, silicone sheets, and/or compression garments may be used to decrease tension within the wound/scar, reduce perfusion and vascularization, and control inflammation, thereby improving wound healing and decreasing scar formation.[97] Early movement, stretching, and exercise (resistance and aerobic) likely influence these processes as well, although the mechanisms underlying the improvement in scarring outcomes with exercise are unknown. In light of these findings, the need for additional well-designed studies designed to elucidate the effects of resistance and aerobic exercise on scar severity, range of motion, social participation and reintegration, and patient quality of life in larger groups of burn survivors is warranted. Studies that link the effects of exercise at the molecular or cellular level with whole-body physiology or function would advance the field by allowing the identification of pharmacologic targets or biomarkers of recovery. In addition, the determination of the mechanisms underlying the positive effects of exercise on burn recovery and rehabilitation is an unmet need.

## FUTURE DIRECTIONS

The benefits of exercise for the burn survivor are numerous, but should be extended beyond current knowledge, especially with respect to determining underlying mechanisms. With improvements in clinical care over the past 50 years,[87] more patients now survive burns, necessitating increased focus on ameliorating long-term function and quality of life (QoL).[98] Large longitudinal studies revealed poorer long-term outcomes for burn survivors compared to age-matched non-burn cohorts, including significant increases in morbidity and mortality beginning as soon as a year after injury and continuing for decades.[21,45,46,98–101] Incidence of long-term organ damage (eg, musculoskeletal, cardiac)[45,46,102] and mortality (all-cause,[45,46,102] disease-specific,[21] and premature[103]) increases while QoL remains poor.[98] In comparison to the general US population, adult burn survivors are disproportionately less fit.[104] Survivors 3–30 years after injury continue to report weak hands, arms, legs, and feet, and difficulty walking or running.[104] Survivors engage in infrequent exercise (eg, walking one time per week or less), and compliance with stretching and strengthening programs is low.[104] Finally, there is evidence that nutritional and exercise strategies benefit pediatric and young adult burn survivors.[105] Thus, a multidisciplinary approach or study to incorporate wellness strategies and lifestyle changes may improve long-term outcomes and QoL for the burn survivor. Such studies should be sought.

## CLINICS CARE POINTS

---

- Participation in an exercise training program as an outpatient with severe burns is beneficial in counteracting burn-induced effects.

- Exercising indoor is recommended to avoid excessive strain on the thermoregulatory and cardiovascular system.

- In the heat an effective and practical method to mitigate rises in core temperature in burn survivors may be to intermittently spritz the grafted skin with lukewarm (not cold, not hot) water using a spray bottle.

- Participation in an exercise program alongside physical/occupational therapy may reduce the need for subsequent surgeries.

- Scar severity may be reduced as a result of participating in an exercise program.

---

## DISCLOSURE

The authors have no relationship with a commercial company that has a direct financial interest in the subject matter or materials discussed in this article or with a company making a competing product

## FUNDING

NIH: R01GM068865; R01 HD049471; P50 GM060338DOD: W81XWH-15-1-0647; W81XWH-14-2-0160; W81XWH-09-2-0194.

## REFERENCES

1. Cucuzzo NA, Ferrando A, Herndon DN. The effects of exercise programming vs traditional outpatient therapy in the rehabilitation of severely burned children. J Burn Care Rehabil 2001;22(3):214–20.

2. Suman OE, Herndon DN. Effects of cessation of a structured and supervised exercise conditioning program on lean mass and muscle strength in severely burned children. Arch Phys Med Rehabil 2007;88(12 Suppl):S24–9.

3. Suman OE, et al. Effects of a 12-wk resistance exercise program on skeletal muscle strength in children with burn injuries. J Appl Physiol 2001;91(3): 1168–75.

4. Ishizaki Y, et al. Psychological effects of bed rest in young healthy subjects. Acta Physiol Scand Suppl 1994;616:83–7.
5. Convertino VA, et al. Cardiorespiratory responses to exercise after bed rest in men and women. Acta Astronaut 1977;4(7–8):895–905.
6. Dirks ML, et al. One Week of Bed Rest Leads to Substantial Muscle Atrophy and Induces Whole-Body Insulin Resistance in the Absence of Skeletal Muscle Lipid Accumulation. Diabetes 2016;65(10):2862–75.
7. Buehlmeier J, et al. Markers of bone metabolism during 14 days of bed rest in young and older men. J Musculoskelet Neuronal Interact 2017;17(1):399–408.
8. Schweickert WD, et al. Early physical and occupational therapy in mechanically ventilated, critically ill patients: a randomised controlled trial. Lancet 2009; 373(9678):1874–82.
9. Stiller K. Safety issues that should be considered when mobilizing critically ill patients. Crit Care Clin 2007;23(1):35–53.
10. Diego AM, et al. Exercise training after burn injury: a survey of practice. J Burn Care Res 2013;34(6):e311–7.
11. Porter C, et al. The role of exercise in the rehabilitation of patients with severe burns. Exerc Sport Sci Rev 2015;43(1):34–40.
12. Hardee JP, et al. Early rehabilitative exercise training in the recovery from pediatric burn. Med Sci Sports Exerc 2014;46(9):1710–6.
13. Celis MM, et al. Effect of a supervised exercise and physiotherapy program on surgical interventions in children with thermal injury. J Burn Care Rehabil 2003; 24(1):57–61, discussion 56.
14. Rivas E, et al. Short-term Metformin and Exercise Training Effects on Strength, Aerobic Capacity, Glycemic Control, and Mitochondrial Function in Children with Burn Injury. Am J Physiol Endocrinol Metab 2017;314(3):E232–40.
15. Harden NG, Luster SH. Rehabilitation considerations in the care of the acute burn patient. Crit Care Nurs Clin North Am 1991;3(2):245–53.
16. Richard R, Staley M. Burn care and rehabilitation : principles and practice. Philadelphia: F.A. Davis. xxviii; 1994. p. 711.
17. Jeschke MG, et al. Long-term persistance of the pathophysiologic response to severe burn injury. PLoS One 2011;6(7):e21245.
18. Williams FN, et al. Changes in cardiac physiology after severe burn injury. J Burn Care Res 2011;32(2):269–74.
19. Gauglitz GG, et al. Abnormal insulin sensitivity persists up to three years in pediatric patients post-burn. J Clin Endocrinol Metab 2009;94(5):1656–64.
20. Herndon DN, et al. Long-term propranolol use in severely burned pediatric patients: a randomized controlled study. Ann Surg 2012;256(3):402–11.
21. Duke JM, et al. Understanding the long-term impacts of burn on the cardiovascular system. Burns 2016;42(2):366–74.
22. Chao T, et al. Skeletal Muscle Protein Breakdown Remains Elevated in Pediatric Burn Survivors up to One-Year Post-Injury. Shock 2015;44(5):397–401.
23. Chang DW, DeSanti L, Demling RH. Anticatabolic and anabolic strategies in critical illness: a review of current treatment modalities. Shock 1998;10(3):155–60.
24. Suman OE, Mlcak RP, Herndon DN. Effect of exercise training on pulmonary function in children with thermal injury. J Burn Care Rehabil 2002;23(4): 288–93, discussion 287.
25. Clayton RP, et al. Effects of different duration exercise programs in children with severe burns. Burns 2016;43(4):796–803.
26. Wurzer P, et al. Long-term effects of physical exercise during rehabilitation in patients with severe burns. Surgery 2016;160(3):781–8.

27. Przkora R, Herndon DN, Suman OE. The effects of oxandrolone and exercise on muscle mass and function in children with severe burns. Pediatrics 2007;119(1): e109–16.

28. Suman OE, et al. Effect of exogenous growth hormone and exercise on lean mass and muscle function in children with burns. J Appl Physiol 2003;94(6): 2273–81.

29. Rivas E, et al. Quantification of an Exercise Rehabilitation Program for Severely Burned Children: The Standard of Care at Shriners Hospitals for Children(R)-Galveston. J Burn Care Res 2018;39(6):889–96.

30. Romero SA, et al. Progressive exercise training improves maximal aerobic capacity in individuals with well-healed burn injuries. Am J Physiol Regul Integr Comp Physiol 2019;317(4):R563–70.

31. Rivas E, et al. Burn Injury May Have Age-Dependent Effects on Strength and Aerobic Exercise Capacity in Males. J Burn Care Res 2018;39(5):815–22.

32. Al-Mousawi AM, et al. Effects of exercise training on resting energy expenditure and lean mass during pediatric burn rehabilitation. J Burn Care Res 2010;31(3): 400–8.

33. Wilmore DW, et al. Catecholamines: mediator of the hypermetabolic response to thermal injury. Ann Surg 1974;180(4):653–69.

34. American College of Sports Medicine, et al. ACSM's guidelines for exercise testing and prescription. 11th edition. Philadelphia: Wolters Kluwer; 2021.

35. Ganio MS, et al. Aerobic Fitness Is Disproportionately Low in Adult Burn Survivors Years After Injury. J Burn Care Res 2015;36(4):513–9.

36. Cambiaso-Daniel J, et al. Cardiorespiratory Capacity and Strength Remain Attenuated in Children with Severe Burn Injuries at Over 3 Years Postburn. J Pediatr 2018;192:152–8.

37. Rosenberg M, et al. Effects of a hospital based Wellness and Exercise program on quality of life of children with severe burns. Burns 2013;39(4):599–609.

38. Ebid AA, Omar MT, Abd El Baky AM. Effect of 12-week isokinetic training on muscle strength in adult with healed thermal burn. Burns 2012;38(1):61–8.

39. Van den Kerckhove EAM. Compression Therapy and Conservative Strategies in Scar Management After Burn Injury. In: Teot MT, Middelkoop E, Gauglitz GG, editors. Textbook on scar management: state of the art management and emerging technologies. 2020. p. 227–31.

40. Jacobson K, et al. Current Concepts Burn Rehabilitation, Part I: Care During Hospitalization. Clin Plast Surg 2017;44(4):703–12.

41. Grisbrook TL, et al. The effect of exercise training on pulmonary function and aerobic capacity in adults with burn. Burns 2012;38(4):607–13.

42. Grisbrook TL, et al. Burn-injured adults with long term functional impairments demonstrate the same response to resistance training as uninjured controls. Burns 2013;39(4):680–6.

43. Grisbrook TL, et al. Exercise training to improve health related quality of life in long term survivors of major burn injury: a matched controlled study. Burns 2012;38(8):1165–73.

44. Palackic A, et al. Rehabilitative Exercise Training for Burn Injury. Sports Med 2021;51(12):2469–82.

45. Duke JM, et al. Long-term mortality among older adults with burn injury: a population-based study in Australia. Bull World Health Organ 2015;93(6):400–6.

46. Duke JM, et al. Mortality after burn injury in children: a 33-year population-based study. Pediatrics 2015;135(4):e903–10.

47. Hung T-Y, et al. Increased risk of ischemic stroke in patients with burn injury: a nationwide cohort study in Taiwan. Scand J Trauma Resuscitation Emerg Med 2016;24(1):1–8.
48. Ben-Simchon C, et al. Heat tolerance in patients with extensive healed burns. Plast Reconstr Surg 1981;67(4):499–504.
49. Dyster-Aas J, Kildal M, Willebrand M. Return to work and health-related quality of life after burn injury. J Rehabil Med 2007;39(1):49–55.
50. Holavanahalli RK, Helm PA, Kowalske KJ. Long-term outcomes in patients surviving large burns: the skin. J Burn Care Res 2010;31(4):631–9.
51. Klein MB, et al. Functional and psychosocial outcomes of older adults after burn injury: results from a multicenter database of severe burn injury. J Burn Care Res 2011;32(1):66–78.
52. Roskind JL, et al. Quantitation of thermoregulatory impairment in patients with healed burns. Ann Plast Surg 1978;1(2):172–6.
53. Shapiro Y, et al. Thermoregulatory responses of patients with extensive healed burns. J Appl Physiol 1982;53(4):1019–22.
54. Holavanahalli R, Kowalske K, Helm P. Long-term neuro-musculoskeletal outcomes in patients surviving severe burns. J Burn Care Res 2009;30:S109.
55. Fletcher GF, et al. Exercise standards for testing and training: a statement for healthcare professionals from the American Heart Association. Circulation 2001;104(14):1694–740.
56. Aspenes ST, et al. Peak oxygen uptake and cardiovascular risk factors in 4631 healthy women and men. Med Sci Sports Exerc 2011;43(8):1465–73.
57. Blair SN, et al. Physical fitness and all-cause mortality: a prospective study of healthy men and women. JAMA 1989;262(17):2395–401.
58. Erikssen G, et al. Changes in physical fitness and changes in mortality. Lancet 1998;352(9130):759–62.
59. Peters RK, et al. Physical fitness and subsequent myocardial infarction in healthy workers. JAMA 1983;249(22):3052–6.
60. Sandvik L, et al. Physical fitness as a predictor of mortality among healthy, middle-aged Norwegian men. N Engl J Med 1993;328(8):533–7.
61. Watso JC, et al. Six Months of Exercise Training Improves Ventilatory Responses During Exercise in Adults with Well-healed Burn Injuries. Med Sci Sports Exerc 2022;55(5):765–76.
62. Watso JC, et al. Six months of unsupervised exercise training lowers blood pressure during moderate, but not vigorous, aerobic exercise in adults with well-healed burn injuries. J Appl Physiol 2022;133(3):742–54.
63. Perhonen MA, et al. Cardiac atrophy after bed rest and spaceflight. Journal of applied physiology 2001;91(2):645–53.
64. Nybo L, Rasmussen P, Sawka MN. Performance in the heat-physiological factors of importance for hyperthermia-induced fatigue. Compr Physiol 2014; 4(2):657–89.
65. Cramer MN, Gagnon D, Laitano O, et al. Human temperature regulation under heat stress in health, disease, and injury. Physiol Rev 2022;102(4):1907–89.
66. Lucas RA, et al. Skin cooling aids cerebrovascular function more effectively under severe than moderate heat stress. Eur J Appl Physiol 2010;109(1):101–8.
67. Lucas RA, et al. The effects of ageing and passive heating on cardiorespiratory and cerebrovascular responses to orthostatic stress in humans. Exp Physiol 2008;93(10):1104–17.
68. Lucas RA, et al. Age-related changes to cardiac systolic and diastolic function during whole-body passive hyperthermia. Exp Physiol 2015;100(4):422–34.

69. Cramer MN, Jay O. Biophysical aspects of human thermoregulation during heat stress. Auton Neurosci 2016;196:3–13.
70. Crandall CG, Davis SL. Cutaneous vascular and sudomotor responses in human skin grafts. J Appl Physiol 2010;109(5):1524–30.
71. Ganio MS, et al. Nongrafted skin area best predicts exercise core temperature responses in burned humans. Med Sci Sports Exerc 2015;47(10):2224.
72. Schlader ZJ, et al. Heat acclimation improves heat exercise tolerance and heat dissipation in individuals with extensive skin grafts. J Appl Physiol 2015;119(1): 69–76.
73. Cramer MN, et al. Exercise Thermoregulation with a Simulated Burn Injury: Impact of Air Temperature. Med Sci Sports Exerc 2020;52(3):712–9.
74. Belval LN, et al. Interaction of Exercise Intensity and Simulated Burn Injury Size on Thermoregulation. Med Sci Sports Exerc 2021;53(2):367–74.
75. Foster J, et al. Individual Responses to Heat Stress: Implications for Hyperthermia and Physical Work Capacity. Front Physiol 2020;11:541483.
76. Armstrong CG, Kenney WL. Effects of age and acclimation on responses to passive heat exposure. J Appl Physiol 1993;75(5):2162–7.
77. Gibson OR, et al. Isothermic and fixed intensity heat acclimation methods induce similar heat adaptation following short and long-term timescales. J Therm Biol 2015;49-50:55–65.
78. Havenith G. Individualized model of human thermoregulation for the simulation of heat stress response. J Appl Physiol 2001;90(5):1943–54.
79. Inoue Y, et al. Exercise- and methylcholine-induced sweating responses in older and younger men: effect of heat acclimation and aerobic fitness. Int J Biometeorol 1999;42(4):210–6.
80. Foster J, et al. Quantifying the impact of heat on human physical work capacity; part II: the observed interaction of air velocity with temperature, humidity, sweat rate, and clothing is not captured by most heat stress indices. Int J Biometeorol 2022;66(3):507–20.
81. Cramer M, et al. Keeping older individuals cool in hot and moderately humid conditions: wetted clothing with and without an electric fan. J Appl Physiol 2020;128(1):604–11.
82. Peña R, et al. Effects of community-based exercise in children with severe burns: a randomized trial. Burns 2016;42(1):41–7.
83. Paratz JD, et al. Intensive exercise after thermal injury improves physical, functional, and psychological outcomes. J Trauma Acute Care Surg 2012;73(1): 186–94.
84. Foster J, et al. Quantifying the impact of heat on human physical work capacity; part III: the impact of solar radiation varies with air temperature, humidity, and clothing coverage. Int J Biometeorol 2022;66(1):175–88.
85. Goverman J, et al. Satisfaction with life after burn: A Burn Model System National Database Study. Burns 2016;42(5):1067–73.
86. Wurzer P, et al. Two-year follow-up of outcomes related to scarring and distress in children with severe burns. Disabil Rehabil 2017;39(16):1639–43.
87. Finnerty CC, et al. Hypertrophic scarring: the greatest unmet challenge after burn injury. Lancet 2016;388(10052):1427–36.
88. Survivors TPSfB. State of the Survivor. 2022; Available from: https://resources. phoenix-society.org/hubfs/Phoenix%20Society%20for%20Burn%20Survivors% 20-%20State%20of%20the%20Survivor%20Report.pdf?hsCtaTracking=e883ff06- 189d-4241-b812-8db2a9d4b541%7C2c38431b-b2a4-4599-92a7-027dda49f988.

89. Dodd H, et al. Current Concepts Burn Rehabilitation, Part II: Long-Term Recovery. Clin Plast Surg 2017;44(4):713–28.
90. Anthonissen M, et al. The effects of conservative treatments on burn scars: A systematic review. Burns 2016;42(3):508–18.
91. Bayuo J, Wong FKY. Intervention Content and Outcomes of Postdischarge Rehabilitation Programs for Adults Surviving Major Burns: A Systematic Scoping Review. J Burn Care Res 2021;42(4):651–710.
92. Godleski M, et al. Treating burn-associated joint contracture: results of an inpatient rehabilitation stretching protocol. J Burn Care Res 2013;34(4):420–6.
93. Richard R, et al. Burn rehabilitation and research: proceedings of a consensus summit. J Burn Care Res 2009;30(4):543–73.
94. Young AW, Dewey WS, King BT. Rehabilitation of Burn Injuries: An Update. Phys Med Rehabil Clin N Am 2019;30(1):111–32.
95. Karimi H, Mobayen M, Alijanpour A. Management of Hypertrophic Burn Scar: A Comparison between the Efficacy of Exercise-Physiotherapy and Pressure Garment-Silicone on Hypertrophic Scar. Asian J Sports Med 2013;4(1):70–5.
96. Lee JO, et al. Effect of Exercise Training on the Frequency of Contracture-Release Surgeries in Burned Children. Ann Plast Surg 2017;79(4):346–9.
97. Mony MP, et al. An Updated Review of Hypertrophic Scarring. Cells 2023; 12(5):678.
98. Haug VF, et al. Long-term sequelae of critical illness in sepsis, trauma and burns: A systematic review and meta-analysis. J Trauma Acute Care Surg 2021;91(4):736–47.
99. Duke JM, et al. Long-term Effects of Pediatric Burns on the Circulatory System. Pediatrics 2015;136(5):e1323–30.
100. Duke JM, et al. Long term cardiovascular impacts after burn and non-burn trauma: A comparative population-based study. Burns 2017;43(8):1662–72.
101. Hundeshagen G, et al. Long-term effect of critical illness after severe paediatric burn injury on cardiac function in adolescent survivors: an observational study. Lancet Child Adolesc Health 2017;1(4):293–301.
102. Duke JM, et al. Long term mortality in a population-based cohort of adolescents, and young and middle-aged adults with burn injury in Western Australia: A 33-year study. Accid Anal Prev 2015;85:118–24.
103. Firchal EW, et al. Long-term survival among elderly after burns compared with national mean remaining life expectancy. Burns 2021;47(6):1252–8.
104. Holavanahalli RK, Helm PA, Kowalske KJ. Long-Term Outcomes in Patients Surviving Large Burns: The Musculoskeletal System. J Burn Care Res 2016;37(4): 243–54.
105. Finnerty CC, et al. The P50 Research Center in Perioperative Sciences: How the investment by the National Institute of General Medical Sciences in team science has reduced postburn mortality. J Trauma Acute Care Surg 2017;83(3): 532–42.

# Special Considerations for Pediatric Burn Injuries

Miranda Yelvington, MS, OTR/L, BT-C[a],*,
Christopher Whitehead, PT[b], Lori Turgeon, PT, DPT[c]

## KEYWORDS

- Pediatric • Burns • Developmental • Children • Family-centered care
- Community reintegration • School re-entry • Skeletal maturity

## KEY POINTS

- Physiological, developmental, and psychosocial differences exist between pediatric and adult burn survivors. While there are similarities in treatment methods, special considerations must be considered for children with burns.
- Severe burn injuries can result in deficits in strength and endurance, regression in fine and gross motor skills, and cognitive changes in young burn survivors.
- Children require engagement and distraction techniques to combat the fear of pain and movement, which may limit burn rehabilitation. This can be mitigated by the incorporation of caregivers through a family-centered care model.
- Directed purposeful play can be used as a therapeutic tool for ADL and functional mobility rehabilitation and should consider the developmental stage of the child.
- Developmentally appropriate physical, psychological, and community-based reintegration is critical in the long-term success of the child both in the acute phase and throughout their lifetime.

## INTRODUCTION

Burns are the fifth leading cause of non-fatal childhood injuries.[1] Children account for more than 41% of all scald burns, most sustained between the ages of one and two years.[2–4] For children over the age of five, flame burns are the most common cause of injury.[2] Risk factors, including living in a single-parent home, young maternal age, lower maternal education level, preexisting mental health diagnoses in the patient or caregiver, immigration status and lower socioeconomic status have been identified as contributing to increased burn risk in pediatrics.[5,6] The child's developmental level can also impact risk. Advanced gross motor skills in children under 2 years of age and coordination difficulties in older children create a greater risk of burn injury.[6]

[a] Arkansas Children's Hospital, 1 Children's Way, Slot 104, Little Rock, AR 72202, USA; [b] Shriners Children's Texas, 815 Market Street, Galveston, TX 77550, USA; [c] Shriners Children's Boston, 51 Blossom Street, Boston, MA 02114, USA
* Corresponding author.
*E-mail address:* yelvingtonml@archildrens.org

Phys Med Rehabil Clin N Am 34 (2023) 825–837
https://doi.org/10.1016/j.pmr.2023.05.004

The assertion that children are not just small adults certainly holds true in pediatric burn rehabilitation, which must consider the physiological differences in the skin and body morphology. Body size can vary considerably from birth to adulthood, with significant morphological changes. Children have a greater body surface area compared to their weight and experience significant changes in proportions as they grow.[7] These changes make the standard "Rule of Nines" assessment of body surface area inaccurate for patients under the age of 14. In children, the body surface area is greater in the head and neck and smaller in the extremities when compared to adults.[8] Pediatric Lund and Browder charts were designed to assess body surface area more accurately, considering the changes in proportions that occur from birth to physical maturation.[9] Additionally, the epidermis is thinner in children than in adults, making them more susceptible to burn injury.[10]

### Developmental Considerations

Successful rehabilitation of pediatric patients with burn injuries requires attention to the medical concerns inherent in all burn injuries. Additionally, it must consider the developmental stage of the child, any preexisting or emerging developmental delays or associated conditions, and the impact of scaring on growth and skill attainment. Children progress through developmental milestones in the first 5 years of life.[11] Successful attainment of these milestones impacts lifelong fine and gross motor functioning, cognitive development, socialization, and communication.

In the first 2 years of life, children develop prehension patterns which continue to be refined through fine motor development.[12] Transitional and gross motor skills such as sitting, pulling to stand, crawling, and walking are often delayed or regressed in hospitalized children whose medical status prevents normal environmental exploration. The ability to walk generally emerges at twelve to 14 months of age, with immature gait patterns continuing until around the age of three when heel-toe gait pattern develops. Gait continues progressing in speed and cadence until age seven.[13] Burn injury-related gait and mobility restrictions may limit a child's ability to explore and interact with their environment.

For children with severe burns, medically required equipment such as ventilators, critical monitoring devices, medical lines, and procedures such as skin grafting can necessitate periods of sedation and immobilization. In children with no preexisting developmental concerns, resulting deficits in physical strength and endurance, regression in fine and gross motor skills, and cognitive changes may be seen in the post-acute stages of burn recovery.

Even years beyond the injury, the maturation of grasping and fine motor skills and the progression of gross motor abilities can be hindered by burn-related scar contractures. The severity of these contractures and deficits have been associated with the burn injury's size and severity, the child's age, and overall hospital length of stay.[14–16]

Preexisting physical or psychosocial diagnoses can further complicate pediatric burn recovery. More than 30% of children who sustain burn injuries experienced neurodevelopmental concerns before their burn.[17] For these children, functional recovery following their injury presents even greater challenges. These children may require adaptations in care delivery and may have more difficulty with treatment adherence, resulting in worsened recovery outcomes.[17] It can often be difficult to differentiate behaviors relating to preexisting conditions from burn-related pain and anxiety behaviors, complicating burn treatments, pain control, and rehabilitation.

Therapists treating pediatric burn survivors should utilize developmental surveillance tools and testing to ensure children meet milestone targets.[18] Children should be given every opportunity to be exposed to normal developmental stimuli and play to facilitate the progression of developmental milestones, even in the presence of severe burn injuries.

### Play and Purposeful Activity

Kinesiophobia is an excessive, irrational, and debilitating fear of physical movement and activity due to the feeling of vulnerability to pain.[19] Kinesiophobia has been found when burn-related pain develops into fear and avoidance behaviors, increasing pain perception and reducing treatment compliance.[20,21] While still developing cognitively, children may display decreased coping with pain and anxiety and have a limited understanding of the benefits of rehabilitation.[22]

Engaging and distracting children can be a powerful force to combat the fear of movement. In pediatric burn rehabilitation, the use of purposeful activity and play has been shown to decrease pain and increase active range of motion, grip strength, function, and enjoyment during treatment sessions.[22–27]

### Scar Management

Scar management interventions in children follow much the same trajectory as with adults, beginning with an assessment of burn wound depth and size, any preexisting scars, and family characteristics of skin maturation.[28–30] Pediatric skin physiology results in a risk for deeper injuries which increases the risk of developing thick, raised, contractile scars that can limit mobility.[31] Additionally, any personal or family history of hypertrophic or keloid scarring, with prolonged wound closure of equal to or greater than 14 to 21 days, can affect scar development.[32,33] Areas most impacted by scar contracture include the shoulder, elbow, wrist, hand, knees and ankles.[16,28] Itch is also a complicated issue for children, presenting with a wide range of severity.

Traditional scar and itch management interventions are applicable in pediatrics; however, therapists must be creative in their execution. These include deep soft tissue massage with moisturizing emollients, compression wraps and garments, and adjunctive materials such as foam padding, silicone, and custom splinting.[33,34] Early intervention is also important; however, given the increased sensitivity to touch experienced by patients, therapists can encounter challenges engaging children in massage. Gentle initiation of touch and desensitization are helpful, beginning immediately after wound closure or graft adherence and progressing to deeper tissue compression as tolerated.[34] Encouraging age-appropriate participation and engaging caregivers in this process will also increase success.

Despite mixed evidence of efficacy, pressure garments remain a first-line agent in scar management.[32,35,36] Patients still follow a progression from non-sheering to sheering or custom garments, with the assessment and adjustment of garments for revisions or total re-fabrication every few months to ensure fit.[32] Education of care providers on optimal response to compression, such as localized tissue hypoxia and softening of scar, versus inappropriate, such as blistering and open wounds, is fundamental.[35]

Special consideration is needed for the toddler and preschool age groups when initiating compression garments. These children are developing mastery of independent skills, including dressing and toileting. Adding compression clothing is often a significant barrier to achieving these milestones. Younger children will have difficulty helping don garments, resulting in significant challenges fitting tight gloves, socks, pants, and sleeves without causing stress or discomfort. Creatively using zipper and Velcro closures, button or Velcro diaper straps, front fly flap pants, and suspenders are all options to improve patient independence with garments as they develop autonomy. Utilizing interim materials can improve tolerance in the early stages.

Additionally, younger children's body shapes can create a challenge in achieving the proper fit of garments with equal pressure in all areas. Developing creativity with adjunctive materials, including inserts to optimize compression, can aid therapists in achieving desired outcomes and increase tolerance and compliance. Insert materials include foam padding, silicone gels and sheeting, moldable putty, thin, flexible splint material, and padded strapping.[33,34] Imaginative use of these materials in web spaces of the hands and feet, palmar surface of the hand, and natural concavities of the torso and face can improve compression conformity for the management of scars. However, closely monitoring skin response to these adjunctive materials is important, as children will be more prone to skin irritation and rashes with non-porous materials.[34,35]

Injuries to the face present a unique challenge due to their high visibility, dynamic facial movements, and the limited ability of children to understand and tolerate pressure on the face. Special focus on age-appropriate education and engaging children in their recovery will optimize compliance with recommendations. Though custom clear facemasks are the ideal solution to pressure and cosmetic challenges, they can be cost-prohibitive. Creatively using silicone gels, thin moldable splint materials, custom fabric masks, and various inserts can also promote optimal outcomes.[33,35] With adolescents, using special cosmetics during the day may be a preferred option. However, education should be provided on the impact of decreased use of compression materials on the long-term outcome of scars.

Basic sun protection is also critical in managing the cosmetic outcomes of maturing skin. During the maturation phase, skin can be highly susceptible to ultraviolet light, causing permanent changes in pigmentation.[34] Sun protection factor lotions, sun protective clothing, and hats can facilitate optimal scar cosmesis.

### Burn Orthoses

Burn orthoses are used for many reasons, including supporting or immobilizing joints, increasing range of motion and movement, or protecting grafted areas. In healing burn wounds, orthoses elongate healing tissue and work against the contraction of wounds.[37] The desired purpose of each device determines the type and design of the orthoses.

A burn expert consensus report recommends individualizing devices to meet each patient's specific needs.[38] In addition to adhering to basic principles of burn splinting and positioning, pediatric orthoses must consider the more fragile skin and more prominent pressure points that may present in children.[37] Securement of an orthosis can be challenging with children and may require larger or longer devices, additional strapping material or coverings to prevent the child from removing a needed device.[39] Pediatric patients require closer monitoring to ensure each orthosis continues to provide appropriate fit and function, especially during periods of rapid growth.[38]

### Activities of Daily Living

For the youngest patients, activities of daily living (ADL) are often play and school-based skills, which facilitate the attainment of developmental milestones. As the child grows, ADL requirements evolve to include self-care and higher levels of motoric demand. Associations have been found between movement recovery and the size of the burn injury, burn depth, and hospital length of stay.[14,15] Loss of ability to perform ADLs can be linked to the range of motion losses. Adult-based studies have quantified range of motion necessary to complete ADL tasks. While it is important to consider the small but significant age-related differences in the range of motion values, these studies can be used as guidelines for goal setting in relation to ADLs.[40,41]

In addition to physical challenges, psychosocial maturation may also impact ADL performance. Pediatric burn survivors show statistically worse psychosocial health and school functioning than a normative sample. They may exhibit more challenges with conduct, hyperactivity, socialization, and emotional regulation than their non-burned peers.[42] Following a burn injury, children may often participate in more informal play and socialization activities than structured tasks. Formal and structured activities such as team sports or extracurricular play are important parts of growth and development and should be encouraged as part of the return to normal ADL performance and can help children establish coping and social skills.[43]

In children who are burned at a young age, ADL limitations may present well after the burn has matured. Normal growth requires recruitment and stretching of skin, which may be hindered by the presence of burn scars. Caregivers of children with burns should be educated to recognize when burns scars are causing difficulty with performing age-appropriate ADL tasks. Pediatric patients should be followed throughout their developmental stages by burn professionals who recognize signs that burn-related sequelae are hindering age-appropriate attainment of ADL skills.

### Therapeutic Exercise, Mobility, and Gait

Children admitted to an intensive care unit (ICU) may develop multiple adverse effects, including ICU-acquired weakness, muscle loss, delirium, and fatigue.[44] Significant muscle loss associated with immobility commences within 48 hours and is greatest from initial injury to the first 3 weeks of admission, with long-lasting effects.[45] Burn-related complications include kinesiophobia, hypermetabolism, and long-lasting development.[46]

A comprehensive rehabilitation program, including exercise and early mobility, is necessary to combat the harmful effects of a severe burn injury. Rehabilitation begins immediately after admission and continues throughout recovery and long after the patient returns home. Active exercises are recommended to maintain range of motion (ROM) and combat muscle wasting; however, cognitive development, medical status, sedation, pain, and kinesiophobia can all hinder active movement in pediatric burn survivors. In instances where active movement is not achievable, active-assistive and passive ROM provide lessening strengthening benefits but can prevent loss of ROM. Isometric and resistive exercises can be incorporated as tolerated.[47]

Exercise programs should be curated to address impairments and limitations and coupled with functional activities to progress toward pre-burn activity levels. A stretching program, including low-load prolonged stretches, can combat the effects of decreased ROM, which may result from scar tissue formation.[48,49] Components of an early mobilization program, including bed mobility, sitting at the edge of the bed, transferring to a bedside chair, weight-bearing in sitting and standing, and ambulation, can be performed with minimal adverse effects.[44,50] A tilt table or stander may be used to mobilize pediatric patients who cannot stand due to strength limitations or medical status or for those limited by pain and anxiety.[47] Rehabilitation incorporating weight-bearing and active movement can progress toward independent mobility and ambulation as the patient recovers.

Mobility and gait should be continually assessed throughout recovery. Common gait abnormalities after a burn injury include decreased hip extension at terminal stance, decreased knee extension throughout stance, and decreased dorsiflexion in late stance.[51] Pediatric burn patients have also demonstrated decreases in stride length, step length, cadence, and velocity compared to non-burned children.[46,52] A wide base of support, gait asymmetry, and decreased stance time on affected limbs have also been noted in patients with lower extremity burns.[53] Continual refinement of gait patterns is essential to prevent long-term compensatory strategies and accommodations. Children may have more difficulty following verbal cueing to correct deviations and often require more tactile cueing and correction. As a child becomes more independent, more challenging environments can be introduced, including stairs, curbs, ramps, and other uneven surfaces, preparing the patients for return to home, school, and the community.

In the outpatient phase, aerobic conditioning, strength training, and interval training significantly benefit pediatric burn patients. Improvements in functional outcomes, mobility, aerobic capacity, lean body mass, strength, and pulmonary function have all been documented.[52,54–56]

### Prosthetic Training

In burn-related amputations, maximizing limb length may be complicated by poor vascularity and tissue quality in the surrounding area. The use of skin grafting or flaps to provide adequate coverage of the residual limb can cause poor healing, hypertrophic scarring, and increased time to successfully fit prosthetics.[57–59] Optimizing durability, limb length, and scarring is critical to successful prosthetic socket fitting, training, and long-term use by the pediatric patient.[57–59] Expected growth should be considered when planning for prosthetic use at skeletal maturity.[60] Working with a prosthetist familiar with the challenges associated with burn reconstruction can be beneficial to identifying prosthetic components with low-sheering suspension and even-pressure distribution to promote optimal fit and tolerance. Additionally, patients with amputations resulting from burns are not immune to experiencing phantom limb sensation, neuromas, and pain. Management of these symptoms, especially in pediatrics, can subsequently be a challenge and overall barrier to a patient's therapeutic progress.[60]

Therapeutic interventions follow the established course of early mobility and strengthening, compression wrapping to shape residual limbs and toughen the skin, but additional challenges are present in pediatric prosthetic rehabilitation.[60,61] Upper or lower limb amputation can affect gross (ie, crawling, standing, and ambulation) and fine motor development (bimanual dexterity, ADLs, and fine motor skill acquisition).[62,63] Promoting early use of the residual limb can reduce this effect, with interventions varying based on age, cognitive level, location and length of the residual limb. Focusing on play and function while incorporating games, prizes, and sensory activities can help patient engagement. Learning to use their limb as a helper in bimanual tasks or for weight-bearing support in balance activities can also be rewarding.

Early application prosthetic devices, custom-fabricated orthoses, and advances in 3D printing allow for improved experimentation with low-cost terminal devices. Trial devices for upper and lower extremities can assess the potential for success with a custom-fabricated prosthetic,[63] reinforce residual limb use[64,65] and promote weight bearing. Encouraging appropriate transition through developmental progressions (ie, floor to stand), standing using foam blocks, or pediatric stander with the limb can all promote successful acceptance of a definitive prosthetic device.

A uniquely pediatric complication with amputation is boney overgrowth, often requiring surgical revision, especially in lower extremity amputations. Patients with intact, uninjured proximal growth plates are at risk for long bone growth and perforation of soft tissue, including muscle and skin, of the distal end of the limb.[59,60,66] Typical treatment for this complication is the surgical revision of the amputation and possibly epiphysiodesis. The presence of scarring, poor skin quality, and vascularity can result in poor healing of surgical revision or significant shortening of the limb to ensure good closure.[57,58] These challenges can create substantial emotional and physical setbacks during rehabilitation.

Pediatric patients can also experience psychological trauma surrounding the loss of a limb. Feelings of depression, grief, stress, and anxiety are as common as in adult populations.[60] Additionally, limb revisions and shortening can re-traumatize a patient and hinder rehabilitation. Early rehabilitation to optimize prosthetic fitting and training, promoting a quick return to pre-injury activities, can benefit a patient's overall psychological outlook.[59] Therapists can also aid patients by coordinating with child life specialists and psychologists to support appropriate coping strategies.

### Community Reintegration

Reintegration following a burn injury is vital to the patient's long-term success and is infinitely complex with children.[67] Age at the time of injury plays an enormous role in how patients view themselves and how they return to the community. Emotions of fear, anxiety, depression, and grief can limit a child's desire to return to preferred activities, including school and sports.[68] Coping strategies of the primary caregivers will influence the patient's ability to assimilate back into their community, as children look for guidance from trusted family members. If families develop maladaptive strategies, this can negatively affect psychosocial recovery, potentially resulting in an increased experience of post-traumatic stress symptoms.[68-70] A dedicated support system and education for caregivers early and throughout a patient's recovery are needed to optimize functional outcomes and promote successful reintegration to age-appropriate activities.

Equally important is a focus on the stages of development, not only at the time of injury but planning for needs as they grow. For infants and toddlers, the focus is on bonding and trust, ensuring a caring and dedicated individual supports them through difficult interventions. In addition to a consistent medical and rehabilitation team, this group includes close and extended family members, daycare providers, and other primary caregivers. With consistent emotional support and high-quality rehabilitation, these patients can seamlessly integrate their injury and subsequent changes in appearance into their developing sense of self.

Reintegration can be more challenging for older patients. Preschool and school-age children have already begun to form a sense of self-identity, are building peer relationships, and have acquired functional skills allowing for independence from primary caregivers. A burn injury, with subsequent functional and cosmetic changes, can significantly influence how these children see themselves and their role in their world. They may experience isolation from peers at school, sports, and community activities due to a perceived inability to participate or concern that they will get hurt.[68] Reintegration challenges are especially common when patients have visible scars, compression garments, splints, or amputations. Older school-age children and teens can experience isolation and are susceptible to body image issues, anxiety, and depression.[68] As children age, issues with peer bullying, both in person and through social media, can become a prominent concern.

Dedicated community reintegration activities are important, both in the early stages of recovery and in the long term. Initial support and education of the family is a primary intervention, but as children age, this should expand to include daycare providers, teachers, and peers. Services such as school re-entry programming can support the child and family while providing education and guidance to those in their community.[71-73] Adaptive sports programs, burn-specific camps, and burn community mentorship programs are also integral in helping patients recover a sense of self and independence while demonstrating to their families how a return to normalcy is possible.[74,75]

### Family-Centered Care and Psychosocial Considerations

Fostering trust and supporting caregivers is crucial to optimizing the patient's care. Given the variability in developmental age and cognitive levels in pediatrics, trusted caregivers are important burn team members with a distinctive role as a constant in the patient's life.[76] They provide insight into the patient's pre-injury level of function and play an important role in supporting acute and long-term care delivery. Their presence also allows clinicians to build rapport with these young patients.[77] Understanding individual family dynamics will help clinicians set appropriate goals and role expectations so primary caregivers can feel confident in best supporting the child. Burn team members must be sensitive to the impact this injury has on the family to ensure comprehensive support.[76] A wide diversity in family makeup exists, but primary caregivers should be identified and engaged in the patient's recovery through focused, family-centered care is important to ensure optimal patient outcomes.

Preliminary data demonstrate that including caregivers in regular family rounding with the team improves communication and caregiver satisfaction. As caregivers may be experiencing a range of emotions, including fear and guilt, open and supportive dialogue goes a long way in gaining their trust and easing their worries.[76,77] In addition to early and consistent education, discipline-specific support will help caregivers focus their energy when supporting patients.

Rehabilitation interventions often present a significant challenge to the patient and family and may increase experiences of anxiety, pain, and grief.[76] Focused education by occupational, physical, and speech therapists ensures caregivers understand how providers' roles, knowledge, and unique skills are essential in supporting the patient's recovery. Building a partnership with trusted caregivers encourages compliance with treatment plans and eventual successful carryover of home programs. The caregiver's education level, cultural norms, family dynamics, and coping strategies should be considered during the education process.

The family's response to the burn injury varies greatly and can impact their ability to engage effectively in the child's recovery.[76] Many factors may limit caregiver involvement in recovery, including occupational or family responsibilities beyond caring for their hospitalized child. The caregiver may have also been injured and may be faced with their own recovery. Even when present, caregivers may have ineffective coping strategies or external stressors that limit their involvement in their child's care.

A small but significant percentage of burn injuries in young children result from neglect or abuse. Approximately 3.3% of all burn injuries in patients under 20 years of age were related to suspected child abuse. These situations may require the involvement of family assistance agencies and can result in the removal of the primary caregiver from the bedside, or a child discharged to foster care. Overall, burn therapists must provide consistent and clear education to all caregivers, including written materials and images to support consistent carryover of interventions.

### SUMMARY

Physical rehabilitation for burn survivors of any age can pose unique challenges to the treating therapist. For children who sustain burns early in life, treatment and long-term follow-up should be conducted under the guidance of a burn center for the early identification of needed interventions during periods of growth and development. It is important to respond not just to the immediate physical needs of the patient but also to consider the fine and gross motor skill progression, future implications of growth and development, the need for family involvement in the entire care process, and the innate need for children to play and explore, even during recovery from a life-altering injury.

## CLINICS CARE POINTS

- Burns sustained early in life may inhibit the attainment of developmental milestones.
- Pediatric burn survivors show statistically worse psychosocial health and school functioning than their non-burned peers, including challenges with conduct, hyperactivity, socialization, and emotional regulation.
- Following a burn injury, fear, anxiety, depression, and grief can limit a child's desire to return to preferred activities, including school and sports.
- Children with preexisting neurodevelopmental concerns may require further adaptations in care delivery and are at risk for worsened recovery outcomes.
- Fostering trust with the caregivers of pediatric burn survivors is crucial to optimize care and outcomes and promote successful reintegration.
- Children who sustained burns early in life require long-term follow-up under the guidance of a burn center.

## DISCLOSURE

The authors have nothing to disclose.

## REFERENCES

1. Burns. World Health Organization. Published 2023. http://www.who.int/news-room/fact-sheets/detail/burns. Accessed February 10, 2023.
2. ABA. American burn association, annual burn injury summary report 2022 update: report of data from 2016-2022. Chicago, IL: American Burn Association; 2022.
3. Padalko A, Cristall N, Gawaziuk JP, et al. Social complexity and risk for pediatric burn injury: A systematic review. J Burn Care Res 2019;40(4):478–99.
4. Sheridan RL. Burn care for children. Pediatr Rev 2018;39(6):273–86.
5. Ohgi S, Gu S. Pediatric burn rehabilitation: Philosophy and strategies. Burns Trauma 2013;1(2):73–9.
6. Schiestl C, Beynon C, Balmer B. What are the differences?-Treatment of burns in children compared to treatment in adults. Osteosynth Trauma Care 2007;15:26–8.
7. Wachtel TL, Berry CC, Wachtel EE, et al. The inter-rater reliability of estimating the size of burns from various burn area chart drawings. Burns 2000;26(2):156–70.
8. Sharma R, Parashar A. Special considerations in paediatric burn patients. Indian J Plast Surg 2010;43(3):43.
9. Centers for Disease Control and Prevention. Learn the signs. Act Early. CDC's Developmental Milestones. Published December 29, 2022. https://www.cdc.gov/ncbddd/actearly/index.html. Accessed February 10, 2023.
10. Graber EG. Childhood Development. Merck Manuals Professional Edition. https://www.merckmanuals.com/professional/pediatrics/growth-and-development/childhood-development. Accessed April 5, 2023.

11. Johnston L, Eastwood D, Jacobs B. Variations in normal gait development. Paediatr Child Health 2014;24(5):204–7.

12. Lensing J, Wibbenmeyer L, Liao J, et al. Demographic and burn injury-specific variables associated with limited joint mobility at discharge in a multicenter study. J Burn Care Res 2020;41(2):363–70.

13. Taylor SL, Sen S, Greenhalgh DG, et al. A competing risk analysis for hospital length of stay in patients with burns. JAMA Surg 2015;150:450–6.

14. Yelvington M, Godleski M, Lee AF, et al. Contracture severity at hospital discharge in children: A Burn Model System database study. J Burn Care Res 2021;42(3):425–33.

15. Sadeq F, Riobueno-Naylor A, DePamphilis MA, et al. Evaluating burn recovery outcomes in children with neurodevelopmental symptoms. J Burn Care Res 2022;43(3):679–84.

16. Zubler JM, Wiggins LD, Macias MM, et al. Evidence-informed milestones for developmental surveillance tools. Pediatrics 2022;149(3). https://doi.org/10.1542/peds.2021-052138.

17. Miller RP, Kori SH, Todd DD. The Tampa Scale: a measure of kinesiophobia. Clin J Pain 1991;7(1).

18. Jeong WJ, Holavanahalli RK, Kowalske KJ. Evaluation of kinesiophobia in survivors of major burn injury. J Burn Care Res 2022;43(6):1380–5.

19. Seyyah M, Topuz S. The effect of physiotherapy and rehabilitation on pain, kinesiophobia and functionality in upper extremity burns. Hand Microsurg 2021;0:1.

20. Parry I, Painting L, Bagley A, et al. A pilot prospective randomized control trial comparing exercises using videogame therapy to standard physical therapy. J Burn Care Res 2015;36(5):534–44.

21. Ali RR, Selim AO, Abdel Ghafar MA, et al. Virtual reality as a pain distractor during physical rehabilitation in pediatric burns. Burns 2021. https://doi.org/10.1016/j.burns.2021.04.031.

22. Kamel FAH, Basha MA. Effects of virtual reality and task-oriented training on hand function and activity performance in pediatric hand burns: A randomized controlled trial. Arch Phys Med Rehabil 2021;102(6):1059–66.

23. Lan X, Tan Z, Zhou T, et al. Use of virtual reality in burn rehabilitation: A systematic review and meta-analysis. Arch Phys Med Rehabil 2023;104(3):502–13.

24. Melchert-McKearnan K, Deitz J, Engel JM, et al. Children with burn injuries: purposeful activity versus rote exercise. Am J Occup Ther 2000;54(4):381–90.

25. Omar MTA, Hegazy FA, Mokashi SP. Influences of purposeful activity versus rote exercise on improving pain and hand function in pediatric burn. Burns 2012;38(2):261–8.

26. Goverman J, Mathews K, Goldstein R, et al. Pediatric contractures in burn injury: A burn model system national database study. J Burn Care Res 2017;38(1):e192–9.

27. van der Wal MBA, Vloemans JFPM, Tuinebreijer WE, et al. Outcome after burns: an observational study on burn scar maturation and predictors for severe scarring: Burn scar outcome. Wound Repair Regen 2012;20(5):676–87.

28. Wallace HJ, Fear MW, Crowe MM, et al. Identification of factors predicting scar outcome after burn injury in children: a prospective case-control study. Burns Trauma 2017;5(1):19.

29. Brownstein BPM, Snook APM. Burns in Children. Burns in Children CINAHL Rehabilitation Guide. Published online 2021.

30. Sharp PA, Pan B, Yakuboff KP, et al. Development of a best evidence statement for the use of pressure therapy for management of hypertrophic scarring. J Burn Care Res 2016;37(4):255–64.

31. Nast A, Carreras M, Thompson AR, et al. Scar management: Using silicone-based products in primary health care. Wounds International 2016;7(4):23–7.

32. Edwards J. Hypertrophic scar management. Br J Nurs 2022;31(20):S24–31.

33. Wiseman J, Ware RS, Simons M, et al. Effectiveness of topical silicone gel and pressure garment therapy for burn scar prevention and management in children: a randomized controlled trial. Clin Rehabil 2020;34(1):120–31.

34. Zuccaro J, Kelly C, Perez M, et al. The effectiveness of laser therapy for hypertrophic burn scars in pediatric patients: A prospective investigation. J Burn Care Res 2021;42(5):847–56.

35. Moore ML, Dewey WS, Richard RL. Rehabilitation of the burned hand. Hand Clin 2009;25(4):529–41.

36. Parry IS, Schneider JC, Yelvington M, et al. Systematic review and expert consensus on the use of orthoses (splints and casts) with adults and children after burn injury to determine practice guidelines. J Burn Care Res 2019;41(3):503–34.

37. Wilton J. Hand splinting/orthotic intervention: principles of design and fabrication. Fremantle (Western Australia): Vivid Publishing; 2015.

38. Oosterwijk AM, Nieuwenhuis MK, van der Schans CP, et al. Shoulder and elbow range of motion for the performance of activities of daily living: A systematic review. Physiother Theory Pract 2018;34(7):505–28.

39. Petuskey K, Bagley A, Abdala E, et al. Upper extremity kinematics during functional activities: three-dimensional studies in a normal pediatric population. Gait Posture 2007;25(4):573–9.

40. Maskell J, Newcombe P, Martin G, et al. Psychosocial functioning differences in pediatric burn survivors compared with healthy norms. J Burn Care Res 2013;34(4):465–76.

41. Grice KO, Barnes KJ, Vogel KA. Influence of burn injury on activity participation of children. J Burn Care Res 2015;36(3):414–20.

42. Colwell BRL, Williams CN, Kelly SP, et al. Mobilization therapy in the pediatric intensive care unit: A multidisciplinary quality improvement initiative. Am J Crit Care 2018;27(3):194–203.

43. Cameron S, Ball I, Cepinskas G, et al. Early mobilization in the critical care unit: A review of adult and pediatric literature. J Crit Care 2015;30(4):664–72.

44. Ebid AA, El-Shamy SM, Draz AH. Effect of isokinetic training on muscle strength, size and gait after healed pediatric burn: a randomized controlled study. Burns 2014;40(1):97–105.

45. Serghiou MA, Ott S, Cowan A. et. In: Herndon D, et al, editors. Burn care, burn rehabilitation along the continuum of care. New York: Elsevier; 2018. p. 476–508.

46. Godleski M, Oeffling A, Bruflat AK, et al. Treating burn-associated joint contracture: Results of an inpatient rehabilitation stretching protocol. J Burn Care Res 2013;34(4):420–6.

47. Usuba M, Akai M, Shirasaki Y, et al. Experimental joint contracture correction with low torque-long duration repeated stretching. Clin Orthop Relat Res 2007;456:70–8.

48. Cartotto R, Johnson L, Rood JM, et al. Clinical Practice Guideline: Early mobilization and rehabilitation of critically ill burn patients. J Burn Care Res 2023;44(1):1–15.

49. Grisbrook TL, Reid SL, Elliott CM, et al. Lower limb functional outcome assessment following burn injury: A novel use for 3D laboratory-based movement analysis. Burns 2010;36(3):e24–30.

50. Ebid AA, El-Shamy SM, Amer MA. Effect of vitamin D supplementation and isokinetic training on muscle strength, explosive strength, lean body mass and gait in severely burned children: A randomized controlled trial. Burns 2017; 43(2):357–65.

51. Özkal Ö, Kısmet K, Konan A, et al. Treadmill versus overground gait training in patients with lower limb burn injury: A matched control study. Burns 2022; 48(1):51–8.

52. ISBI Practice Guidelines Committee, Advisory Subcommittee, Steering Subcommittee. ISBI practice guidelines for burn care, part 2. Burns 2018;44(7):1617–706.

53. Tapking C, Popp D, Herndon DN, et al. Cardiovascular effect of varying interval training frequency in rehabilitation of severely burned children. J Burn Care Res 2019;40(1):34–8.

54. Clayton RP, Wurzer P, Andersen CR, et al. Effects of different duration exercise programs in children with severe burns. Burns 2017;43(4):796–803.

55. Bartley CN, Atwell K, Purcell L, et al. Amputation following burn injury. J Burn Care Res 2019;40(4):430–6.

56. Singh M, Li H, Nuutila K, et al. Innovative techniques for maximizing limb salvage and function. J Burn Care Res 2017;38(3):e670–7.

57. Parry IS, Mooney KN, Chau C, et al. Effects of skin grafting on successful prosthetic use in children with lower extremity amputation. J Burn Care Res 2008; 29(6):949–54.

58. Khan MAA, Javed AA, Rao DJ, et al. Pediatric traumatic limb amputation: The principles of management and optimal residual limb lengths. World J Plast Surg 2016;5(1):7–14.

59. Foncerrada G, Capek KD, Peña R, et al. 343 mental and physical changes after an exercise program in burn children with extensive limb amputations. J Burn Care Res 2018;39(suppl_1):S141.

60. Thornby MA, Krebs DE. Bimanual skill development in pediatric below-elbow amputation: a multicenter, cross-sectional study. Archives of physical medicine and rehabilitation 1992;73:697–702.

61. Whitehead C, Begnaud E. 319 clinical observations using 3D printed hand and finger devices in pediatric burn rehabilitation. J Burn Care Res 2019; 40(Supplement_1):S137.

62. Newman C. Adaptive cuff for early stage hand amputees. Burns Open 2021;5(4): 59–61.

63. Romero YLM. Adaptive device for lower extremity prosthetics. Burns Open 2021; 5(4):206–10.

64. Horsch A, Gleichauf S, Lehner B, et al. Lower-limb amputation in children and adolescents-A rare encounter with unique and special challenges. Children 2022;9(7):1004.

65. McMullen K, Bamer AM, Gibran NS, et al. 25 social integration in the first 2 years after moderate to severe burn injury: A Burn Model System national database study. J Burn Care Res 2020;41(Supplement_1):S19–20.

66. Patel KF, Rodríguez-Mercedes SL, Grant GG, et al. Physical, psychological, and social outcomes in pediatric burn survivors ages 5 to 18 years: A systematic review. J Burn Care Res 2022;43(2):343–52.

67. Enlow PT, Brown Kirschman KJ, Mentrikoski J, et al. The role of youth coping strategies and caregiver psychopathology in predicting post-traumatic stress symptoms in pediatric burn survivors. J Burn Care Res 2019;40(5):620–6.
68. Odar C, Kirschman KJB, Pelley TJ, et al. Prevalence and correlates of post-traumatic stress in parents of young children postburn. J Burn Care Res 2013; 34(3):299–306.
69. Holavanahalli RK, Badger K, Acton A. Community Reintegration. J Burn Care Res 2017;38(3):e632–4.
70. McCartney DM, Fowler L, James L, et al. 424 School re-entry presentations - A faculty and staff perspective. J Burn Care Res 2018;39(suppl_1):S184.
71. Turgeon L, Bradbury C, Weed V, et al. 122 The efficacy of community reintegration programming in the physical and psychosocial recovery of pediatric burn survivors. J Burn Care Res 2019;40(Supplement_1):S77.
72. Won P, Bello MS, Stoycos SA, et al. The impact of peer support group programs on psychosocial outcomes for burn survivors and caregivers: A review of the literature. J Burn Care Res 2021;42(4):600–9.
73. Radics-Johnson JB, Chacon DW, Zhang L. 570 Who benefits the most from burn camps? J Burn Care Res 2020;41(Supplement_1):S125–6.
74. Bayuo J, Wong FKY. Issues and concerns of family members of burn patients: A scoping review. Burns 2020. https://doi.org/10.1016/j.burns.2020.04.023.
75. Rimmer RB, Bay RC, Alam NB, et al. Measuring the burden of pediatric burn injury for parents and caregivers: informed burn center staff can help to lighten the load. J Burn Care Res 2015;36(3):421–7.
76. Arredondo O, Day M, Martens SA, et al. 777 Improving parent communication with family rounds in the pediatric critical care unit (PICU). J Burn Care Res 2022;43(Supplement_1):S196.
77. Campos JK, Wong YM, Hasty BN, et al. The effect of socioeconomic status and parental demographics on activation of Department of child and Family Services in pediatric burn injury. J Burn Care Res 2017;38(4):e722–33.

# Factors Associated with the Rehabilitation of the Older Adult Burn Patient

Kathleen S. Romanowski, MD, MAS, FCCM

## KEYWORDS

- Burn • Older adults • Frailty • Rehabilitation • Surgery

## KEY POINTS

- The population is aging, and the number of older adults sustaining burn injuries is also increasing.
- As skin ages, it becomes thinner and more susceptible to full-thickness injury, therefore requiring surgical intervention.
- There are no studies looking at the optimum timing for surgery in older adult patients.
- Frailty is an important determinant of outcomes in older adult burn patients and may be able to predict rehabilitation potential and rehabilitation outcomes, but this has yet to be studied.

## BACKGROUND

The older adult population is growing. As of 2019, 54.1 million Americans are older than 65 years, and by 2060 it is estimated that this number will grow to almost 95 million people.[1] With this population growth there will also be a corresponding increase in the number of older burn-injured patients and an increase in the economic burden associated with these injuries.[2] Older adult patients are also at increased risk of severe burn injury with larger total body surface area (TBSA) for multiple reasons, including impaired vision, decreased coordination, preexisting comorbidities, and medication side effects.[3]

Severe burn injuries can worsen preexisting conditions, decrease mobility, and worsen the patient's nutritional status, making older adult burn patients more likely to require or benefit from rehabilitation.[4,5] Older adult burn patients are at increased risk for having adverse outcomes (eg, mortality, longer hospital stays, and discharge to a skilled nursing facility [SNF]) when they are compared with younger patients.[6] The

Department of Surgery, University of California, Davis and Shriners Children's Northern California, 2425 Stockton Boulevard, Suite 718, Sacramento, CA 95817, USA
*E-mail address:* ksromanowski@ucdavis.edu
Twitter: @KSRomanowski (K.S.R.)

Phys Med Rehabil Clin N Am 34 (2023) 839–848
https://doi.org/10.1016/j.pmr.2023.06.032
1047-9651/23/© 2023 Elsevier Inc. All rights reserved.

cutoff for burn-injury size over which patients are at an increased risk for complications and mortality is 40% TBSA in younger adult patients (aged ≤65 years) and 30% TBSA in older adult patients (aged >65 years).[7] In addition, older adult burn patients are at an increased risk of readmission to the hospital and an increased risk of mortality in the first 2 years following hospital discharge.[4,5,8–10] Mandell and colleagues[5] found that patients who were 65 to 74 years old had an adjusted odds ratio (OR) for mortality of 2.51 (95% confidence interval [CI], 2.03–3.09) and patients aged 75 years or older had an adjusted OR of 2.90 (95% CI, 2.36–3.55) when compared with patients who were 45 to 54 years old.

All patients who sustain a significant burn injury, irrespective of patient age, have some amount of disability following their injury and benefit from rehabilitation to regain and maintain optimal functioning. When thinking about the care of older adults, geriatric rehabilitation is defined as a set of evaluative, diagnostic, and therapeutic interventions whose purpose is to restore functional ability or enhance residual functional capability in older adults with physical impairments.[11] There have been few, if any, studies examining postburn rehabilitation in older adults, but when rehabilitation of older adult patients in general is examined, it is found to have a positive effect on outcomes for improved functioning, decreased risk of admission to an SNF, and decreased mortality.[12] Although rehabilitation in older adults is not well studied, there are multiple factors that can influence patient outcomes, including the need for surgical treatment secondary to the physiology of older adult skin and frailty.

## EFFECTS OF AGE ON BURN DEPTH AND WOUND HEALING
### Aging Skin

The integrity and function of the skin deteriorates as patients age, which leads to diminished neurosensory perception, altered skin permeability, and a compromised healing in response to injury.[13] The number of cell layers remains constant as people age, but as they get older, the skin flattens at the dermoepidermal junction by more than one-third due to thinning of the dermal papillae and decreased interdigitation between the epidermis and the dermis.[13,14] The flattening of the skin begins at around 60 years of age and leads to increased susceptibility to injury, decreased resistance to shearing, and reduced oxygen and nutrient delivery.[13,14] For older adults with burn injuries, these skin changes can lead to clinically significant deeper burn wounds with prolonged healing time and the potential for reduced reepithelialization, which can in turn lead to increased likelihood of requiring skin grafting for healing of burn wounds.[14]

### Burn Depth and Need for Surgery

Burn depth is a significant determinant of the acute management of severe burn injuries. The depth of the burn defines the extent and complexity of the treatment required and contributes to each patient's long-term functional and aesthetic outcomes as well as determining their need for extensive rehabilitation.[15–17] Burn wounds that initially seem to be superficial partial thickness can undergo secondary burn wound progression during the initial postburn period, which leads to conversion of these wounds to deep partial-thickness (DPT) or full-thickness (FT) wounds.[18] When wounds progress to either DPT or FT they are at increased risk of developing hypertrophic scarring, requiring surgical excision and grafting, and developing wound infections or other wound complications.[18] Older adult patients with burn injury are at increased risk for burn wound conversion due to the changes in the skin that were previously discussed such as the thinning of the dermis, decreased number and density of skin adnexa (hair follicles, sweat and sebaceous glands), making healing of superficial partial-thickness (SPT) and DPT wounds more challenging, age-related immune dysregulation, and other comorbidities such as vascular disease and diabetes.[18–21] Patients who require surgery often require more extensive rehabilitation than those who heal without surgery. Despite the obvious potential problems with wound healing in older adults, there have not been any studies looking specifically at time to burn wound closure in older adult patients, instead the available studies use hospital length of stay (LOS) and number of operations required as surrogate markers for time to wound healing. These studies suggest that although older age is associated with longer LOS, it is not associated with an increased number of operative procedures.[22–27]

### Future Directions for Surgery in Older Burn Patients

Although it is documented that older adult burn patients have longer LOS, but no difference in number of operations when compared with their younger counterparts, there have not been any studies done that examine the optimal surgical management of older adult patients. Early excision and grafting of burn wounds are well accepted as the standard of care for younger adult patients,[28,29] but it is unknown whether the same principles are appropriate for older adult patients. In addition, it is not yet known if primary skin grafting is the best treatment option for older adults or if they would benefit from a staged operative approach using either allograft or a dermal substitute. Both are areas where future research is needed and in fact a multicenter retrospective study is underway to examine how older adult patients are currently being treated in burn centers.

### FRAILTY

The traditional model for predicting mortality in burn patients is the Baux score, which is based on patient age and burn size (%TBSA). Updated models have moved beyond only using these 2 factors to include presence/amount of full-thickness burns, inhalation injury, and sex in their predictions.[30,31] Unfortunately, these models fail to fully account for the individual difference between patients. Individuals with the same chronological age can have widely different states of health and functional status, making age alone a poor predictor of outcome.[32] The idea that age alone is not a good predictor of outcomes has been tested in an older adult burn patients by Alpert and colleagues.[33] This study used Trauma Quality Improvement Program data to examine 282 patients who were older than 65 years. They divided the patients into those who were 65 to 79 years (209 patients) and those who were older than 80 years (73 patients). They found that octogenarians have similar injuries with respect to TBSA when compared with the younger patients as well as similar comorbidities. They also found that older age was not associated with increased complications or increased mortality when compared with patients who were 65 to 79 years old.

Frailty has been suggested as an alternative to age alone for predicting outcomes in older adults with burn injury. Frailty, present in 10% to 20% of the population older than 65 years, has been defined as age-related vulnerability related to multiple physiologic systems that can either coexist with or be independent of disability and chronic disease.[32] Initial studies looking at the importance of frailty in burn patients have been conducted. These studies have examined choice/development of frailty scores for a burn population, the combination of frailty and sarcopenia, and the ability to use frailty as an outcome measure in burn patients.

## Frailty Score Development and Choice of Frailty Score in the Burn Population

More than 70 tools exist for measuring frailty, but generally there is not a scale that is considered a gold standard because most have been used only within one area of medicine and have not been widely tested across patient populations.[34] Tools for measuring frailty range from single-item measurements to frailty scores that include 90 items.

Because of its ease of use and ability to be used in retrospective studies, the most commonly used frailty score in a burn population has been the Canadian Study on Health and Aging Clinical Frailty Score (CSHA CFS) (**Table 1**). The development of the CSHA CFS came out of the Canadian Study on Health and Aging (CSHA), which was a 10-year study designed to examine the epidemiology of dementia that followed older adults from 1991 to 2001. The initial study was a 5-year prospective cohort study that included 9008 people older than 65 years and led to their initial development of a rules-based frailty score.[35] A secondary analysis of 2914 patients validated a 20-item frailty index of observed deficits, which was eventually simplified to the CSHA CFS.[36,37] It is a 7-point clinical opinion scale (see **Table 1**) that was validated in 2305 patients. The CHSA CFS was highly correlated with the previously developed frailty index and, as its predecessors, was predictive of institutionalization and death.[37]

The CSHA CFS was the first frailty score that was studied in a burn population. Masud and colleagues[38] examined 42 patients who were older than 65 years and had sustained at least 10% TBSA burns. They retrospectively assigned a CHSA CFS score to each patient based on their admission assessment. They found that patients with better preinjury functional status (lower frailty scores) and those who had surgical treatment of their burns were more likely to survive their burn injuries. The survivors had a median CSHA CFS of 3, whereas those who died had a median CSHA CFS of 5. The study concluded that CSHA CFS was a useful adjunct in predicting outcome in burns requiring admission to the hospital and that CSHA CFS may be able to predict which patients will benefit from surgery.

Masud and colleagues'[38] study was an important proof of concept for the use of frailty scoring in an older adult burn population. Despite the success of CSHA CFS in predicting outcomes in the burn population, some researchers have started to examine the utility of moving from general frailty scores (such as CSHA CFS) to specialty specific scales that are designed to be used in a specific patient population. The Trauma-Specific Frailty Index (TSFI) was designed for and is validated for the

| Table 1 Canadian study on health and aging clinical frailty score | |
|---|---|
| 1-Very fit | Robust, active, energetic, well motivated, and fit |
| 2-Well | Without active disease but less fit than people in category 1 |
| 3-Well with treated comorbid disease | Disease symptoms are well controlled compared with those in category 4 |
| 4-Apparently vulnerable | Although not frankly dependent, these people commonly complain of being "slowed up" or have disease symptoms |
| 5-Mildly frail | With limited dependence on others for instrumental activities of daily living |
| 6-Moderately frail | Help is needed with both instrumental and noninstrumental activities of daily living |
| 7-Severely frail | Completely dependent on others for the activities of daily living or terminally ill |

prediction of an unfavorable discharge (death or discharge to an SNF) in a trauma population. The TSFI is made up of 15 variables that examine the domains of comorbidities, daily activities, health attitudes, and nutrition.[39] The TSFI and the Emergency General Surgery Frailty Index, which was subsequently created, both served as the inspiration for the development of the Burn Frailty Index (BFI)[40,41] (**Table 2**). Maxwell and colleagues[41] used a randomized cohort of 100 patients older than 65 years to create the BFI. In their study they found that frail patients had more complications ($p < 0.001$), more discharges to nonhome locations ($p < 0.001$), longer hospital stays ($p < 0.001$), and lower rates of survival at both 1 and 3 years ($p < 0.001$).

In the older adult burn population, there has not been a study that compares the BFI and the CSHA CFS. Currently there is not one frailty score that is considered the gold standard in burn research. In choosing a scale for burn research and burn clinical use there are several factors to consider. The BFI includes injury-related factors such as TBSA and requires patient interaction to complete, which could be either helpful or a hindrance depending on the goals of a particular study. The CSHA CFS is a generic scale that can be used even with minimal patient participation. Depending on the goals associated with the use of the frailty score, either BFI or CSHA CFS might be a reasonable choice in an older burn patient population.

### Frailty and Sarcopenia

Beyond simply looking at frailty there has been some work done to look at the intersection between frailty and sarcopenia. Sarcopenia is described as the loss of muscle mass, resulting in loss of strength, mobility, and function.[42] The prevalence of sarcopenia increases with age, increasing from 5% to 13% in the seventh decade of life to 11% to 50% by the age of 80 years.[43] Although clearly related, sarcopenia and frailty are different. Although the decreased muscle mass observed in sarcopenia can lead to the physical function impairment that is observed with frailty, frailty is more complex and is defined as a clinically recognizable state of increased vulnerability resulting from aging-associated decline in reserve and function across multiple physiologic systems, resulting in fatigue, weight loss, cognitive impairment, and social isolation.[44]

Romanowski and colleagues[45] conducted a study that aimed to look at the interaction between sarcopenia as measured by chest or abdomen computed tomography (CT) scans and frailty as measured by CSHA CFS in burn patients older than 60 years. Sarcopenia was assessed on CT examinations by measuring skeletal muscle index of paraspinal muscles at T12 and all skeletal muscles at L3. The sample size for this study was very small with only 50 patients having chest CT scans and 60 patients having abdominal CT scans, making it underpowered to examine the relationship between frailty scores and sarcopenia with LOS and mortality. CT-derived measurement of muscle mass at T12 was associated with LOS ($p < .05$) but not with mortality ($p = 0.561$). CT-derived metrics of sarcopenia at L3 were associated with mortality or LOS. One of the significant limitations of using CT measurements of sarcopenia in a burn population is that most patients do not undergo a CT scan as part of routine care. Alternative methods for measuring muscle mass will need to be assessed if this is to become part of predictive modeling for older adult burn patients. The intersection of frailty and sarcopenia could be an important indicator of rehabilitation potential as well as serving as a maker of rehabilitation success.

### Frailty as a Predictor of Outcomes

As previously described, Masud and colleagues' was the first study to look at the correlation between CSHA CFS and mortality.[38] One of the limitations of their study was that they only looked at burns that were greater than 10% TBSA. Romanowski and

**Table 2**
**Burn frailty score**

| | | | |
|---|---|---|---|
| 1. Cancer history | No (0) | | Yes (1) |
| 2. Diabetes | No (0) | | Yes (1) |
| 3. Need help with grooming | No (0) | | Yes (1) |
| 4. Need help with managing money | No (0) | | Yes (1) |
| 5. Need help doing household work | No (0) | | Yes (1) |
| 6. Need to be sexually active | No (0) | | Yes (1) |
| 7. Coronary artery disease | Medication (0.25) | PCI (0.50) | CABG (0.75) | MI (1) |
| 8. Dementia | None (0) | Mild (0.25) | Moderate (0.5) | Severe (1) |
| 9. Need help with walking | None (0) | Cane (0.25) | Walker (0.75) | Wheelchair (1) |
| 10. Feel sad | Rarely (0) | Sometimes (0.5) | | Most of the time (1) |
| 11. Feel lonely | Rarely (0) | Sometimes (0.5) | | Most of the time (1) |
| 12. GCS on admission | ≥ 14 (0) | | <14 (1) |
| 13. Albumin level on admission | ≥ 3 mg/dL (0) | | A |
| 14. Creatinine level on admission | < 1.0 mg/dL (0) | 1.0–1.49 mg/dL (1) | 1.5–1.99 mg/dL (1.5) | ≥ 2.0 mg/dL (2) |
| 15. TBSA in admission | < 5.0% (0) | 5.0%–9.9% (0.25) | 10%–14.9% (1.00) | 15%–199% (1.50) | 20%–24.9% (1.75) | ≥25% (2) |

colleagues repeated their study but included all patients irrespective of burn size.[46] A total of 89 patients were admitted during the study period. This study also found that patients who died had significantly higher CHSA CFS compared with survivors (5.2±1.2 vs 4.4±1.2). It was also found that CSHA CFS was significantly higher in patients discharged to an SNF (5.34±0.9) compared with those who were discharged home (4.1±1.2). Multivariate logistic regression found that CSHA CFS was independently associated with increased risk of discharge to SNF and increased risk of mortality.

Given that frailty is not restricted to those older than 65 years, Romanowski and colleagues also examined frailty in patients 50 years and older.[47] A total of 502 patients were examined in this study. Again, higher CSHA CFS was found to be associated with increased risk of death and discharge to an SNF. In looking at patients aged 50 to 64 years, multivariate logistic analysis found that the OR for death in this group was 2.5 (95% CI 1.4–4.6); this was even higher than the OR for patients 65 years and older of 1.63 (95% CI 1.003–2.7).

All the previously discussed studies examined admission CSHA CFS scores but did not consider the effects that hospitalization would have on frailty. To quantify the change in frailty that occurs over the course of a hospitalization, a recent study measured both admission CSHA CFS and discharge CSHA CFS.[48] The change in frailty over the course of admission was also calculated. In this study the mean CHSA CFS on admission and discharge was 4.3±1.2 and 5.1±1.2, respectively. The mean change in CHSA CFS was 0.55 worse than on admission. Over the course of the study 46 patients (59%) had no change or an improvement in their CSHA CFS, whereas 32 patients (41%) had a worsened CSHA CFS. Multivariate analysis found that patients with lower CSHA CFS on admission were at the greatest risk of worsened scores at discharge; this suggests that these patients may represent a target for future inpatient frailty prevention programs and inpatient and outpatient rehabilitation programs by being able to potentially use frailty as both a predictor of and measurement of success as part of a rehabilitation program after burn injury.

### Future Directions for Frailty

Previous studies have established the correlation between frailty and outcomes such as mortality, discharge to an SNF, and likelihood of undergoing a goals-of-care discussion. Research now needs to move beyond examining the correlation of frailty with outcomes and begin using frailty to plan care and make decisions for patients. Studies in the general medical and hip fracture populations have shown that frailty is a predictor of poor rehabilitation outcomes.[49,50] Frailty has not been studied as a factor for determining rehabilitation potential in an older adult burn patient population or if frailty can be altered through intense rehabilitation programs, but this could certainly be an area of future research that would benefit older adult burn patients.

### SUMMARY

Given the aging of the population, more older adult patients and more frail patients are presenting with burn injuries than ever before. Despite this, there has been relatively few studies examining how these patients differ from their younger counterparts with respect to wound healing, wound care, surgical treatment, nutrition, and rehabilitation. It is known that older skin is thinner and more susceptible to burn wound conversion, but how these changes affect the need for surgery, how surgery is performed, and recovery after surgery have not been widely examined. More research is needed on how to determine how rehabilitation potential and rehabilitation success are determined in an older adult burn population.

## CLINICS CARE POINTS

- When older patients sustain burns their wounds are more likely to convert from superficial partial thickness to either DPT or FT.
- Frailty can predict outcomes in older adult burn patients and should be measured in all adult burn patients to assist with prognostication and setting of expectations with families.
- There has been minimal work done examining rehabilitation potential, techniques, and definitions of success in older adult burn patients. More research is needed to better determine best practices for these patients.

## DISCLOSURE

The authors have nothing to disclose.

## REFERENCES

1. U.S. Census Bureau. n.d. Population Estimates and Projections. U.S. Department of Commerce. Available at: https://www.census.gov/programs-surveys/popproj.html. Accessed December 2021.
2. American Burn Association. *National Burn Repository Report of Data from 2009-2018. 2019*, American Burn Association; Chicago, IL.
3. Klein MB, Lezotte DC, Heltshe S, et al. Functional and psychosocial outcomes of older adults after burn injury: results from a multicenter database of severe burn injury. J Burn Care Res 2011;32(1):66–78.
4. Duke JM, Boyd JH, Rea S, et al. Long-term mortality among older adults with burn injury: a population-based study in Australia. Bull World Health Organ 2015;93(6):400–6.
5. Mandell SP, Pham T, Klein MB. Repeat hospitalization and mortality in older adult burn patients. J Burn Care Res 2013;34(1):e36–41.
6. Lundgren RS, Kramer CB, Rivara FP, et al. Influence of comorbidities and age on outcome following burn injury in older adults. J Burn Care Res 2009;30(2):307–14.
7. Jeschke MG, Pinto R, Kraft R, et al. Morbidity and survival probability in burn patients in modern burn care. Crit Care Med 2015;43(4):808–15.
8. Pomahac B, Matros E, Semel M, et al. Predictors of survival and length of stay in burn patients older than 80 years of age: does age really matter? J Burn Care Res 2006;27(3):265–9.
9. McGwin G, Cross JM, Ford JW, et al. Long-term trends in mortality according to age among adult burn patients. J Burn Care Rehabil 2003;24(1):21–5.
10. Lionelli GT, Pickus EJ, Beckum OK, et al. A three decade analysis of factors affecting burn mortality in the elderly. Burns 2005;31(8):958–63.
11. Boston working group on improving health care outcomes through geriatric rehabilitation. Med Care 1997;35(Supplement):JS4–20.
12. Bachmann S, Finger C, Huss A, et al. Inpatient rehabilitation specifically designed for geriatric patients: systematic review and meta-analysis of randomised controlled trials. BMJ 2010;340(apr20 2):c1718.
13. Farage MA, Miller KW, Elsner P, et al. Functional and physiological characteristics of the aging skin. Aging Clin Exp Res 2008;20(3):195–200.
14. Abu-Sittah GS, Chahine FM, Janom H. Management of burns in the elderly. Ann Burns Fire Disasters 2016;29. 249-245.

15. Shupp JW, Nasabzadeh TJ, Rosenthal DS, et al. A review of the local pathophysiologic bases of burn wound progression. J Burn Care Res 2010;31(6):849–73.

16. Asuku ME, Milner SM. Burn surgery. In: Granick MS, editor. Iuc teot. Surgical wound Healing and management. Boca Raton, FL, USA: CRC Press; 2012.

17. Singer AJ, Boyce ST. Burn Wound healing and tissue engineering. J Burn Care Res 2017;38(3):e605–13.

18. Rani M, Schwacha MG. Aging and the pathogenic response to burn. Aging Dis 2012;3(2):171–80.

19. Farinas AF, Bamba R, Pollins AC, et al. Burn wounds in the young versus the aged patient display differential immunological responses. Burns 2018;44(6): 1475–81.

20. Greenhalgh DG. Burns in the geriatric population. In: Greenhalgh DG, editor. Burn Care for general Surgeons and general practitioners. Cham, Switzerland: Cham Springer International Publishing; 2016. p. 189–92.

21. Greenhalgh DG. Management of the skin and soft tissue in the geriatric surgical patient. Surg Clin North Am 2015;95(1):103–14.

22. Goei H, van Baar ME, Dokter J, et al. Burns in the elderly: a nationwide study on management and clinical outcomes. Burns & Trauma 2020;8. https://doi.org/10. 1093/burnst/tkaa027.

23. Nitzschke SL, Aden JK, Serio-Melvin ML, et al. Wound healing trajectories in burn patients and their impact on mortality. J Burn Care Res 2014;35(6):474–9.

24. Li H, Yao Z, Tan J, et al. Epidemiology and outcome analysis of 6325 burn patients: a five-year retrospective study in a major burn center in Southwest China. Sci Rep 2017;7(1). https://doi.org/10.1038/srep46066.

25. Palmieri TL, Molitor F, Chan G, et al. Long-term functional outcomes in the elderly after burn injury. J Burn Care Res 2012;33(4):497–503. https://doi.org/10.1097/bcr.0b013e31825aeaac.

26. Stylianou N, Buchan I, Dunn KW. A review of the international Burn Injury Database (iBID) for England and Wales: descriptive analysis of burn injuries 2003-2011. BMJ Open 2015;5(2):e006184.

27. Taylor SL, Sen S, Greenhalgh DG, et al. A competing risk analysis for hospital length of stay in patients with burns. JAMA Surgery 2015;150(5):450.

28. Janzekovic Z. A new concept in the early excision and immediate grafting of burns. J Trauma Inj Infect Crit Care 1970;10(12):1103–8.

29. Herndon DN, Barrow RE, Rutan RL, et al. A comparison of conservative versus early excision. Therapies in severely burned patients. Ann Surg 1989;209(5): 547–53. https://doi.org/10.1007/00000658-198905000-00006.

30. Werner CA. The older population: 2010," 2010 census brief. Washington, DC: U.S. Census Bureau; 2011.

31. Hussain A, Choukairi F, Dunn K. Predicting survival in thermal injury: a systematic review of methodology of composite prediction models. Burns 2013;39(5): 835–50.

32. Robinson TN, Walston JD, Brummel NE, et al. Frailty for surgeons: review of a national institute on aging conference on frailty for specialists. J Am Coll Surg 2015; 221(6):1083–92.

33. Alpert M, Grigorian A, Joe V, et al. No difference in morbidity or mortality between octogenarians and other geriatric burn trauma patients. Am Surg 2022;88(12): 2907–12.

34. Rodríguez-Mañas L, Féart C, Mann G, et al. Searching for an operational definition of frailty: a delphi method based consensus statement. The frailty operative definition-consensus conference project. J Gerontol: Series A 2012;68(1):62–7.

35. Rockwood K, Stadnyk K, MacKnight C, et al. A brief clinical instrument to classify frailty in elderly people. Lancet 1999;353(9148):205–6.
36. Mitnitski AB, Graham JE, Mogilner AJ, et al. Frailty, fitness and late-life mortality in relation to chronological and biological age. BMC Geriatr 2002;2(1). https://doi.org/10.1186/1471-2318-2-1.
37. Rockwood K. A global clinical measure of fitness and frailty in elderly people. Can Med Assoc J 2005;173(5):489–95.
38. Masud D, Norton S, Smailes ST, et al. The use of a frailty scoring system for burns in the elderly. Burns 2013;39(1):30–6.
39. Joseph B, Pandit V, Zangbar B, et al. Validating trauma-specific frailty index for geriatric trauma patients: a prospective analysis. J Am Coll Surg 2014;219(1):10–7.e1.
40. Orouji Jokar T, Ibraheem K, Rhee P, et al. Emergency general surgery specific frailty index: a validation study. J Trauma Acute Care Surg 2016;81(2):254–60.
41. Maxwell D, Rhee P, Drake M, et al. Development of the burn frailty index: a prognostication index for elderly patients sustaining burn injuries. Am J Surg 2019;218(1):87–94.
42. Boutin RD, Yao L, Canter RJ, et al. Sarcopenia: current concepts and imaging implications. Am J Roentgenol 2015;205(3):W255–66.
43. Morley JE, Anker SD, von Haehling S. Prevalence, incidence, and clinical impact of sarcopenia: facts, numbers, and epidemiology-update 2014. Journal of Cachexia, Sarcopenia and Muscle 2014;5(4):253–9.
44. Cesari M, Landi F, Vellas B, et al. Sarcopenia and physical frailty: two sides of the same coin. Front Aging Neurosci 2014;6.
45. Romanowski KS, Fuanga P, Siddiqui S, et al. Computed tomography measurements of sarcopenia predict length of stay in older burn patients. J Burn Care Res 2020;42(1):3–8.
46. Romanowski KS, Barsun A, Pamlieri TL, et al. Frailty score on admission predicts outcomes in elderly burn injury. J Burn Care Res 2015;36(1):1–6.
47. Romanowski KS, Curtis E, Palmieri TL, et al. Frailty is associated with mortality in patients aged 50 years and older. J Burn Care Res 2017;39(5):703–7.
48. Romanowski K, Curtis E, Barsun A, et al. The frailty tipping point: determining which patients are targets for intervention in a burn population. Burns 2019;45(5):1051–6.
49. Singh I, Gallacher J, Davis K, et al. Predictors of adverse outcomes on an acute geriatric rehabilitation ward. Age Ageing 2012;41(2):242–6.
50. Kawryshanker S, Raymond W, Ingram K, et al. Effect of frailty on functional gain, resource utilisation, and discharge destination: an observational prospective study in a GEM ward. Current Gerontology and Geriatrics Research 2014;2014:e357857.

# Psychological Issues

Emma Turner, BA*, Diana M. Robinson, MD, Kimberly Roaten, PhD

## KEYWORDS

- Psychological concerns • Anxiety • Depression • Trauma related disorders • Pain
- Delirium • Assessment • Psychiatric disorders • Community reintegration
- Long-term psychological sequalae • Body image • Social skills

## KEY POINTS

- Psychological distress is common following a burn injury, and many burn survivors have pre-morbid psychiatric illnesses including mood and trauma-related disorders, and substance and alcohol use.
- Early recognition of psychological distress is important for developing effective treatment plans and determining long-term care needs. Standardized screening tools can be used for symptom detection among burn survivors in various settings at all points of recovery.
- Multimodal treatment and support options including psychotherapy, medication, and community engagement are important components of burn recovery.

## PRACTICAL APPLICATION

Psychological distress is common following a burn injury, and many burn survivors have pre-morbid psychiatric illnesses including mood and trauma-related disorders, and substance and alcohol use.[1] This article is intended to be used by all interdisciplinary health care team members to improve the identification and treatment of common psychological concerns experienced by survivors and is organized to follow the general recovery timeline.

## ACUTE PHASE

The acute phase of treatment is characterized by procedures such as debridement and surgery to treat wound(s) and may require hospital and intensive care unit (ICU) admission.[2] Psychosocial challenges during this phase may include fear/anxiety, pain, delirium, and grief. The treatment team should focus on building rapport and providing education as components of addressing pain and distress. Adopting a collaborative treatment style and emphasizing clear communication helps to provide

The University of Texas Southwestern Medical Center, 5323 Harry Hines Boulevard, Suite CS6.
104B, Dallas, TX 75390, USA
* Corresponding author.
*E-mail addresses:* emma.turner@utsouthwestern.edu (E.T.); diana.robinson@utsouthwestern.
edu (D.M.R.); kimberly.roaten@utsouthwestern.edu (K.R.)

Phys Med Rehabil Clin N Am 34 (2023) 849–866
https://doi.org/10.1016/j.pmr.2023.05.005
1047-9651/23/© 2023 Elsevier Inc. All rights reserved.
pmr.theclinics.com

a foundation for intervention. It is also recommended to normalize a wide range of emotional reactions and provide education about symptoms that require treatment.

### Fear and Anxiety

Fear and anxiety may manifest in response to the trauma leading to the injuries but also the associated social stressors and unknowns while recovering. Patients should be provided with information about the anticipated course of recovery, hospital routines, and availability of behavioral health support. Maintaining a consistent schedule and keeping patients informed about changes to daily activities or care is essential to addressing anxiety while hospitalized. As heightened anxiety impacts comprehension, patients and their families may benefit from the repetition of information.[2]

Providers should consistently assess and treat anxiety before procedures to help minimize anticipatory anxiety. The process of assessing anxiety and pain may provide validation to patients of their concerns and normalize these experiences.[2] Addressing treatment anxiety may also help mitigate pain intensity. Undergoing painful procedures often creates a positive feedback loop: procedural pain elicits anxiety, in turn fostering anticipatory anxiety before the next procedure, and more anxiety during the procedure may increase pain perception.[3] If left unrecognized/untreated, these symptoms may develop into anxiety disorders which will be discussed in more detail later in discussion.

### Pain

During the acute phase, patients commonly experience two primary types of pain: procedural and breakthrough. Procedural, or acute, pain is intense, brief pain that occurs during treatment procedures such as dressing changes or early rehabilitation. Breakthrough pain is intermittent, with intensity increasing rapidly during procedures but also occurring when patients are at rest.[4] Untreated/undertreated pain during hospitalization is correlated with long-term negative psychological outcomes.[5]

#### Assessment
Several validated assessment tools for pain are available, including the Numeric Rating Scale (NRS) and the Visual Analog Scale (VAS).[6] For a thorough review, refer to Loehr and colleagues[7]

#### Treatment recommendations
Interdisciplinary, multimodal pain management is recommended, including both pharmacological and non-pharmacological interventions.[8] Non-pharmacological options with the strongest evidence include cognitive-behavioral therapy (CBT), hypnosis, and distraction via virtual reality. Relaxation techniques (eg, deep breathing, music therapy) are effective for pain reduction in some patients and do not require behavioral health expertise. There is also evidence for involving family in wound care in both pediatric[9] and adult burn populations.[10]

When choosing medication routes of administration during the acute phase, pharmacokinetic and pharmacodynamic medication alterations should be considered. Intravenous medications are generally preferred. In the immediate post-burn injury, there is peripheral and splanchnic vasoconstriction that significantly impairs drug absorption. Treatments and direct complications of burns including IV fluid resuscitation, respiratory support, surgical intervention, end-organ dysfunction, metabolic derangement, and nutritional deficiencies further impair oral (PO) administration via the GI tract.[11]

For additional information including practical, patient-friendly materials on treating pain, refer to fact sheets available through the Burn Injury Model Systems (BIMS) Knowledge and Translation Center.[12]

### Delirium

Delirium is a common neuropsychiatric syndrome characterized by acute changes in cognition, attention, awareness, circadian rhythm dysregulation, and psychomotor dysregulation that are the direct physiological consequence of another medical condition.[13] Symptoms develop rapidly and are a change from previous functioning, with severity often fluctuating throughout the day.[14] The incidence of delirium in adult burn patients varies, with higher rates in those requiring ICU admission (47%) compared to those who do not (5%).[15] For burn patients requiring ventilation, the prevalence of delirium is even higher at 77%.[16] Monitoring for symptoms is particularly important, as delirium can result in negative outcomes for ICU patients, including increased mortality and longer ICU/hospital length of stay.[17] Delirium risk factors include older age ($\geq$65 years old), male sex, pre-morbid cognitive deficits, severity of medical illness, isolation and sensory deprivation, restraints, and immobility.[13]

Delirium can result from a myriad of medical conditions, so a broad differential should consider contributions of multiple sources including infectious, withdrawal, metabolic, trauma, neurological, hypoxia, endocrine, vascular, and intoxication/poisoning.[17] Sleep cycle disruptions can contribute to the development of delirium. Delirium can be mistaken for psychiatric conditions such as posttraumatic stress disorder (PTSD), psychosis, or depression. It is important to recognize delirium early and identify the cause to implement effective treatment.

There are three psychomotoric subtypes of delirium: hyperactive, hypoactive, and normal arousal.[18] Hyperactive delirium is distinguished by psychomotor agitation, wandering, and/or hallucinations and delusions.[19] Patients may suddenly become uncooperative, aggressive, or emotionally labile. Hypoactive symptoms include psychomotor retardation, decreased responsiveness, or a sudden decrease in treatment engagement which may be overlooked or mistaken for depressive symptoms. Symptoms should be monitored throughout the day, as patients commonly fluctuate between subtypes.[19]

While it has been shown that scheduled neuroleptics do not treat or decrease delirium days, the judicious use of psychotropic medications has a role in the symptomatic management of delirium. Neuroleptics can be considered on an individual basis in patients with distressing hallucinations or paranoia or who have agitation that is an imminent risk of harm to the patient or staff. There may be specific considerations for the use of different first or second-generation antipsychotics based on the route of administrations available to the patient (eg, orally, parenteral, intramuscular), medical comorbidities (including impacts on renal and hepatic function and cardiac complications with QT prolongation), severity of agitation, and the desired time to onset of action. In severe agitation due to delirium one of the most common agents of choice is haloperidol due to its lower risks of blood pressure, pulmonary artery pressure, heart rate, delirium, and respiration side effects compared to benzodiazepines.[20] In general, for the treatment of severe agitation, intravenous medications are preferred to have faster drug absorption, lower trauma to the patient, and are lower risk to administer by the staff. Intramuscular injections can complicate interpretations of muscle enzyme studies. Intravenous haloperidol is less likely to cause extrapyramidal symptoms than when given IM or by mouth.[21,22]

*Assessment*
Several validated options are available for assessing delirium, including the Confusion Assessment Method (CAM).[23] ICU-specific assessments include the CAM for the Intensive Care Unit (CAM-ICU)[24] and the Intensive Care Delirium Screening Checklist (ICCDSC).[25] Additional assessment information can be found in Loehr and colleagues[7]

*Treatment recommendations*

- Work-up to determine the etiology of delirium[26]
- Reinforce behavioral strategies for improving the sleep-wake cycle26:
  ○ Minimize and consolidate daytime sleep. Lights on/blinds open throughout the day.
  ○ Minimize nighttime disruptions (eg, vital sign checks, blood draws).
  ○ Optimize the timing of medication to support uninterrupted sleep.
  ○ Utilize eye mask/earplugs to reduce environmental noise.
  ○ Increase time out of bed and mobilizing during daytime hours, as medically appropriate.
- Provide assistive devices such as hearing aids/glasses to improve recognition and orientation.[26]
- Provide a visible clock/calendar for orientation.[26]
- Optimize pain management and minimize the use of deliriogenic medications.[16]
- Provide the patient, family, and visitors with education[26]:
  ○ Information about common symptoms and how to respond.
  ○ Explanation of possible causes and treatment options.
  ○ Involve family in helping patients stay awake during the day, moving about the room, and providing staff with information about baseline functioning and routines.
- For critically ill patients, the intensive care team should implement the ABCDEF bundle of evidence-based interventions.[27]

### Bereavement and Grief

Burn patients may have experienced losses including the death of family, friends, or pets as well as amputation and the loss of belongings/shelter. It is generally recommended that patients are notified about losses as soon as they can understand the information. Ideally the treatment team schedules a time for supportive family or trusted staff members to be present when the news is shared and adapts a plan such as the GRIEV-ING death notification protocol for the discussion.[28]

### MIDDLE PHASE

During the middle phase of treatment, burn patients progress from acute medical care to the early rehabilitation stage. This transition may be associated with new or increased distress as the patient begins to physically heal and understand the extent of injuries, functional limitations, and changes to appearance.[2] Common psychosocial issues during this time may include changes in pain, development of psychiatric symptoms/disorders, and viewing injuries for the first time.

### Changes in Pain from the Acute Phase

Many burn patients continue to experience pain during rehabilitation and ongoing wound care. Pain intensity is associated with numerous factors including depth of burn and number of burn locations.[29] Background pain may continue until the wound is closed. This pain occurs even when the patient is resting and remains consistent throughout the day.[4] Discomfort due to itching and neuropathic pain may occur and be associated with persistent psychological distress.[30] Strategies for assessing pain and effective non-pharmacological interventions remain the same during this phase of recovery. Before discharge, clinicians should adjust pain management plans to outpatient protocols to monitor efficacy and reduce fear about poorly controlled pain at home.

### Psychiatric Disorders

As discussed previously, it is well established that burn patients often have pre-morbid psychiatric disorders and are at risk for the exacerbation/development of symptoms and disorders post-injury.[1,31,32] Common diagnoses include adjustment disorder, acute stress disorder (ASD), posttraumatic stress disorder (PTSD), and substance use disorders (SUDs). In addition, patients may develop symptoms of depressive and anxiety disorders and experience suicidality.

#### Assessment
Few tools have been validated with burn patients but may still be used with appropriate caution and recognition of limitations. Commonly used options are described later in discussion. For a full review of screening and assessment tools to assess psychiatric symptoms after burn injury, please refer to Loehr and colleagues[7]

#### Treatment recommendations
The combination of medication and psychotherapy is typically most effective for moderate to severe disorders. Mild to moderate symptoms may be effectively treated with psychotherapy and other non-pharmacological options such as relaxation and distraction. CBT has the most research supporting its efficacy for reducing the symptoms of major psychiatric disorders experienced by burn patients such as PTSD and Major Depressive Disorder (MDD).[12] Motivational Interviewing-informed techniques may also be helpful for addressing SUD symptoms and enhancing treatment engagement and can be used by all members of the interdisciplinary team.[33,34] It is important to note that some people may experience a variety of symptoms without meeting full diagnostic criteria. Many of the non-pharmacological and supportive treatment recommendations below are still indicated for these patients. In general, when treatment with medication is indicated, the choice of medication and dosage are the same as they would be for a patient without a burn injury.

The following sections consist of brief summaries of the most frequently identified psychiatric disorders among burn patients including information about symptoms, prevalence, assessment, and medication recommendations.

#### Acute stress disorder/posttraumatic stress disorder
- Primary symptoms[14]:
  - 3-30 days post-trauma (ASD), 1-month post-trauma (PTSD)
  - Avoidance, re-experiencing, hyperarousal, negative changes in cognition/mood
- Screening/assessment:
  - PTSD Checklist for DSM-V (PCL-5)[35]
  - Injured Trauma Survivor Screen (ITSS)[36]
- Prevalence:
  - Prevalence of ASD ranges from 10 to 23%.[2]

- ○ Prevalence of PTSD varies greatly over time since injury: 3-35% while hospitalized, 2-40% between 3-6 months, 9-45% at one year, and 7-25% at two or more years post injury.[37]
- Outcomes:
  - ○ Greater difficulty adjusting to injury[38]
  - ○ Longer hospital stays[39]
  - ○ Symptoms of ASD while hospitalized are predictive of PTSD even up to two years post-injury.[40]
- *Medication Treatment*:
  - ○ For patients unable to swallow pills, consider liquid and orally disintegrating formulations[21]:
    - ■ Antidepressants:
      - • Liquid formulations:
        - ○ SSRIs: Citalopram, Escitalopram, fluoxetine, paroxetine, sertraline
      - • Orally disintegrating tablet (ODT):
        - ○ NaSSA (noradrenergic and selective serotonin antagonist): Mirtazapine
    - ■ Anxiolytics (benzodiazepines):
      - • Benzodiazepines are relatively contraindicated for patients with ASD or recent trauma. Although benzodiazepines are commonly used in the symptomatic management of ASD, the long-term risks of benzodiazepines frequently outweigh their short-term benefit. Studies have shown that they are associated with an increased risk of developing PTSD with the use after a recent trauma, paradoxical agitation, and dependence.[41]

### Depressive disorders

- Primary symptoms[14]:
  - ○ Two or more weeks, nearly every day
  - ○ Sad or irritable mood, anhedonia, somatic and cognitive changes (eg, fatigue, appetite/weight changes, difficulty concentrating)
- Screening/assessment:
  - ○ Patient Health Questionnaire-9 (PHQ-9)[42]
  - ○ Hamilton Depression Rating Scale (HAM-D)[43]
- Prevalence:
  - ○ Prevalence of significant MDD symptoms (mild to severe) in adult burn patients has been estimated to be between 13-54% within the year after hospital discharge.[44]
- Outcomes:
  - ○ Greater depressive symptoms in the month following discharge may negatively influence physical functioning within the year after injury.[45]
- Medication Treatment:
  - ○ For patients that are unable to swallow pills there are additional liquid and orally disintegrating formulations to consider[21]:
    - ■ Antidepressants:
      - • As above in the ASD/PTSD Medication Treatment section
      - • Liquid formulations:
        - ○ TCAs: Doxepin
      - • Sublingual:
        - ○ Monoamine oxidase inhibitor (MAOI): Selegiline
      - • Rectal:
        - ○ TCAs: Amitriptyline, doxepin
      - • Transdermal:
        - ○ Monoamine oxidase inhibitor (MAOI): Selegiline

### Anxiety Disorders

- Primary symptoms[14]:
  - Persistent, typically at least six months
  - Restlessness, muscle tension, irritability, difficulty concentrating, sleep disturbances
  - May include panic-like symptoms such as shortness of breath, heart palpitations, nausea, dizziness, and chest pain.
- Screening/assessment:
  - Hospital Anxiety and Depression Scale (HADS)[46]
  - Generalized Anxiety Disorder Assessment (GAD-7)[47]
- Prevalence:
  - Estimated to be 21% at 6-months post burn injury.[48]
- Outcomes:
  - Anxiety symptoms continuing over 2 years post injury may impact levels of pain, fatigue, and physical functioning.[49]
- Medication Treatment:
  - For patients that are unable to swallow pills there are additional liquid and orally disintegrating formulations to consider[21]:
    - Antidepressants:
      - As above in the ASD/PTSD Medication Treatment section
    - Anxiolytics:
      - Liquid formulations:
        - Alprazolam, lorazepam
      - ODTs:
        - Alprazolam, clonazepam
      - Intravenous: Diazepam, lorazepam, midazolam
      - Intramuscular: Chlordiazepoxide, diazepam, lorazepam, midazolam
      - Rectal: Diazepam
    - Antipsychotics:
      - Liquid formulations:
        - Aripiprazole, risperidone, fluphenazine, thioridazine
      - ODTs:
      - Aripiprazole, clozapine, olanzapine
      - Intravenous:
        - Typical antipsychotics: Chlorpromazine, haloperidol, olanzapine, perphenazine
        - Atypical antipsychotics: Chlorpromazine, fluphenazine, haloperidol, loxapine, perphenazine, prochlorperazine, thiothixene
      - Intramuscular:
        - Atypical antipsychotics: Aripiprazole, olanzapine, ziprasidone
      - Sublingual:
        - Asenapine

### Substance/Alcohol Use Disorders

- Primary symptoms[14]:
  - Impaired control, risky use, social impairment, tolerance, and/or withdrawal symptoms
- Screening/assessment:
  - Alcohol Use Disorders Identification Test (AUDIT)[50]
  - Drug Abuse Screen Test (DAST-10)[51]

- Prevalence:
  - For patients admitted to the hospital for a burn injury, rates of substance abuse may be over 50%.[52]
  - Drug/alcohol abuse are among the most common comorbidities in burn patients.[53]
- Outcomes:
  - Longer hospital length of stay, greater number of surgeries, and greater daily use of morphine are associated with SUD.[54]
- Medication Treatment:
  - Acute, severe alcohol, benzodiazepine, or barbiturate withdrawal may lead to seizures and potentially death. Treatment of uncomplicated withdrawal, most commonly with GABA-agonists such as benzodiazepines and less often with phenobarbital, can be completed on a fixed scheduled or symptom-triggered basis with scales such as the Clinical Institute Withdrawal Assessment (CIWA).[55]
  - In addition to medication management, all patients treated for alcohol withdrawal should be given thiamine nutritional supplementation due to increased risk for Wernicke encephalopathy and Korsakoff psychosis, typically at doses of 100 mg PO for low-risk patients. High-risk patients may require high-dose IV repletion (typically 500 mg IV three times daily for three days, though other protocols exist).[56]
  - Screen for low risk versus high risk with the Caine criteria and if there are two of more of the following four signs, then treat with high dose IV thiamine repletion: 1) dietary deficiencies, 2) oculomotor abnormalities, 3) cerebellar dysfunction, and 4) either an altered mental state or mild memory impairment.[57] Patients with a history of opioid misuse experience challenges with pain control due to higher opioid debt leading to the potential need for more opioid analgesia than patients without opioid use. Undertreatment of pain may lead to pain medication-seeking behaviors. Acute opioid withdrawal should be managed with symptomatic medications and opioid agonist medications including buprenorphine and methadone.
  - After the initial treatment of alcohol and opioid withdrawal, patients should be screened for an underlying moderate-severe use disorder and offered medication assistant treatment of alcohol use disorder (typically with naltrexone or acamprosate) and opioid use disorder (typically with buprenorphine, methadone, or naltrexone).
  - Patients should be referred to evidence-based outpatient substance treatment on discharge.

*Suicidality*

- Primary symptoms:
  - Talking about or threatening to kill themselves; seeking access to suicide means (eg, pills, weapons); feeling hopeless and/or trapped; experiencing anger, anxiety, or other sudden mood changes; increasing use of drugs/alcohol; withdrawing from social support[58]
- Screening/assessment:
  - Ask Suicide-Screening Questions (ASQ)[59]
  - Columbia-Suicide Severity Rating Scale (C-SSRS)[60]
- Prevalence:
  - Prevalence of some level of suicidal ideation at both 6- and 12-months post-injury is between 25-33% in adults burn patients.[49]

○ Self-immolation, intentionally setting oneself on fire, as a method of suicide ranges from 1 to 6% of all suicides in the United States and Europe vs. as high as 11% in lower income countries.[61,62]
- *Outcomes*[63]:
  ○ Compared to the general population, burn survivors endorse more suicidal ideation and have a greater lifetime prevalence of suicide attempts.
  ○ Greater risk for suicidality associated with comorbid psychiatric disorders, prior attempts, lack of social support, greater TBSA, and greater pain.

### Viewing Injuries and Changes in Appearance

Body image dissatisfaction is linked to many factors including burn size, importance of appearance, and sex, reinforcing the need for adequate recognition and support.[64] Burn patients may be fearful about viewing their injuries and their overall appearance. The treatment team can first clarify what the patient has seen and then develop a plan for viewing the changed skin with support from family members or hospital staff. A behavioral health clinician can elicit the patient's concerns and expectations related to changes in appearance and generate adaptive coping strategies to reduce and prevent distress. The Phoenix Society for Burn Survivors (The Phoenix Society) is a national organization for the burn community that offers online resources specifically for burn patients, including information about body image changes.[65]

## REINTEGRATION PHASE

Reintegration is the last stage of recovery and is marked by treatment transitions such as hospital discharge, initiation of outpatient care, and returning to school/work.[2] Psychosocial challenges during this phase may include community reintegration, persistent difficulties with sleep and pain, long-term psychological sequelae, and adjustment to body image and sexuality changes.

### Community Reintegration

Reintegrating into the community is an important milestone for burn survivors and their families.[66] Integration outcomes vary based on many factors including sex, age, race/ethnicity, and marital status.[67,68]

Returning to work is a significant part of reintegration associated with functional outcomes and requiring a holistic approach involving areas outside of work itself such as social support, rehabilitation, and survivors' personal characteristics.[69] Research has shown that within approximately 3.5 years, 72% of burn survivors resume some form of work.[70] Factors negatively impacting return to work include greater TBSA, longer hospitalization, greater reported pain, and premorbid psychiatric or physical comorbidities. Additional barriers may include insurance coverage limitations, changes in physical ability, and workplace conditions.[70] A survivor's previous occupation and functional changes following injury may also negatively impact return to work if physical limitations exist. Addressing barriers early is beneficial, including educating survivors about options for vocational rehabilitation or supporting requests for workplace accommodations. Finally, it may be helpful to explore with survivors whether the injury occurred at work; addressing this early may help ease distress and prevent avoidance.

Most pediatric burn survivors enrolled in school will return within 1-2 weeks after discharge.[71] It is recommended to begin planning for transition back to school while the child is still hospitalized and to adjust the timeline based on the social and educational context for each individual.[72] Implementing school re-entry programs has been found to decrease the time it takes to return to school after discharge. Scheduling time for survivors to visit the school and providing education for staff and other students may help ease the transition for all.[73] The Phoenix Society[65] and the Burn Injury BIMS Knowledge and Translation Center[12] offer resources for school re-entry.

### Assessment
Burn survivors' experiences of community integration can be assessed using the Community Integration Questionnaire (CIQ).[74]

### Treatment Recommendations
During this phase, it is important to assist survivors to find or create strong social support networks. Survivors and families can check with their local hospital and/or the nearest American Burn Association-verified burn center to determine if a support group is available. Support groups may help reduce psychological distress[75] and improve outcomes regarding social and work interactions.[76] The Phoenix Society offers formal peer support training through the *Survivors Offering Assistance and Recovery (SOAR)* program. The program links volunteer peers with hospitalized burn survivors to facilitate emotional adjustment.[65] The Phoenix Society also provides educational resources for burn survivors and families, virtual support options, and hosts an annual meeting for survivors, families, and health care providers.[65]

Providing education to families specifically about the transition home can be beneficial, particularly when the survivor's role at home has changed. Recommendations for family members include reinforcing the use of relaxation to manage pain and improve sleep for survivors, listening to the experience/feelings of survivors regarding the injury, and asking for their own support when needed.[77]

For pediatric burn survivors, burn camps are another way to receive peer support in a safe environment. Locations are often near a burn center and staff include professionals with experience treating burns.[78] Qualitative research suggests that the benefits of camp attendance include improved self-esteem, social skills, and coping skills.[77-79]

### Pain and itching/pruritis

Pain during the reintegration phase often meets the threshold for chronic pain, continuing for six or more months following wound healing. The etiology of chronic pain is unknown but hypothesized to be the result of neuropathic pain, which occurs when there is damage to nerve endings in the skin and/or regeneration of nerve endings.[4,80] Continued pain endorsed by outpatients impacts many domains of functioning including work, interpersonal relationships, and sexual functioning. The impact of pain on these areas may be mediated by psychological symptoms, highlighting the need to continue addressing these symptoms during long-term treatment.[81]

Itching, or pruritus, continues to impact more than 40% of burn survivors long-term.[82] Itch can worsen psychological distress by interrupting sleep, making concentration and physical activities difficult, and worsening anxiety.[12]

### Assessment
See recommendations for pain assessments under "Acute Phase." The 4-D Itch Scale is an assessment of itching/pruritus validated with burn patients.[83] Additional assessment information for pruritus can be found in Loehr and colleagues[7]

### Treatment recommendations
Many pharmacological treatments are available for itching and pain, including oral medications and creams/lotions.[12] Additionally, non-pharmacological treatments

are effective for both conditions, including interventions described above (eg, hypnosis, CBT, virtual reality).[8]

## Sleep

The prevalence of sleep disturbances reported by burn survivors following discharge is between 40 and 73%.[84] A strong inverse relationship exists between insomnia and pain, itch, and emotional distress. Dysregulated sleep often improves from the acute phase but continues to be impaired for many survivors in the months to years after discharge.[84]

### Assessment
Several validated sleep assessment tools are publicly available, including the Pittsburg Sleep Quality Index (PSQI)[85] and the Richards-Campbell Sleep Questionnaire (RCSQ).[86]

### Treatment Recommendations
Addressing sleep concerns is particularly important due to its impact on physical and psychological healing. While specific therapeutic interventions exist for disrupted sleep (eg, CBT for Insomnia), any treatment team member can provide psychoeducation on sleep-hygiene practices.

- Consistent sleep/wake schedule
- Restrict activities in bed to sleep and sex
- Allow sunlight in during the day, keep blinds/curtains open
- Do not consume substances containing caffeine, alcohol, or nicotine 4-6 hours before going to bed
- Regular exercise and healthy diet
- Reduce naps (ideally <1 hour)

Research also supports utilizing progressive muscle relaxation to improve sleep quality for burn survivors.[87]

### Medication Treatment
If behavioral techniques are not effective, brief, intermittent use of a sedative-hypnotic agent may be appropriate. Commonly used sedative-hypnotics include several classes, such as sedating antidepressants, benzodiazepines, benzodiazepine receptor agonists, melatonin receptor agonists, antihistamines, and atypical antipsychotics. Melatonin, a hormonal supplement (not FDA approved), decreases sleep latency and improves the quality of sleep.[88] Trazodone, a sedating antidepressant, is one of the most used agents due to improving total sleep time, decreasing sleep latency, decreasing waking after sleep onset, and increasing the quality of sleep (not FDA approved for insomnia).[88] It is commonly used for patients with a history of substance abuse or sedative-hypnotic abuse. The use of benzodiazepines and sedating antihistamines should only be considered with caution in burn patients and only for the briefest duration possible, , due to the risk of delirium.

## Long-term Psychological Sequalae

The treatment team should continue evaluating burn survivors' psychosocial function across the lifespan. Survivors have reported decreased quality of life and poorer physical and mental health years after their injury.[89,90]

Long-term symptoms of depression and anxiety have also been associated with self-reported fatigue, pain, and physical dysfunction.[49] Six months post-injury, research has found that 55% of burn survivors met the criteria for at least one psychiatric disorder.[48]

### Body image

Dissatisfaction with body image may be influenced by gender, race/ethnicity, TBSA, and personal value of appearance.[64,91] Pre-existing fear of negative evaluation by others and greater perceived stigmatization due to the burn injury may also play a role in body image concerns.[92]

Burns that are not visible, or "hidden" burns, can also lead to distress regarding body image. Anecdotal accounts from burn survivors cite difficulties such as knowing if, when, or how to reveal a hidden burn injury.[93]

### Assessment

The Satisfaction with Appearance Scale (SWAP) is a publicly available self-report tool validated for burn survivors.[94]

### Treatment Recommendations

Body image concerns may be exacerbated by negative social interactions such as people staring, avoiding, or asking intrusive questions. Resources and training provided by The Phoenix Society can help survivors prepare for these interactions to reduce anticipatory anxiety and improve confidence.[95] In addition, cognitive-behavioral strategies such as cognitive restructuring and psychoeducation regarding the development of body image are effective for burn survivors.[95]

### Sexuality

In addition to body image, concerns about sexuality are common. Survivors may experience pain or changes in sensation, as well as low libido due to pharmacological side effects, fear of rejection, or low self-esteem. Education may include partners of survivors, who are often balancing the role of caregiver and intimate partner. Difficulties regarding relationships, body image, and sexuality seem to persist in the year following discharge and greatly impact the overall quality of life.[96,97]

Members of the burn team should address these concerns early with burn survivors and/or their partner. Different aspects of sexuality education can be addressed collaboratively by the interdisciplinary team; for example, occupational therapists may address functional changes for comfort and safety and behavioral health clinicians may address emotional concerns and communication. Bringing up sexuality as a possible concern helps to normalize discussion of these issues as an important part of the recovery process. The Phoenix Society provides additional strategies and tools to discuss sexuality with burn survivors.[65]

### Social Skills

As part of preparing patients and families for reintegration into the community, treatment team members should provide education to enhance social skills throughout recovery. Current literature is limited regarding the efficacy of formal social skills training to assist survivors and families with reintegration, but anecdotal evidence suggests that these skills may ease the transition by promoting increased confidence and reducing avoidance. For example, providers can assist survivors in generating rehearsed responses to questions regarding their injuries. Burn survivors have reported these practiced responses are helpful and may include the use of humor, redirection, reassurance, or a brief explanation. Additional training can include strategies such as role-playing commonly faced social situations. The Phoenix Society provides training and materials for building social skills.[65]

## CLINICS CARE POINTS

- Monitor closely for psychological distress and assess the history of psychiatric illness and treatment, including substance and alcohol use disorders
  - Utilize validated screening and assessment tools for monitoring symptoms
  - Consider medication for moderate to severe symptomatology
  - Refer for psychotherapy and normalize the role of behavioral health clinicians in recovery
- Monitor closely for delirium during the acute phase of recovery and after significant procedures or illness
  - Identify and treat the cause of delirium
  - Reinforce behavioral strategies including sleep hygiene and mobilization
  - Educate patients and families about the etiology of symptoms and strategies for mitigation
- Assess sleep during all phases of recovery
  - Provide education regarding sleep hygiene
  - Monitor for the effect of sleep dysfunction on physical and mental health
  - Avoid nighttime interruptions
- Use multimodal strategies to assess and treat pain and itch
  - Proactively discuss and address pain management early and often during recovery
  - Implement and/or recommend non-pharmacological strategies for pain management
- Be aware of evidence-based/informed community support resources
  - The Phoenix Society and ABA verified burn center support groups
  - Burn camps
  - BIMS fact sheets

## ACKNOWLEDGEMENT

The contents of this article were developed under a grant from the National Institute on Disability, Independent Living, and Rehabilitation Research (NIDILRR grant number 90DPBU0006). NIDILRR is a Center within the Administration for Community Living (ACL), Department of Health and Human Services (HHS). The contents of this article do not necessarily represent the policy of NIDILRR, ACL, or HHS, and you should not assume endorsement by the Federal Government.

## REFERENCES

1. Patterson DR, Finch CP, Wiechman SA, et al. Premorbid mental health status of adult burn patients: comparison with a normative sample. J Burn Care Rehabil 2003;24(5):347–50.
2. Rosenberg L, Rosenberg M, Rimmer RB, et al. 66 - Psychosocial recovery and reintegration of patients with burn injuries. In: Herndon DN, editor. Total burn care. Fifth Edition. Elsevier; 2018. p. 709–20.e4.
3. Summer GJ, Puntillo KA, Miaskowski C, et al. Burn injury pain: the continuing challenge. J Pain 2007;8(7):533–48.
4. Wiechman Askay S, Patterson DR, Sharar SR, et al. Pain management in patients with burn injuries. Int Rev Psychiatry 2009;21(6):522–30.
5. Patterson DR, Tininenko J, Ptacek JT. Pain during burn hospitalization predicts long-term outcome. J Burn Care Res 2006;27(5):719–26.
6. Wibbenmeyer L, Sevier A, Liao J, et al. Evaluation of the usefulness of two established pain assessment tools in a burn population. J Burn Care Res 2011;32(1): 52–60.

7. Loehr VGG WF, Roaten K. Screening and assessment for psychological distress among burn survivors. European Burn Journal 2022;3(1):57–88.
8. Romanowski KS, Carson J, Pape K, et al. American burn association guidelines on the management of acute pain in the adult burn patient: a review of the literature, a compilation of expert opinion, and next steps. J Burn Care Res 2020; 41(6):1129–51.
9. Egberts MR, de Jong AEE, Hofland HWC, et al. Parental presence or absence during paediatric burn wound care procedures. Burns 2018;44(4):850–60.
10. Bishop SM, Walker MD, Spivak IM. Family presence in the adult burn intensive care unit during dressing changes. Crit Care Nurse 2013;33(1):14–24.
11. Bittner EA, Shank E, Woodson L, et al. Acute and perioperative care of the burn-injured patient. Anesthesiology 2015;122(2):448–64.
12. Burn Injury Factsheets. Model Systems Knowledge Translation Center. Available at: https://msktc.org/burn/factsheets. Accessed February 25, 2023.
13. Maldonado JR. Delirium pathophysiology: An updated hypothesis of the etiology of acute brain failure. Int J Geriatr Psychiatry 2018;33(11):1428–57.
14. American Psychiatric Association. Diagnostic and statistical manual of mental disorders. 5th edition. American Psychiatric Association; 2013.
15. Abdelrahman I, Vieweg R, Irschik S, et al. Development of delirium: association with old age, severe burns, and intensive care. Burns 2020;46(4):797–803.
16. Agarwal V, O'Neill PJ, Cotton BA, et al. Prevalence and risk factors for development of delirium in burn intensive care unit patients. J Burn Care Res 2010;31(5): 706–15.
17. Barr J, Fraser GL, Puntillo K, et al. Clinical practice guidelines for the management of pain, agitation, and delirium in adult patients in the intensive care unit. Crit Care Med 2013;41(1):263–306.
18. Han JH, Hayhurst CJ, Chandrasekhar R, et al. Delirium's arousal subtypes and their relationship with 6-month functional status and cognition. Psychosomatics 2019;60(1):27–36.
19. Meagher D. Motor subtypes of delirium: past, present and future. Int Rev Psychiatry 2009;21(1):59–73.
20. Cassem N, Sos J. Intravenous use of haloperidol for acute delirium in intensive care settings. Thieme; 1978. p. 196–9.
21. Stern TA. Massachusetts general hospital handbook of general hospital psychiatry. Stuttgart (Germany): Elsevier Inc.; 2018.
22. Girard TD, Exline MC, Carson SS, et al. Haloperidol and ziprasidone for treatment of delirium in critical illness. N Engl J Med 2018;379(26):2506–16.
23. Shi Q, Warren L, Saposnik G, et al. Confusion assessment method: a systematic review and meta-analysis of diagnostic accuracy. Neuropsychiatr Dis Treat 2013; 9:1359–70.
24. Ely EW, Margolin R, Francis J, et al. Evaluation of delirium in critically ill patients: validation of the confusion assessment method for the intensive care unit (CAM-ICU). Crit Care Med 2001;29(7):1370–9.
25. Bergeron N, Dubois MJ, Dumont M, et al. Intensive care delirium screening checklist: evaluation of a new screening tool. Intensive Care Med 2001;27(5): 859–64.
26. Rieck KM, Pagali S, Miller DM. Delirium in hospitalized older adults. Hosp Pract 2020;48(sup1):3–16.
27. Ely EW. The ABCDEF bundle: science and philosophy of how ICU liberation serves patients and families. Crit Care Med 2017;45(2):321–30.

28. Hobgood C, Woodyard J, Sawning S, et al. Delivering the news with compassion: the GRIEV_ING death notification protocol. MedEdPORTAL 2010;6:8210.
29. Singer AJ, Beto L, Singer DD, et al. Association between burn characteristics and pain severity. Am J Emerg Med 2015;33(9):1229–31.
30. Van Loey NEE, de Jong AEE, Hofland HWC, et al. Role of burn severity and post-traumatic stress symptoms in the co-occurrence of itch and neuropathic pain after burns: a longitudinal study. Front Med 2022;9:997183.
31. Fauerbach JA, McKibben J, Bienvenu OJ, et al. Psychological distress after major burn injury. Psychosom Med 2007;69(5):473–82.
32. Logsetty S, Shamlou A, Gawaziuk JP, et al. Mental health outcomes of burn: a longitudinal population-based study of adults hospitalized for burns. Burns 2016; 42(4):738–44.
33. Rollnick S, Miller WR, Butler CC, et al. Motivational interviewing in health care: helping patients change behavior. COPD. Journal of Chronic Obstructive Pulmonary Disease 2008;5(3):203.
34. Goans CRR, Meltzer KJ, Martin B, et al. Treatment adherence interventions for burn patients: what works and what role can motivational interviewing play? European Burn Journal 2022;3(2):309–19.
35. Blevins CA, Weathers FW, Davis MT, et al. The posttraumatic stress disorder checklist for DSM-5 (PCL-5): development and initial psychometric evaluation. J Trauma Stress 2015;28(6):489–98.
36. Hunt JC, Sapp M, Walker C, et al. Utility of the injured trauma survivor screen to predict PTSD and depression during hospital admission. J Trauma Acute Care Surg 2017;82(1):93–101.
37. Giannoni-Pastor A, Eiroa-Orosa FJ, Fidel Kinori SG, et al. Prevalence and predictors of posttraumatic stress symptomatology among burn survivors: a systematic review and meta-analysis. J Burn Care Res 2016;37(1):e79–89.
38. Fauerbach JA, Lawrence JW, Munster AM, et al. Prolonged adjustment difficulties among those with acute posttrauma distress following burn injury. J Behav Med 1999;22(4):359–78.
39. Fauerbach JA, Lawrence J, Haythornthwaite J, et al. Preburn psychiatric history affects posttrauma morbidity. Psychosomatics 1997;38(4):374–85.
40. McKibben JB, Bresnick MG, Wiechman Askay SA, et al. Acute stress disorder and posttraumatic stress disorder: a prospective study of prevalence, course, and predictors in a sample with major burn injuries. J Burn Care Res 2008; 29(1):22–35.
41. Guina J, Rossetter SR, De RB, et al. Benzodiazepines for PTSD: a systematic review and meta-analysis. J Psychiatr Pract 2015;21(4):281–303.
42. Spitzer RL, Kroenke K, Williams JB. Validation and utility of a self-report version of PRIME-MD: the PHQ primary care study. Primary Care Evaluation of Mental Disorders. Patient Health Questionnaire. JAMA 1999;282(18):1737–44.
43. Hamilton M. A rating scale for depression. J Neurol Neurosurg Psychiatr 1960; 23(1):56–62.
44. Thombs BD, Bresnick MG, Magyar-Russell G. Depression in survivors of burn injury: a systematic review. Gen Hosp Psychiatry 2006;28(6):494–502.
45. Ullrich PM, Askay SW, Patterson DR. Pain, depression, and physical functioning following burn injury. Rehabil Psychol 2009;54(2):211–6.
46. Zigmond AS, Snaith RP. The hospital anxiety and depression scale. Acta Psychiatr Scand 1983;67(6):361–70.
47. Spitzer RL, Kroenke K, Williams JB, et al. A brief measure for assessing generalized anxiety disorder: the GAD-7. Arch Intern Med 2006;166(10):1092–7.

48. Palmu R, Suominen K, Vuola J, et al. Mental disorders after burn injury: a prospective study. Burns 2011;37(4):601–9.
49. Edwards RR, Smith MT, Klick B, et al. Symptoms of depression and anxiety as unique predictors of pain-related outcomes following burn injury. Ann Behav Med 2007;34(3):313–22.
50. Babor TF, Higgins-Biddle JC, Saunders JB, et al. AUDIT: the alcohol use disorders identification test : guidelines for use in primary health care. 2nd ed. Geneva: World Health Organization; 2001.
51. Skinner HA. The drug abuse screening test. Addict Behav 1982;7(4):363–71.
52. Hodgman EI, Subramanian M, Wolf SE, et al. The effect of illicit drug use on outcomes following burn injury. J Burn Care Res 2017;38(1):e89–94.
53. Thombs BD, Singh VA, Halonen J, et al. The effects of preexisting medical comorbidities on mortality and length of hospital stay in acute burn injury: evidence from a national sample of 31,338 adult patients. Ann Surg 2007;245(4):629–34.
54. Duraes EFR, Hung Y-C, Asif M, et al. Acute burn treatment and history of drug and alcohol addiction: treatment outcomes and opioid use. European Burn Journal 2022;3(1):10–7.
55. Wiehl WO, Hayner G, Galloway G. Haight Ashbury Free Clinics' drug detoxification protocols–Part 4: Alcohol. J Psychoactive Drugs 1994;26(1):57–9.
56. Thomson AD, Guerrini I, Marshall EJ. The evolution and treatment of Korsakoff's syndrome: out of sight, out of mind? Neuropsychol Rev 2012;22(2):81–92.
57. Caine D, Halliday GM, Kril JJ, et al. Operational criteria for the classification of chronic alcoholics: identification of Wernicke's encephalopathy. J Neurol Neurosurg Psychiatr 1997;62(1):51–60.
58. Rudd MD, Berman AL, Joiner TE Jr, et al. Warning signs for suicide: theory, research, and clinical applications. Suicide Life Threat Behav 2006;36(3):255–62.
59. Horowitz LM, Snyder DJ, Boudreaux ED, et al. Validation of the ask suicide-screening questions for adult medical inpatients: a brief tool for all ages. Psychosomatics 2020;61(6):713–22.
60. Posner K, Brown GK, Stanley B, et al. The columbia-suicide severity rating scale: initial validity and internal consistency findings from three multisite studies with adolescents and adults. Am J Psychiatry 2011;168(12):1266–77.
61. Peck MD. Epidemiology of burns throughout the World. Part II: intentional burns in adults. Burns 2012;38(5):630–7.
62. Nisavic M, Nejad SH, Beach SR. Intentional self-inflicted burn injuries: review of the literature. Psychosomatics 2017;58(6):581–91.
63. Lerman SF, Sylvester S, Hultman CS, et al. Suicidality after burn injuries: a systematic review. J Burn Care Res 2021;42(3):357–64.
64. Thombs BD, Notes LD, Lawrence JW, et al. From survival to socialization: a longitudinal study of body image in survivors of severe burn injury. J Psychosom Res 2008;64(2):205–12.
65. Phoenix Society for Burn Survivors. Phoenix Society for Burn Survivors. Available at: https://www.phoenix-society.org. Accessed February 27, 2023.
66. Blakeney P, Partridge J, Rumsey N. Community integration. J Burn Care Res 2007;28(4):598–601.
67. Esselman PC, Ptacek JT, Kowalske K, et al. Community integration after burn injuries. J Burn Care Rehabil 2001;22(3):221–7.
68. Pierce BS, Perrin PB, Pugh M, et al. Racial/ethnic disparities in longitudinal trajectories of community integration after burn injury. Am J Phys Med Rehabil 2020;99(7):602–7.

69. Oster C, Kildal M, Ekselius L. Return to work after burn injury: burn-injured individuals' perception of barriers and facilitators. J Burn Care Res 2010;31(4): 540–50.

70. Mason ST, Esselman P, Fraser R, et al. Return to work after burn injury: a systematic review. J Burn Care Res 2012;33(1):101–9.

71. Christiansen M, Carrougher GJ, Engrav LH, et al. Time to school re-entry after burn injury is quite short. J Burn Care Res 2007;28(3):478–81 [discussion: 482-3].

72. Pan R, Dos Santos BD, Nascimento LC, et al. School reintegration of pediatric burn survivors: an integrative literature review. Burns 2018;44(3):494–511.

73. Arshad SN, Gaskell SL, Baker C, et al. Measuring the impact of a burns school reintegration programme on the time taken to return to school: a multidisciplinary team intervention for children returning to school after a significant burn injury. Burns 2015;41(4):727–34.

74. Willer B, Ottenbacher KJ, Coad ML. The community integration questionnaire. A comparative examination. Am J Phys Med Rehabil 1994;73(2):103–11.

75. Won P, Bello MS, Stoycos SA, et al. The impact of peer support group programs on psychosocial outcomes for burn survivors and caregivers: a review of the literature. J Burn Care Res 2021;42(4):600–9.

76. Grieve B, Shapiro GD, Wibbenmeyer L, et al. Long-term social reintegration outcomes for burn survivors with and without peer support attendance: a life impact burn recovery evaluation (LIBRE) study. Arch Phys Med Rehabil 2020;101(1s): S92–s98.

77. Rimmer RB, Fornaciari GM, Foster KN, et al. Impact of a pediatric residential burn camp experience on burn survivors' perceptions of self and attitudes regarding the camp community. J Burn Care Res 2007;28(2):334–41.

78. Maslow GR, Lobato D. Summer camps for children with burn injuries: a literature review. J Burn Care Res 2010;31(5):740–9.

79. Kornhaber R, Visentin D, Kaji Thapa D, et al. Burn camps for burns survivors—Realising the benefits for early adjustment: a systematic review. Burns 2020; 46(1):33–43.

80. Schneider JC, Harris NL, El Shami A, et al. A descriptive review of neuropathic-like pain after burn injury. J Burn Care Res 2006;27(4):524–8.

81. Cariello AN, Perrin PB, Tyler CM, et al. Mediational models of pain, mental health, and functioning in individuals with burn injury. Rehabil Psychol 2021;66(1):1–9.

82. Carrougher GJ, Martinez EM, McMullen KS, et al. Pruritus in adult burn survivors: postburn prevalence and risk factors associated with increased intensity. J Burn Care Res 2013;34(1):94–101.

83. Amtmann D, McMullen K, Kim J, et al. Psychometric properties of the Modified 5-D Itch scale in a burn model system sample of people with burn injury. J Burn Care Res 2017;38(1):e402–8.

84. Lerman SF, Owens MA, Liu T, et al. Sleep after burn injuries: a systematic review and meta-analysis. Sleep Med Rev 2022;65:101662.

85. Buysse DJ, Reynolds CF 3rd, Monk TH, et al. The pittsburgh sleep quality index: a new instrument for psychiatric practice and research. Psychiatry Res 1989; 28(2):193–213.

86. Richards KC, O'Sullivan PS, Phillips RL. Measurement of sleep in critically ill patients. J Nurs Meas 2000;8(2):131–44. Fall-Winter.

87. Harorani M, Davodabady F, Masmouei B, et al. The effect of progressive muscle relaxation on anxiety and sleep quality in burn patients: A randomized clinical trial. Burns 2020;46(5):1107–13.

88. Sateia MJ, Buysse DJ, Krystal AD, et al. Clinical practice guideline for the pharmacologic treatment of chronic insomnia in adults: an american academy of sleep medicine clinical practice guideline. J Clin Sleep Med 2017;13(2):307–49.

89. Bich CS, Kostev K, Baus A, et al. Burn injury and incidence of psychiatric disorders: a retrospective cohort study of 18,198 patients from Germany. Burns 2021; 47(5):1110–7.

90. Abouzeid CA, Wolfe AE, Ni P, et al. Are burns a chronic condition? Examining patient reported outcomes up to 20 years after burn injury-A Burn Model System National Database investigation. J Trauma Acute Care Surg 2022;92(6):1066–74.

91. Mata-Greve F, Wiechman SA, McMullen K, et al. The relation between satisfaction with appearance and race and ethnicity: a National Institute on Disability, Independent Living, and Rehabilitation Research burn model system study. Burns 2022;48(2):345–54.

92. Willemse H, Geenen R, Egberts MR, et al. Perceived stigmatization and fear of negative evaluation: Two distinct pathways to body image dissatisfaction and self-esteem in burn survivors. Psychol Health 2021;1–14. https://doi.org/10.1080/08870446.2021.1970160.

93. Edwards KJ. Learning to Live with Hidden Burns. Phoenix Society for Burn Survivors. Available at: https://www.phoenix-society.org/resources/learning-to-live-with-hidden-burns. Accessed February 27, 2023.

94. Lawrence JW, Heinberg LJ, Roca R, et al. Development and validation of the Satisfaction with appearance scale: assessing body image among burn-injured patients. Psychol Assess 1998;10:64–70.

95. Wiechman Askay S. Gaining and Maintaining a Healthy Body Image. December 3, 2019. Available at: https://www.phoenix-society.org/resources/gaining-and-maintaining-a-healthy-body-image. Accessed February 27, 2023.

96. Connell KM, Coates R, Doherty-Poirier M, et al. A literature review to determine the impact of sexuality and body image changes following burn injuries. Sex Disabil 2013;31:403–12.

97. Connell KM, Phillips M, Coates R, et al. Sexuality, body image and relationships following burns: analysis of BSHS-B outcome measures. Burns 2014;40(7): 1329–37.

# A Narrative Review of Outcomes in Burn Rehabilitation Based on the International Classification of Functioning, Disability, and Health

Huan Deng, PhD[a,1], Timothy J. Genovese, MD, MPH[a,1],
Jeffrey C. Schneider, MD[a,b,c],*

## KEYWORDS

- Burn injury • Outcomes • Rehabilitation • International classification of functioning
- Disability and health • Function • Participation

## KEY POINTS

- Burn injury commonly causes chronic impairments ranging from anatomical structures and physiological functions to activities of daily living and social integration.
- The International Classification of Functioning, Disability, and Health (ICF) is increasingly being used to comprehensively survey the long-term impairments and related needs of burn survivors; subsequent research has resulted in the publication of diverse patient-centered outcomes.
- Primary long-term functional impairments, particularly in skin functions, sensory functions, joint and muscle functions, and mental function, are associated with burn survivors' ability to perform prior essential activities and participation in social activities. These long-term challenges faced by survivors drive the increasing recognition of burn injury as a chronic condition.
- Greater burn severity, older patient age, and psychosocial barriers such as lack of support and insurance are associated with poorer outcomes across domains.
- Future research may clarify impairments in specific functional activities and examine subtle engagement limitations in prior social roles as well as potential interventions to address such problems.

[a] Department of Physical Medicine and Rehabilitation, Spaulding Rehabilitation Hospital, Harvard Medical School, 300 1st Avenue, Boston, MA 02129, USA; [b] Rehabilitation Outcomes Center at Spaulding, Boston, MA, USA; [c] Massachusetts General Hospital, Harvard Medical School, Boston, MA, USA
[1] Huan Deng and Timothy J. Genovese contributed equally to this article.
* Corresponding author.
*E-mail address:* jcschneider@mgh.harvard.edu

Phys Med Rehabil Clin N Am 34 (2023) 867–881
https://doi.org/10.1016/j.pmr.2023.05.006
1047-9651/23/© 2023 Elsevier Inc. All rights reserved.
pmr.theclinics.com

## INTRODUCTION

Approximately 486,000 individuals in the United States (US) receive medical treatment in a hospital or emergency department for burn injury annually.[1] Burn injuries are increasingly recognized as causing diverse and dynamic biopsychosocial challenges that can persist throughout survivorship. There is growing evidence regarding burn survivor outcomes being reported from larger datasets. It is important to summarize common impairments after burn injury that will guide future rehabilitation for comprehensive burn recovery.

The International Classification of Functioning, Disability, and Health (ICF) model developed by the World Health Organization (WHO) in 2001 is a framework for comprehensively assessing the array of biopsychosocial impairments after injuries.[2,3] As shown in **Fig. 1**, the ICF considers not only the effects of disease on body structure and function, but also effects on activities and participation in societal roles. This article is organized using the domains of the ICF to present an update on adult burn rehabilitation outcomes with a focus on common long-term functional limitations and participation restrictions.

## BODY FUNCTIONS AND STRUCTURES

This section combines body functions with corresponding body structures in the ICF model, and highlights the long-term functional impairments after burn injuries **(Table 1)**.

### *Skin and Related Structures*

Skin is the organ primarily involved in a burn injury. Burn severity, determined by the size of the total body surface area (TBSA) involved and depth of damaged skin and subcutaneous tissues, is strongly associated with many long-term outcomes. Based on studies published from 2001 to 2016, burn injury severity globally shows a decreasing trend over time likely related to an increase in burn prevention education.[4]

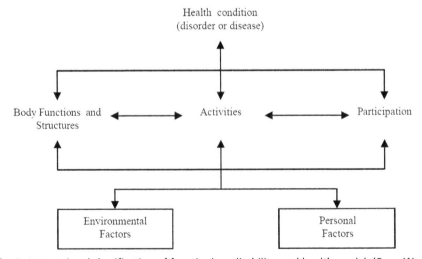

**Fig. 1.** International classification of functioning, disability, and health model. (*From* World Health Organization. (2001). ICF: International Classification of Functioning, Disability and Health. Available at: http://www.who.int/icf.)

**Table 1**
**Common long-term functional impairments after burn injury using the world health organization international classification of functioning, disability, and health framework**

| ICF Category | Example of Functional Impairment after Burn Injury |
|---|---|
| Skin and related structures<br>b810 Protective functions of the skin<br>b820 Repair functions of the skin<br>b830 Other functions of the skin<br>b840 Sensation related to the skin | for example, hypertrophic scarring and pruritus |
| Movement-related structures<br>b710 Mobility of joint functions<br>b730 Muscle power functions<br>b740 Muscle endurance functions | for example, joint contracture and muscle weakness |
| Genitourinary and reproductive systems<br>b640 Sexual functions | for example, erectile dysfunction |
| Digestive, metabolic, and endocrine systems<br>b540 General metabolic functions<br>b550 Thermoregulatory functions | for example, heat and cold intolerance |
| Immunological, cardiovascular, and respiratory systems<br>b410 Heart functions<br>b435 Immunological system functions<br>b455 Exercise tolerance functions | for example, fatigue |
| Voice and speech<br>b310 Voice functions | for example, dysphonia |
| Eye, ear, and related structures, sensory functions, and pain<br>b280 Sensation of pain | for example, chronic pain |
| Nervous system and mental functions<br>b134 Sleep functions<br>b152 Emotional functions | for example, sleep disturbance and anxiety |

At the early stage of a burn injury, the patient is at risk of developing wound infection, sepsis, and multi-organ dysfunction due to loss of skin's protective function.[5] Abnormal or delayed wound healing usually leads to scar formation. It has been reported that the prevalence of hypertrophic scar after burn injury is between 32% and 72%. Patients are more likely to develop hypertrophic scar with younger age, female sex, darker skin tone, greater injury severity, delayed wound healing, involvement of neck or upper extremity, or treatment with surgery or meshed skin grafts. Scarring may continue to worsen for months after the initial injury, and become erythematous, firm, and elevated. Hypertrophic scarring has shown a significant negative influence on survivors' long-term psychosocial outcomes.[6]

Burn injury may cause transient or permanent sensory problems by damaging sensory receptors in the skin. Pruritus is the most common sensory disturbance and has been reported in more than 70% of the survivors at 12 and 24 months after burn injury. Pruritus symptoms are the most significant during the first 3 months post-injury. Similarly, more than 66% of the survivors reported paresthesia. Sensory problems tend to be more severe and chronic for deep burns and grafted skin compared to superficial burns.[7] Furthermore, burn injury may damage cutaneous accessory structures including hair, nails, and sweat and sebaceous glands that can lead to hair loss, skin dryness, and thermoregulation impairment.

### Movement-related Structures

Fourth degree or deep burns of the extremity cause direct damage to muscle, tendon, and bone. Amputation following a burn injury is rare. It has been reported that 1.4% of the 8313 patients admitted to a regional burn center received at least one amputation. Fingers (46.7%) and toes (22%) were the most common amputation locations and were significantly associated with electrical burns.[8]

Joint contracture is a critical physical sequela of burn injury and is defined by a restricted passive range of motion. The major cause of joint contracture is scarring with a prevalence of 38% to 54% at hospital discharge and decreasing during the rehabilitation period. Upper extremity contracture is more common than lower extremity contracture among burn survivors.[9] It is also possible that joint contracture results from immobilization and heterotopic ossification after burn injury, and severe joint contracture may progress to joint deformity with total loss of joint movement.

Skeletal muscle metabolism provides energy for wound healing and is altered by the hypermetabolic response to burn injury, especially after severe injuries. Muscle catabolism may persist after wound closure, and results in muscle wasting and atrophy.[10] One study demonstrated significant losses of lower extremity muscle strength ranging from 20% to 30% at an average of 20 weeks post-injury in patients with severe lower extremity burns compared to healthy controls.[11] Problems related to muscle, tendon and bone will further affect burn survivors' balance, gait, and movement coordination.

### Genitourinary and Reproductive Systems

Burn injury involving the genitalia and perineum has been classified as a major burn injury by the American Burn Association. Genital burns comprise 2.8% to 13% of all hospital admissions for burn injury. Flame and chemical burns are common agents for adult genital burns, whereas scald is the major cause for children genital burns.[12] Genital burns may directly cause sexual dysfunction due to hypoesthesia or erectile dysfunction. It is increasingly recognized that multiple other factors following a burn injury, including alteration in body image, hormonal imbalance, and medication side effects, impact sexual function with possible long-term effects. For pregnant individuals, burn injury also increases the risk of abortion and premature labor.

### Digestive, Metabolic, and Endocrine Systems

Metabolic response following burn injury is possibly present as an increase in the basal metabolic rate, while severe burn injury is associated with a profound hypermetabolic response. Increased metabolism and degradation of muscle protein following the hypermetabolic response can lead to significant weight loss and increased mortality. Patients with more than 40% TBSA showed an average of 10% weight loss at the 2nd week and 22% at the 8th week after injury. The catabolic response can persist for years after severe burns and is associated with insulin resistance, increased infection risk, and multi-organ dysfunction.[13]

Thermoregulation is the ability of maintaining core body temperature. Within 24 hours after a burn injury, 38% of adult patients demonstrated hypothermia that was significantly related to TBSA and inhalation injury.[14] Given changes in metabolic activities and damage to skin structures, burn survivors are prone to temperature sensitivity in the long term, such as heat and cold intolerance. It has been reported that temperature sensitivity is present in 43% of the individuals at discharge, 17% at 1 year, and 9% at 2 years after injury.[15] Moreover, temperature sensitivity is commonly reported by survivors to limit their participation in outdoor activities and physical exercise when they return and live in the community.

## Immunological, Cardiovascular, and Respiratory Systems

In addition to the acute inflammatory response to injury, burn injury has long-term effects on the immune system. The burn population has shown twice the number of hospital admissions and 3.5 times the length of hospital stay compared to the uninjured population due to infectious diseases.[16] Similarly, cardiovascular diseases following burn injuries were significantly associated with 1.46 times of hospital admissions, three times the length of hospital stay, and 1.12 times risk of long-term mortality for those older than 45 years compared to uninjured controls. Ischemic heart disease, congestive heart failure, and cerebrovascular disease accounted for more than 60% of the hospital re-admissions.[17]

For the respiratory system, burn patients may get clinical consequences of acute pulmonary infection, respiratory failure, and long-term functional deficits in exercise tolerance. Even at 5 years after burn injury, survivors with an average of 33.3% TBSA showed a significant lower tolerance for aerobic exercise than the healthy individuals.[18]

## Voice and Speech

Damage to the structures of the upper respiratory tract may result from direct thermal injury after hot gas inhalation, local or systematic chemical injury after toxic gas inhalation, impaired oxygen transportation or utilization, or systematic inflammatory response syndrome after burn injuries. A larynx injury is also reported after an endotracheal intubation with possible sequelae of posterior glottic scarring and arytenoid cartilage dislocation. Cough and dysphonia are the most common clinical symptoms of laryngeal inhalation injuries after burns. Other clinical symptoms include dysphasia, dyspnea, wheezes/rales, and stridor.[19] One study examined the voice function in a group of survivors ranging from 16 to 25 years after burn injuries with varied inhalation injury, smoke exposure, and intubation. The results showed that more than half of the participants had dysphonia and all participants demonstrated different degrees of laryngeal mucosa abnormity.[20]

## Eye, Ear and Related Structures, Sensory Functions, and Pain

Survivors with facial burns are associated with the increased risk of developing psychological problems and experiencing social re-integration challenges during recovery. The eye is commonly involved in facial burns. Among all burn injuries to the eye and its related structures, eyelid burns are the most frequently reported. Possible complications following ocular burns include visual loss, lagophthalmos, and ectropion.[21] The ear is another structure commonly involved in facial burns. One study reviewed the burn patients admitted to a regional burn center in a 4-year period. The results showed that few patients reported damage to the inner and middle ear, whereas 22% of the patients with facial burns had auricle injuries. Due to limited blood perfusion and lack of subcutaneous layer, burns of the ear cartilage may result in chondritis, cartilage infection, and necrosis, as well as subsequent deformation or loss of peripheral auricular structures, which cause cosmetic and functional impacts.[22]

Pain is one of the most frequently reported problems throughout the whole recovery process. At the time of burn injury, patients with partial-thickness burns commonly experience more intensive acute pain than those with full-thickness burns due to the destruction of sensory nerve endings in the affected skin. The burned location may remain painful and sensitive to mechanical and thermal stimulation for days due to the inflammatory response following injury. Survivors also report procedural pain during dressing change, wound cleaning, and early mobilization of the burned areas. Furthermore, approximately 25% to 36% of the burn population develop chronic pain. With direct or indirect damage to peripheral nerves, 7.3% to 18% of the burn patients report chronic neuropathic pain.[23]

### Nervous System and Mental Functions

Burn injury may co-exist with traumatic brain injury (TBI) and cause damage to the nervous system. Approximately 3% of the burn patients in a national trauma database experienced TBIs and 9% of them experienced other traumatic injuries. TBI and burn co-diagnosis appears to be associated with both greater injury severity at hospital admission and higher mortality than burn co-diagnosis with other injuries.[24] Meanwhile, around two-thirds of the patients with high-voltage electrical burns experience neurological sequelae such as confusion, amnesia, and seizures. In an inpatient rehabilitation facility, 79% and 27% of the burn patients showed cognitive deficits at admission and discharge, respectively. Analyses of inpatient rehabilitation facilities across the US demonstrated that patients with burn injuries present different levels of cognitive deficits, especially in the domains of memory and problem solving, that were worse than other traumatic (non-TBI) rehabilitation populations. Furthermore, cognitive function levels in the burn population were significantly related to their rehabilitation outcomes.[25]

Psychological responses following burn injuries may be triggered by multiple factors, such as functional limitations, chronic pain, and disfigurement in visible body parts, that have a detrimental impact on survivors' mental health. Prevalence of depression, generalized anxiety, and post-traumatic stress disorder for inpatients with burn injuries are 23% to 61%, 13% to 47% and 30%, respectively.[26] Within 5 years post-injury, 4%, 3%, and 2% of the burn survivors had a hospital admission due to a mental health problem, a behavioral issue related to drug or alcohol use, and self-harm, respectively. The burn population also showed five times higher likelihood of hospital admission for mental health than the uninjured population.[27]

Likewise, burn survivors commonly experience different types of sleep disturbances. General sleep disturbances have been reported by 12% to 82% of burn inpatients and 40% to 73% of the burn outpatients. Difficulty falling or staying asleep were shown in 54% of burn inpatients and 27% to 37% of burn outpatients, and nightmares occurred in 5% to 82% of burn inpatients and 35% to 46% of burn outpatients. Sleep disturbances and nightmare show improvements with time. However, a significant percentage of burn survivors continue to experience sleep problems long-term.[28]

## ACTIVITIES AND PARTICIPATION

In the ICF model, an activity refers to a task or individual action, whereas participation refers to the performance of activities within a bio-sociocultural context. A single activity limitation may cause several participation restrictions, and conversely different activity limitations could cause a specific participation restriction seen in different burn survivors. For example, temporary inability to walk after a fracture surgery may reduce participation in work and friendships due to difficulty in going places. Even if the walking limitation improves over time, the participation outcomes may remain reduced by other activity limitations, such as inability to afford transportation due to accumulated losses in economic productivity.

The present section focuses on the participation outcomes (self-care, domestic life, interpersonal interactions and relationships, major life areas, and community, social and civic life) and connects to related activity outcomes (learning and applying knowledge, general tasks and demands, communication, and mobility). **Table 2** presents common long-term participation limitations after burn injury.

### Self-care and Domestic Life

### Activities of daily living

Ability to perform self-care, or Activities of Daily Living (ADLs), is essential for the transition to independent living and ultimately re-establishing a daily routine, which was ranked as the single most important activity-related goal for survivors with chronic burns by an expert multidisciplinary panel.[3] Common assessments of burn rehabilitation outcomes, such as the Functional Independence Measure (FIM) and the Modified Barthel Index (MBI), utilize composite ratings to rate performance on a group of discrete tasks. Analysis of the Uniform Data System for Medical Rehabilitation database of US inpatient rehabilitation facilities showed an improvement in average ADL independence from moderate assistance at admission to supervision level at discharge.[29] Similarly, a Chinese non-randomized controlled trial found significant improvements in the ADLs for burn survivors aged 18 to 60 receiving inpatient rehabilitation and changing to moderate dependency, compared to the usual care group remaining at severe dependency.

### Ambulation

Mobility outcomes depend on the premorbid level of mobility, burn severity and location, medical complications and comorbidities, and effective rehabilitation including early mobilization. Ambulation is a significant predictor of discharge to the community. A large national sample showed that almost three-quarters of the burn survivors discharging home from inpatient rehabilitation were completely independent with ambulation, whereas most survivors discharging to supervised living situations had total

| Table 2 Common long-term participation limitations after Burn injury using the world health organization international classification of functioning, disability, and health framework | |
| --- | --- |
| ICF Category | Example of Participation Limitation after Burn Injury |
| Self-care and domestic life<br>d570 Looking after one's health<br>d599 Self care, unspecified<br>d649 Household tasks, other specified and unspecified | for example, requirement of assistance for self-care due to joint contractures |
| Interpersonal interactions and relationships<br>d730 Relating with strangers<br>d740 Formal relationships<br>d750 Informal social relationships<br>d760 Family relationships<br>d770 Intimate relationships | for example, avoidance of interaction with strangers due to discomfort with strangers' reactions to one's facial burns |
| Major life areas<br>d845 Acquiring, keeping, and terminating a job<br>d850 Remunerative employment | for example, inability to work due to upper limb amputation or contracture |
| Community, social and civic life<br>d920 Recreation and leisure<br>d999 Community, social and civic life, unspecified | for example, avoidance of outdoor activities due to heat intolerance |

dependence on others for walking or forward movement.[30,31] Requirement of any hands-on assistance for ambulation appears to be a determinant of discharge to independent or supervised living, and only about 10% of the burn survivors requiring contact guard or greater level of supervision without actual hands-on assistance were discharged to independent community living. The likelihood of independent ambulation at discharge from inpatient care is negatively associated with older age, larger burn size, higher body-mass index (BMI), burns affecting the feet, and lower extremity contracture or amputation.[29,31]

### Other mobility

Meanwhile, the average ability to transfer at discharge from inpatient rehabilitation was slightly better than contact guard level of assistance, indicating most survivors were able to transfer without hands-on assistance. Ability to transfer was specifically impaired by elevated BMI and larger burn size, particularly in females.[31] Inpatient rehabilitation has shown positive effects on overall mobility outcomes and balance with decreased fall risk.[32] Further research into mobility outcomes should focus on more specific components of mobility including balance, transfer mobility, assistive device use, and ability to drive after burn injury.

### Hand function

Hands are frequently involved in burn injury due to their use for interaction with the environment. Hand burns can pose limitations in functional activities including carrying, lifting, and manipulating objects that can impair self-care activities such as bathing or eating. Chronic deficits in hand function are seen in the domains of strength, range of motion, and functional use. During the acute phase of recovery, grip strength is reduced in correlation with the size of the burn injury.[33] In a series of survivors with full-thickness hand burns, almost half were lacking total functional upper extremity range of motion.[34] The strongest predictors of recovery are the depth of injury, burn size, and need for surgery.[33–35] It was reported that greater than 90% of patients with superficial-thickness hand burns maintained normal function in all parts of the hand at follow-up, whereas patients with full-thickness hand injuries involving the bone, joint, or extensor mechanism maintained normal function only 10% of the time.[36] Among the latter group, 10% were limited in hand function that they required assistance for the completion of ADLs. Additionally, hand contracture is a negative outcome that predicts long-term functional impairment and occurs in about 25% of all survivors by discharge from inpatient rehabilitation[32,37] and 44% among those with full-thickness burns.[38] Old age and amputation are other independent risk factors for worse hand function outcomes.[39]

Following inpatient rehabilitation, survivors with major burns demonstrated a mean improvement of 42% in the dominant hand and 33% in the non-dominant hand in performance on simulated ADL tasks from worst post-injury function.[32] Another group demonstrated about 40% to 50% improvement in self-reported function after outpatient rehabilitation in the outpatient setting.[40] Longitudinal studies show that improvement in hand function tends to plateau between 3 and 6 months post-injury. There may be ongoing subtle improvement in hand function beyond the acute rehabilitation period, and about 50% of the lost hand function is expected to be recovered long-term considering both partial- and full-thickness burns.

### Living situation

A significant minority of hospitalized burn survivors are not able to initially discharge home, yet over time most return to independent living. Of all burn patients in acute care, about half discharge to home, about 20% discharge to long-term care facilities, about 16% expire, and about 5% discharge to other acute care. A large US database of burn survivors in inpatient rehabilitation reported 75% were discharged home versus 8.5% to skilled nursing or subacute care and the remainder to other rehabilitation or acute settings.[29] Another study found 80% of acutely hospitalized burn survivors aged 55 years or older were able to discharge to independent living.[41] Of those patients discharged to supervised living, about half were able to later transition to independent living.[41,42] A prospective study of 603 burn survivors noted no significant change in the living situation compared to pre-injury in aggregate but was prone to selection bias.[41,42] Homelessness is a significant problem affecting about 1% to 15% of patients admitted for burn injuries and is associated with greater hospital expenses, more surgical intervention, and longer length of stay.[26,43]

### Interpersonal Interactions and Relationships

Burns have been associated with long-term issues related to interpersonal interactions such as friendships, romantic and sexual relationships.[44] The consequences of major burn injury can introduce new challenges into the patient's existing relationships. Romantic relationship status in burn survivor samples at long-term follow-up have not demonstrated statistically significant change compared to pre-injury; two large studies found that about two-thirds of burn survivors are in romantic relationships at follow-up, which is similar to the rate in the general population.[45] However, more than 10% of a large cohort of survivors reported dissatisfaction with appearance, resulting feelings of embarrassment or discomfort in social situations, and reactive avoidance of participation in social events or situations. More than 20% of the cohort reported that the same difficulties challenged meeting new people or maintaining relationships with friends.

Burn survivors' reports of sexual satisfaction outcomes are not significantly different compared to the general population, and similar to the general population, sexual activity is more common amongst males than females. Male burn survivors are more likely to report being in a sexual relationship than female survivors,[46] and report greater sexual functioning and satisfaction.[47] One sample reported 80% of male burn survivors were in a sexual relationship compared to 52% of females.[46] Involvement of the hands or genitalia is thought to be negatively associated with sexual activity and satisfaction despite inconsistent associations reported across studies.[46,47] Discrepant results are also reported regarding whether there tends to be improvement in sexual function and activity over time.[46,47]

### Major Life Areas

Burn injuries can have lasting effects on each major area of life, which include education, employment, and economics. Patient educational background is highly associated with improved rehabilitation outcomes; however, education has received significant attention as an outcome of childhood burns but not adult burns.[29] This is likely because most major burn survivors are of an age where they would be expected to have attained their maximum education.[29]

Return to work (RTW) is an important rehabilitation outcome to indicate significant functional recovery and community reintegration. A systematic review of 26 studies noted that most previously-employed burn survivors will return to employment and 28% to 33% of burn survivors never return to work.[48] The median time from injury to return to work is about 17 weeks but sometimes is longer than 1 year.[49] Pre-injury employment is the most important predictor of employment post-injury, and those who were employed pre-injury are 171 times more likely to find employment after injury than those who were unemployed.[50] Greater burn depth, larger burn size, involvement of hands or arms, longer length of hospitalization, and older age all associated with lower rates of RTW.[51]

At all timepoints after injury, survivors cite pain as the most common barrier to RTW. Burn injury in the workplace compared to outside the workplace is associated with twice the odds of failure to RTW[52] and decreased self-reported interpersonal participation at the workplace after RTW. The survivor's physical ability was a significant early barrier to RTW, whereas working conditions and the survivor's cognitive and social abilities became stronger predictors of RTW at 1 year post-injury.[50] Among those who successfully return to work, participation is impaired primarily by feelings of fear and decreased performance at work,[53] psychiatric problems, fatigue, pain, impaired mobility,[52] and joint contracture.[54] Despite these limitations, survivors of non-workplace-associated injuries who return to work report more interpersonal engagement in the workplace than non-injured controls, possibly due to resilience or change in perspective.

Burn survivors returning to work after injury may require work accommodations such as activity restrictions, temperature- or moisture-controlled work environments, and assistive devices. Job-specific factors are important for determining a burn survivor's suitability for return to the job and any necessary accommodations. The frequency of workplace accommodations with RTW has been estimated to be from 20% to greater than 50%.[49,55] Some survivors may need to return to jobs with different responsibilities despite accommodations. In the US Burn Model Systems database, about 40% of burn survivors returned to jobs with significantly different responsibilities, whereas studies from Taiwan and the Netherlands reported rates of about 20%.[55,56] About one-quarter of survivors who successfully RTW will experience underemployment, or significant loss in income due to productivity loss, at 24 months post-injury.[57] The finding of significant underemployment among those achieving RTW demonstrates the importance of continued efforts to collect more refined employment outcomes data.

### Community, Social, and Civic Life

The burn rehabilitation literature has been increasingly shifting focus from survival and functional outcomes to outcomes related to societal functions. Burn survivors may face barriers of community reintegration related to distressing symptoms, difficulty in navigating shared spaces, and unwanted attention from others due to aesthetic changes. Generally, many burn survivors continue to report decreased health-related quality of life as far out as 20 years after injury.[58] The outcomes literature is shifting from general, patient-reported outcomes such as quality of life, to more specific domains of impairment. For example, 13% of burn survivors reported significant limitation in leisure activity participation at long-term follow-up.[59]

A study of community reintegration after burn injury found burn survivors reported lower community integration at 1 year compared to non-injured controls, except for female burn survivors, who reported greater home integration but less social activities and interaction outside the home.[60] However, a different sample of 603 burn survivors with a median time since injury of 15 years reported similar or greater participation in each domain of community participation than non-injured controls. The most common specific barriers to participation in social activities were discomfort with participation in activities that attract attention to their appearance and avoidance of outdoor activities; both were reported by more than 30% of the sample.[59] Limitations in social participation and community integration appear more likely to return to pre-injury levels than physical impairments.

There is an association between higher level of education and greater social reintegration after burn injury among the young adult age group.[61] There are also racial disparities; white survivors report significantly higher community reintegration than Black survivors.[62] Another analysis found that larger burn size is associated with decreased social interactions and workplace participation, but increased participation within the home, possibly as a result of greater inter-reliance.[58] Unemployment after injury is associated with limited participation in each of these domains. Of note, alcohol and substance abuse negatively predict community integration and well-being and rates of substance abuse tend to decline compared to pre-injury.[45] Participation in support groups with peer mentors has shown benefits in improving community reintegration related to social interactions, social activities, and work.[63]

## SUMMARY

Burn survivors commonly experience multiple long-term challenges during their recovery. This review used the ICF conceptual model to guide a comprehensive understanding of outcomes from structural and functional impairments to activities and participation restrictions following burn injuries. This review of rehabilitation outcomes may help advance the development of long-term care plans, promote burn recovery, and improve survivors' quality of life. Although there are a growing number of studies examining community and social outcomes after injury, the literature is limited by short follow-up periods and limited sample diversity. Contextual environmental and personal factors in the ICF model are not included in this study and could be examined in future studies.

## CLINICS CARE POINTS

- Burn injury is increasingly recognized as a chronic condition with multi-system functional impairments and participation limitations; long-term regular follow-up is necessary to prevent a multitude of late or cumulative impairments and is critical for comprehensive burn recovery.
- Older patient age, medical and psychosocial comorbidities, greater burn severity, and involvement of critical structures such as face, or genitalia are predictors of impairments across domains.

## DISCLOSURE

The authors have nothing to disclose.

## ACKNOWLEDGEMENT

This work was supported by the National Institute on Disability, Independent Living, and Rehabilitation Research grant (NIDILRR grant #90DPBU0001, 90DPBU0004 and 90DPBU0008). NIDILRR is a Center within the Administration for Community Living (ACL), Department of Health and Human Services (HHS). The contents of this manuscript do not necessarily represent the policy of NIDILRR, ACL, HHS, and you should not assume endorsement by the Federal Government.

## REFERENCES

1. Carrougher GJ, Bamer AM, Mandell SP, et al. Factors Affecting Employment After Burn Injury in the United States: A Burn Model System National Database Investigation. Arch Phys Med Rehabil 2020;101(1S):S71–85.

2. Wong RCP, Yang L, Szeto WY. Wearable fitness trackers and smartphone pedometer apps: Their effect on transport mode choice in a transit-oriented city. Travel Behaviour and Society 2021;22:244–51.

3. Lin YR, Wang JY, Chang SC, et al. Developing a Delphi-Based Comprehensive Core Set from the International Classification of Functioning, Disability, and Health Framework for the Rehabilitation of Patients with Burn Injuries. Int J Environ Res Public Health 2021;18(8). https://doi.org/10.3390/ijerph18083970.

4. Smolle C, Cambiaso-Daniel J, Forbes AA, et al. Recent trends in burn epidemiology worldwide: A systematic review. Burns 2017;43(2):249–57.

5. Abazari M, Ghaffari A, Rashidzadeh H, et al. A Systematic Review on Classification, Identification, and Healing Process of Burn Wound Healing. Int J Low Extrem Wounds 2022;21(1):18–30.

6. Lawrence JW, Mason ST, Schomer K, et al. Epidemiology and impact of scarring after burn injury: a systematic review of the literature. J Burn Care Res 2012;33(1):136–46.

7. Girard D, Laverdet B, Buhé V, et al. Biotechnological Management of Skin Burn Injuries: Challenges and Perspectives in Wound Healing and Sensory Recovery. Tissue Eng B Rev 2017;23(1):59–82.

8. Bartley CN, Atwell K, Purcell L, et al. Amputation Following Burn Injury. J Burn Care Res 2019;40(4):430–6.

9. Oosterwijk AM, Mouton LJ, Schouten H, et al. Prevalence of scar contractures after burn: A systematic review. Burns 2017;43(1):41–9.

10. Knuth CM, Auger C, Jeschke MG. Burn-induced hypermetabolism and skeletal muscle dysfunction. Am J Physiol Cell Physiol 2021;321(1):C58–71.

11. Omar MTA, Abd El Baky AM, Ebid AA. Lower-Limb Muscular Strength, Balance, and Mobility Levels in Adults Following Severe Thermal Burn Injuries. J Burn Care Res 2017;38(5):327–33.

12. Michielsen DP, Lafaire C. Management of genital burns: a review. Int J Urol 2010;17(9):755–8.

13. Williams FN, Herndon DN, Jeschke MG. The hypermetabolic response to burn injury and interventions to modify this response. Clin Plast Surg 2009;36(4):583–96.

14. Lukusa MR, Allorto NL, Wall SL. Hypothermia in acutely presenting burn injuries to a regional burn service: The incidence and impact on outcome. Burns Open 2021;5(1):39–44.

15. Oh J, Madison C, Flott G, et al. Temperature Sensitivity After Burn Injury: A Burn Model System National Database Hot Topic. J Burn Care Res 2021;42(6):1110–9.

16. Duke JM, Randall SM, Wood FM, et al. Burns and long-term infectious disease morbidity: A population-based study. Burns 2017;43(2):273–81.

17. Duke JM, Randall SM, Fear MW, et al. Understanding the long-term impacts of burn on the cardiovascular system. Burns 2016;42(2):366–74.

18. Willis CE, Grisbrook TL, Elliott CM, et al. Pulmonary function, exercise capacity and physical activity participation in adults following burn. Burns 2011;37(8):1326–33.

19. Tang JA, Amadio G, Nagappan L, et al. Laryngeal inhalational injuries: A systematic review. Burns 2022;48(1):23–33.

20. Casper JK, Clark WR, Kelley RT, et al. Laryngeal and phonatory status after burn/inhalation injury: a long term follow-up study. J Burn Care Rehabil 2002;23(4):235–43.

21. Cabalag MS, Wasiak J, Syed Q, et al. Early and late complications of ocular burn injuries. J Plast Reconstr Aesthet Surg 2015;68(3):356–61.

22. Kraenzlin FS, Mushin OP, Ayazi S, et al. Epidemiology and Outcomes of Auricular Burn Injuries. J Burn Care Res 2018;39(3):326–31.

23. Morgan M, Deuis JR, Frøsig-Jørgensen M, et al. Burn Pain: A Systematic and Critical Review of Epidemiology, Pathophysiology, and Treatment. Pain Med 2018; 19(4):708–34.

24. Martin R, Taylor S, Palmieri TL. Mortality following combined burn and traumatic brain injuries: An analysis of the national trauma data bank of the American College of Surgeons. Burns 2020;46(6):1289–96.

25. Bajorek AJ, Slocum C, Goldstein R, et al. Impact of Cognition on Burn Inpatient Rehabilitation Outcomes. PM R 2017;9(1):1–7.

26. Wiechman SA, Patterson DR. ABC of burns. Psychosocial aspects of burn injuries. BMJ 2004;329(7462):391–3.

27. Duke JM, Randall SM, Boyd JH, et al. A population-based retrospective cohort study to assess the mental health of patients after a non-intentional burn compared with uninjured people. Burns 2018;44(6):1417–26.

28. Lerman SF, Owens MA, Liu T, et al. Sleep after burn injuries: A systematic review and meta-analysis. Sleep Med Rev 2022;65:101662.

29. Tan WH, Goldstein R, Gerrard P, et al. Outcomes and predictors in burn rehabilitation. J Burn Care Res 2012;33(1):110–7.

30. Farrell RT, Gamelli RL, Sinacore J. Analysis of functional outcomes in patients discharged from an acute burn center. J Burn Care Res 2006;27(2):189–94.

31. Farrell RT, Gamelli RL, Aleem RF, et al. The relationship of body mass index and functional outcomes in patients with acute burns. J Burn Care Res 2008;29(1): 102–8.

32. Schneider JC, Qu HD, Lowry J, et al. Efficacy of inpatient burn rehabilitation: a prospective pilot study examining range of motion, hand function and balance. Burns 2012;38(2):164–71.

33. Gittings PM, Hince DA, Wand BM, et al. Grip and Muscle Strength Dynamometry in Acute Burn Injury: Evaluation of an Updated Assessment Protocol. J Burn Care Res 2018;39(6):939–47.

34. Holavanahalli RK, Helm PA, Gorman AR, et al. Outcomes after deep full-thickness hand burns. Arch Phys Med Rehabil 2007;88(12 Suppl 2):S30–5.

35. Mata-Ribeiro L, Vieira L, Vilela M. Epidemiology And Outcome Assessment Of Hand Burns: A 3-Year Retrospective Analysis In A Burn Unit. Ann Burns Fire Disasters 2022;35(1):18–25.

36. Sheridan RL, Hurley J, Smith MA, et al. The acutely burned hand: management and outcome based on a ten-year experience with 1047 acute hand burns. J Trauma 1995;38(3):406–11.

37. Schneider JC, Holavanahalli R, Helm P, et al. Contractures in burn injury part II: investigating joints of the hand. J Burn Care Res 2008;29(4):606–13.

38. Dobbs ER, Curreri PW. Burns: analysis of results of physical therapy in 681 patients. J Trauma 1972;12(3):242–8.

39. van Zuijlen PP, Kreis RW, Vloemans AF, et al. The prognostic factors regarding long-term functional outcome of full-thickness hand burns. Burns 1999;25(8): 709–14.

40. Choi JS, Mun JH, Lee JY, et al. Effects of modified dynamic metacarpophalangeal joint flexion orthoses after hand burn. Ann Rehabil Med 2011;35(6):880–6.

41. Pham TN, Carrougher GJ, Martinez E, et al. Predictors of Discharge Disposition in Older Adults With Burns: A Study of the Burn Model Systems. J Burn Care Res 2015;36(6):607–12.

42. McGill V, Kowal-Vern A, Gamelli RL. Outcome for older burn patients. Arch Surg 2000;135(3):320–5.

43. Vrouwe SQ, Johnson MB, Pham CH, et al. The Homelessness Crisis and Burn Injuries: A Cohort Study. J Burn Care Res 2020;41(4):820–7.

44. Kelter BM, Shepler LJ, Ni P, et al. Developing trajectories of social recovery after burn injury: Preliminary results from the LIBRE Journey Study. Burns 2022;48(2): 460–2.

45. Smolle C, Hutter MF, Kamolz LP. Life after Burn, Part II: Substance Abuse, Relationship and Living Situation of Burn Survivors. Medicina (Kaunas) 2022;58(5). https://doi.org/10.3390/medicina58050563.

46. Ohrtman EA, Shapiro GD, Wolfe AE, et al. Sexual activity and romantic relationships after burn injury: A Life Impact Burn Recovery Evaluation (LIBRE) study. Burns 2020;46(7):1556–64.

47. Connell KM, Phillips M, Coates R, et al. Sexuality, body image and relationships following burns: analysis of BSHS-B outcome measures. Burns 2014;40(7): 1329–37.

48. Mason ST, Esselman P, Fraser R, et al. Return to Work After Burn Injury: A Systematic Review. J Burn Care Res 2012;33(1):101–9.

49. Brych SB, Engrav LH, Rivara FP, et al. Time off work and return to work rates after burns: systematic review of the literature and a large two-center series. J Burn Care Rehabil 2001;22(6):401–5.

50. Esselman PC, Askay SW, Carrougher GJ, et al. Barriers to return to work after burn injuries. Arch Phys Med Rehabil 2007;88(12 Suppl 2):S50–6.

51. Wrigley M, Trotman BK, Dimick A, et al. Factors relating to return to work after burn injury. J Burn Care Rehabil 1995;16(4):445–50 [discussion: 444].

52. Schneider JC, Bassi S, Ryan CM. Barriers impacting employment after burn injury. J Burn Care Res 2009;30(2):294–300.

53. Schneider JC, Shie VL, Espinoza LF, et al. Impact of Work-Related Burn Injury on Social Reintegration Outcomes: A Life Impact Burn Recovery Evaluation (LIBRE) Study. Arch Phys Med Rehabil 2020;101(1s):S86–91.

54. Pham TN, Goldstein R, Carrougher GJ, et al. The impact of discharge contracture on return to work after burn injury: A Burn Model System investigation. Burns 2020;46(3):539–45.

55. Hwang YF, Chen-Sea MJ, Chen CL. Factors related to return to work and job modification after a hand burn. J Burn Care Res 2009;30(4):661–7.

56. Spronk I, Van Loey NEE, van der Vlies CH, et al. Activity Impairment, Work Status, and Work Productivity Loss in Adults 5-7 Years After Burn Injuries. J Burn Care Res 2022;43(1):256–62.

57. Sheckter CC, Brych S, Carrougher GJ, et al. Exploring "Return to Productivity" Among People Living With Burn Injury: A Burn Model System National Database Report. J Burn Care Res 2021;42(6):1081–6.

58. Abouzeid CA, Wolfe AE, Ni P, et al. Are burns a chronic condition? Examining patient reported outcomes up to 20 years after burn injury-A Burn Model System National Database investigation. J Trauma Acute Care Surg 2022;92(6):1066–74.

59. Saret CJ, Ni P, Marino M, et al. Social Participation of Burn Survivors and the General Population in Work and Employment: A Life Impact Burn Recovery Evaluation (LIBRE) Profile Study. J Burn Care Res 2019;40(5):669–77.

60. Esselman PC, Ptacek JT, Kowalske K, et al. Community integration after burn injuries. J Burn Care Rehabil 2001;22(3):221–7.

61. Schulz JT, Shapiro GD, Acton A, et al. The Relationship of Level of Education to Social Reintegration after Burn Injury: A LIBRE Study. J Burn Care Res 2019; 40(5):696–702.
62. Mata-Greve F, Wiechman SA, McMullen K, et al. The relation between satisfaction with appearance and race and ethnicity: A National Institute on Disability, Independent Living, and Rehabilitation Research burn model system study. Burns 2022;48(2):345–54.
63. Grieve B, Shapiro GD, Wibbenmeyer L, et al. Long-Term Social Reintegration Outcomes for Burn Survivors With and Without Peer Support Attendance: A Life Impact Burn Recovery Evaluation (LIBRE) Study. Arch Phys Med Rehabil 2020;101(1s):S92–8.

# Holistic Approach to Burn Reconstruction and Scar Rehabilitation

Barclay T. Stewart, MD, PhD[a],*, Clifford C. Sheckter, MD[b],
Kiran K. Nakarmi, MBBS, MS, MCh[c]

## KEYWORDS

- Burn • Surgery • Reconstruction • Rehabilitation

## KEY POINTS

- Principles of burn reconstruction should be incorporated into acute care, while scar rehabilitation should occur with maturing or matured scars and focus on improving function.
- The timing and intensity of burn reconstruction should be aligned with patients' deficits, goals, life events, and current ability to cope with perioperative requirements.
- All techniques along the reconstructive ladder can be useful for burn reconstruction (eg, scar release and skin graft, local tissue rearrangements, regional and distant flaps).
- Outcomes of burn reconstruction and scar rehabilitation should be patient-centered and include patient-reported measures to assess individual recoveries and system-level benchmarks.
- Successful reconstruction programs include strategies to track patient needs, range of motion and functional gains, timing of staged procedures, and key milestones in functional recovery.

## INTRODUCTION

More than 11 million burn injuries occur each year across the world.[1] Many people with burn injuries, regardless of injury size, develop hypertrophic scar, contracture, heterotopic ossification (HO), and disability resulting from these sequelae.[2] Advances in trauma systems, critical care, safe surgery, and multidisciplinary burn care have markedly improved the survival of people who have experienced extensive burn

[a] UW Medicine Regional Burn Center at Harborview Medical Center, University of Washington, 325 9th Avenue, Box 359796, Seattle, WA 98104, USA; [b] The Burn Center at Santa Clara Valley Medical Center, Stanford University, 751 South Bascom Avenue, San Jose, CA 95128, USA; [c] Nepal Cleft and Burn Center at Kirtipur Hospital, National Academy of Medical Sciences, Kirtipur Ring Road, Kathmandu 44618, Nepal
* Corresponding author. Department of Surgery, Division of Trauma, Burn and Critical Care Surgery, Harborview Medical Center, 325 9th Avenue, Box 359796, Seattle, WA 98104
*E-mail address:* barclays@uw.edu

Phys Med Rehabil Clin N Am 34 (2023) 883–904
https://doi.org/10.1016/j.pmr.2023.06.018
1047-9651/23/© 2023 Elsevier Inc. All rights reserved.

injuries. However, it should be noted that 90% of burn injuries globally occur in countries without organized trauma systems or advanced burn care capacity.[1] While some low- and middle-income countries have well-planned and organized emergency care systems, many have not prioritized care for the injured and experience unsatisfactory outcomes despite exhausting efforts by individual clinicians.[3,4] As a result, the most complex burn reconstruction challenges are highly prevalent in areas with the most limited resources.[5]

Burn reconstruction refers to the procedures performed, both in acute and rehabilitation phases of care, to improve functional outcomes and appearance.[6] Like acute burn care, burn reconstruction requires thoughtful, coordinated approaches along the continuum of burn injury. Psychological preparedness for surgery, adequate nutrition, postoperative splinting, stretching programs, and overall conditioning require participation from all members of an organized burn team to achieve excellent outcomes. Individual response to reconstruction procedures and system-level burn reconstruction benchmarking is best performed with serial use of patient-reported outcome measures.[7,8]

## TIMING AND READINESS FOR BURN RECONSTRUCTION

Reconstructive procedures can occur days, weeks, months, and years after burn injury (**Table 1**). Acute reconstruction works to achieve wound closure while mitigating the effects of hypertrophic scar and preventing contractures to maximize long-term function (eg, selection of wound closure strategy, use of dermal templates, careful orientation of grafts, interruption of future scar lines) (**Figs. 1–3**).[9] Procedures performed after wound closure are generally done to address hypertrophic scarring (**Fig. 4**), contracture, dyspigmentation, hair loss, pain, and/or itch—these procedures are more aptly described as scar rehabilitation. Several factors are considered when planning reconstructive procedures, namely personal, physical, scar, and psychosocial factors. The most ideal time for burn reconstruction is when the scar has fully

| Table 1 Urgency of burn reconstruction and scar rehabilitation | | |
|---|---|---|
| **Urgent (days – weeks)** | **Semi-urgent (weeks – months)** | **Elective (months and after scar maturation)** |
| Preservation of airway (eg, commissuroplasty for microstomia, neck contracture release and reconstruction) | Unstable scar or ulcer | Contracture affecting range of motion that can be corrected with passive stretch and at low risk of joint deformation |
| Protection of vision (eg, cicatricial ectropion release and skin autograft) | Contracture in children at risk of causing limb length discrepancy (eg, restriction of bone or tendon growth), joint deformity, or impaired neurovascular bundle growth | Hypertrophic scar not causing functional limitations |
| Exposed vital structures (eg, joint, nerve) | Contracture affecting range of motion and with significant functional limitations | |

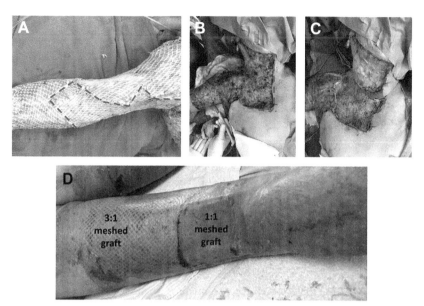

**Fig. 1.** Examples of acute burn reconstruction that aim to improve functional recovery and limit needs for late scar rehabilitation. (*A*) Careful orientation of skin grafts to prevent long, uninterrupted seams along the length of the extremity. (*B, C*) Use of a local rotational flap to interrupt the lateral edge of a neck wound that would otherwise result in a certain contracture. The healthy skin flap will expand or lengthen while the skin graft scar contracts. (*D*) Use of more tightly meshed skin grafts (eg, 1:1 vs 3:1) across flexor surfaces (eg, popliteal fossa) to prevent negative effects of graft contracture on knee extension. (From Papp A, et al. Interrupting the seams: The principle of preventive burn reconstruction. Burns Open. 2019(3):121-125.).

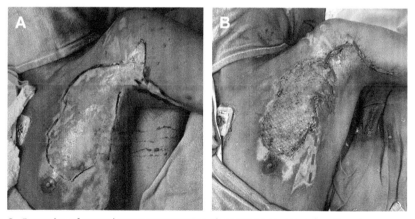

**Fig. 2.** Examples of acute burn reconstruction that aim to improve functional recovery and limit needs for late scar rehabilitation. Dashed red line in (*A*) demonstrates anticipated edge of anterior axillary fold contracture. Efforts to interrupt that edge (dashed red line in (*B*), eg, local rotational flap and local axillary advancement flap) reduce needs for major late reconstruction. The healthy skin flaps will expand or lengthen as the grafts and scars around the flaps contract.

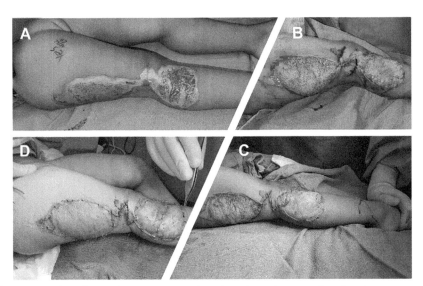

**Fig. 3.** Examples of acute burn reconstruction that aim to improve functional recovery and limit needs for late scar rehabilitation. (*A*) A preoperative image demonstrating wound across the lateral aspect of the right leg in a young child who will grow substantially. (*B*) Excised wound and intraoperative markings for a Z-plasty to interrupt the future scar with healthy skin flaps. (*C*) The completed Z-plasty. (*D*) Placement of sheet skin grafts with a seem oriented transversely to the long axis of the limb to reduce the risk of graft contracture on knee function. Sheets of skin contract less than meshed autografts and do not create the checkered pattern related to the interstices devoid of dermis.

matured, if not urgent or semi-urgent. This allows time for exercise, stretching, and splinting regimens to achieve maximum effects, reduces the risks of operating on active scar (eg, poor wound healing, recurrent contracture), and ensures scar is sufficiently supple for mobilization and rearrangements.

Recovering from burn injury, returning to school or work, and reintegrating into the community can be arduous and require intentional, stepwise efforts by the patient,

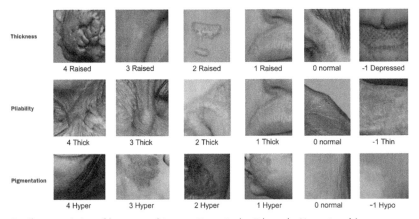

**Fig. 4.** Characteristics of hypertrophic scar. From Jacky Edwards, Hypertrophic scar management, British Journal of Nursing 2022 31:20, S24-S31.

their support system, and their burn team. Initial outpatient visits after injury are designed to address urgent physical and psychosocial problems, establish a rehabilitation regimen, and develop a list of reconstruction needs and procedures to address them. Prioritization of this list and strategies to address them is a continuous process and evolves as people become more active and adjusted in their respective environments. Reconstructive procedures should be planned with the patient, goal-oriented, scaled to the degree of dysfunction, timed around specific rehabilitation milestones, and scheduled to avoid significant disruptions in recovery and life more generally. Since scars mature for up to 18 to 24 months after wound closure, major procedures are typically performed no earlier than 8 to 12 months after injury, as the need for and extent of reconstruction procedures often decrease as scars mature (**Fig. 5**). Additionally, this allows time for the person living with burn injury to adapt to changes in their physical function, habituate stretching and exercise programs, develop comfort and compliance with compression and splinting regimens, and cope with psychosocial stressors of injury.[10] There are problems that require more urgent reconstruction, including exposure of vital structures (eg, joints, nerves), eyelid ectropion that can lead to corneal ulceration and vision loss, and unstable wounds.

In addition to the functional and anatomic indications outlined below, people needing burn reconstruction should be psychosocially prepared for surgery and returning to being "a patient" for a short period. At a basic level, this includes readiness to miss work or school and having coping strategies to manage additional anxiety and pain related to surgery and the recovery process. Complications are common after scar operations, and patients must be prepared for unexpected setbacks. Many patients have stress symptoms or disorders that can be triggered or aggravated by re-exposure to the healthcare environment or pain. Screening for and management of stress symptoms should be done prior to planning reconstructive procedures. After surgery, patients also need an environment and community that support healing (eg, safe and stable housing, caregivers, access to transportation). For people with significant psychosocial challenges, a strategy that uses less invasive, smaller, and less frequent procedures initially is worth consideration. Regardless, reconstructive strategies generally aim to minimize inpatient stays by performing smaller procedures with predictable outcomes and lower postoperative care burdens when possible, particularly for the initial procedures in patients with multiple or significant reconstruction needs. Conversely, some patients will prefer a single, larger procedure rather than multiple, smaller procedures to minimize disruptions in their lives. Efforts should be made to group procedures, when possible, to limit disruptions in the overall recovery process. However, grouping procedures is not always possible as some require

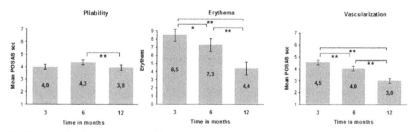

**Fig. 5.** Changes in characteristics of hypertrophic scar over time. Hypertrophic scars improve over 18 months after burn injury. (From van der Wal MB, et al. Outcome after burns: an observational study on burn scar maturation and predictors for severe scarring. Wound Repair and Regeneration. 2012 Sep-Oct;20(5):676-87.)

postoperative mobilization (eg, joint capsulotomy), while others require brief (eg, scar release with skin graft) or prolonged immobilization (eg, arthrodesis). For these reasons, reconstruction on both hands of an independent person is not advisable. In rare cases, there are no reconstructive options, or the patient is unable to endure reconstruction. Major efforts should be dedicated to these patients to ensure maximum possible functional recovery in the absence of surgery.

Expectation management is vital for achieving successful outcomes. Patients often believe or hope that scars can be erased, that their intensive engagement with exercise or splinting regimens will not be required, or that rehabilitation will be complete after reconstructive surgery; none of these are true. Therefore, the importance of relationship and trust building, education around timeline for functional recovery, and shared decision-making are required ahead of reconstruction.

## SPECIAL CONSIDERATIONS WITH CHILDREN

Children between the ages of 6 months and 4 years can experience great stress from medical interventions but lack the developmental tools to understand, cope, and communicate their concerns effectively.[11] However, children and adolescents should be included in the shared decision-making around need for and timing of reconstructive surgery when possible (ie, informed assent). Children have a remarkable healing potential and capability to adapt to functional deficits. However, several additional factors should be considered when determining the need for reconstruction related to their growth and development (eg, scar causing limb-length discrepancy, scar restriction of breast bud development). Given the need for children and adolescents to participate in their postoperative care and recovery, it is vital that they buy into the process, including wound care, immobilization, splinting, stretching, and range of motion exercises. Efforts should be made to time reconstruction procedures and postoperative rehabilitation plans (eg, splinting) around school, sport, and camp schedules when able. Clinicians should be aware that children often outgrow their reconstruction and many need serial procedures until skeletal maturity. Furthermore, clinicians should have vigilance during periods of rapid growth with a focus on loss of range of motion, worsening deformity, joint subluxation, pain, and/or ulcerations in case more urgent reconstruction procedures are required.

## RECONSTRUCTION CHALLENGES AFTER BURN INJURY
### Scars and Contractures

Hypertrophic scar remains the major physical challenge after burn injury and a common source of frustration, functional limitation, discomfort, stigma, and dissatisfaction with appearance (see **Fig. 4**).[12] Burn wounds that take longer than 2 to 3 weeks after injury to heal are at higher risk of hypertrophic scar. Other known risk factors include wound infection and race or ethnicity (eg, patients with more pigmented skin are believed to experience worse hypertrophic scar).[13] Therefore, many efforts have been dedicated to early diagnosis of deeper wounds, early excision and wound closure, and preventing complicated wound healing.[14]

Several nonsurgical treatments for hypertrophic scar are used with additive but moderate benefits (eg, massage, compression, silicone, topical vitamins and steroids). More invasive techniques such as steroid injection, nanofat and microfat grafting, and microneedling with topical vitamins (eg, vitamins A and E) and steroid application have been used to treat thick, painful, and itchy scars. However, these techniques have limited application for large and severe scars. Fractionated ablative laser treatments, often performed 1 to 6 months after stable scar formation and performed serially in 3- to 6-month intervals until no improvements are experienced, have been shown to reduce scar rubor, pain, itch, tightness, and thickness (**Fig. 6**). Some benefits of laser treatment are difficult to evaluate with our current scar assessment systems but can be reported by patients based on their assessment of their scar and changes in sensation and function.

Wounds, skin grafts, and scars all contract. Contractures refer to the deformities and functional limitations of contraction that occur across joints. Contractures may extend well beyond the affected joint and cross multiple body areas (eg, extrinsic contractures such as lower eyelid ectropion caused by a scar band that extends from the cheek to the lower neck). Therefore, cutaneous functional units injured along a limb are as important for contracture formation as a scar across a joint alone.[15]

One of the key factors when deciding surgical approach to correct a contracture is the presence, quality, and recruitability of adjacent skin and soft-tissue. Minor contractures with sufficient neighboring soft tissue are addressed with local tissue rearrangements (eg, Z-plasty, Y-V plasty, local flaps). When neighboring soft tissue is deficient, the scar is released and reconstructed by adding tissue in the form of skin grafts (with or without the use of a dermal template) or flaps. Given that hypertrophic scar is associated with continuous traction of the scar itself, scar release and reconstruction will lead to a gradual decrease in the bulk of the scar postoperatively.

### Dyspigmentation

Hyperpigmentation and hypopigmentation are both commonly reported challenges from people living with hypertrophic scar and can occur in skin that healed primarily,

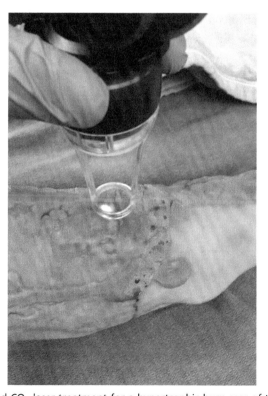

**Fig. 6.** Fractionated $CO_2$ laser treatment for a hypertrophic burn scar of the arm.

areas of autograft, and even donor sites. Dyspigmentation remains one of the most difficult scar challenges to treat. Hyperpigmentation can be mitigated by donor site selection (eg, preauricular or postauricular graft for face, foot instep graft to replace glabrous skin of the palm) and has been treated with whitening agents (eg, intense pulsed light, hydroquinone) after scar maturation with variable results. Deep fractional ablative laser treatments (eg, NdYAG laser) have improved scars with hypervascularity and hyperpigmentation. Macrodermabrasion (ie, removing the epidermis) of mature hypertrophic scars and application of either locally or remotely harvested epidermal cells (eg, suspension epidermal autografts) have been successful in some patients with dyspigmented scars (eg, burn scars, vitiligo). Medical tattooing has been used to treat mature hypopigmented scars with variable satisfaction. Makeup artists can also teach patients how to camouflage areas that do not have significant contour deformity.

### Alopecia and Inappropriate Hair Growth

Alopecia occurs when the reticular dermis is severely injured or replaced with a skin graft. Medical treatments for alopecia in these areas are ineffective given the lack of hair follicles. Small areas of alopecia can be addressed by serial excision of the hairless area and primary closure, or island flaps from the temporal scalp (eg, eyebrow deficits). Larger areas can be addressed with serial taping or tissue expansion, followed by staged excision and closure. Alopecia and these more advanced techniques can be disruptive to patients' lives due to additional stigma and body image challenges and require significant commitment from patients and/or their caregivers. Hair micrografting can be performed to address loss of eyebrows or facial hair (eg, moustache deficits). Inappropriate hair growth on thick or full-thickness grafts or flaps of hair-bearing tissue can be addressed with standard depilation techniques (eg, laser hair removal).

## COMMON TECHNIQUES FOR BURN RECONSTRUCTION

Burn scar reconstruction, like soft-tissue reconstruction more generally, follows the reconstructive ladder (**Fig. 7**).

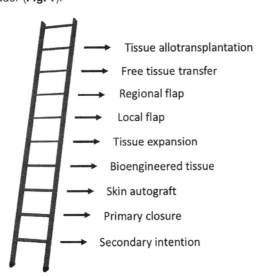

Tissue allotransplantation

Free tissue transfer

Regional flap

Local flap

Tissue expansion

Bioengineered tissue

Skin autograft

Primary closure

Secondary intention

**Fig. 7.** The reconstructive ladder.

### Fractionated Ablative Laser Therapy

Fractionated ablative laser treatments are usually performed with carbon dioxide and deeper-penetrating Nd:YAG lasers. Current theory supports mechanisms of restoring epidermal architecture through the growth of pseudo-rete ridges along with changing fibroblast expression and collagen organization in the deeper scar.[16] While laser treatments do not grow skin or treat contractures, they offer significant symptom relief— pain, itch, and sensations of tension are reduced with serial laser treatments.[17] Given the safety and effectiveness of fractionated ablative laser treatments, these techniques have become first-line therapy for scar symptom relief after healing from a partial thickness burn or skin graft.[18]

### Scar Release

Scar release is most often incisional (ie, incisions are made within the limits of the scar). Incisions must be carried through the entire scar to healthy tissue and sometimes involve the fascia of underlying muscles (eg, latissimus dorsi fascia with posterior axillary release). Additional releasing incisions are created until maximal range of motion or peripheral skin pliability is achieved, which often extend beyond the visible scar. Scar is often dissected free from underlying tissues to allow complete release. Long-standing contractures, particularly those across digits, may also require delicate division of scar from around nerves, tendons, and joint capsules. Furthermore, severe contractures may have resulted in tendon and ligament shortening, adhesive capsulitis, or joint subluxation. The patient and surgical team should obtain x-ray imaging before joint-related contracture surgery and be prepared to perform regional flap techniques to address soft-tissue deficits over joints and tendons.

Scar excision with or without resurfacing is appropriate for some patients with limited scars, particularly those with significant pain and/or itch and no contracture. Scar excision can be extralesional or intralesional. Extralesional excision is performed by incising healthy skin just outside of the scar and excising the scar in its entirety. Healthy, unscarred skin is primarily closed. Intralesional excision is performed by incising immediately within scar and excising the central area. The scar edges are then closed to one another. Since scar maturation has already occurred, additional scar formation related to this new closure is less likely. Serial excisions (ie, every 6– 12 months) can be performed for scars that cannot be excised and closed in one procedure, which allows sufficient time for tissue healing to facilitate additional excision, mobilization, and closure.

### Skin Autograft

When skin defects after scar release are too large to be closed primarily, skin grafts remain the predominant method of wound closure. Skin grafts are either split-thickness (ie, partial dermis and epidermis) or full-thickness (ie, entire dermis and epidermis) and applied as sheets of skin, perforated to facilitate transudate egress, or meshed to allow expansion for coverage of large areas with relatively small donor sites. Full-thickness skin graft donors are generally smaller and closed primarily. Contraction of the graft is proportional to the thickness of the dermis it contains (eg, split-thickness grafts contract more than full-thickness grafts) and the mesh expansion ratio (eg, 2:1 grafts contract more than 1:1 grafts). The dermis deficits within meshed grafts (ie, interstices) do not regenerate, and the mesh pattern is forever visible. Therefore, full-thickness and sheet grafts are preferred when cosmetic appearance is a priority.

Split-thickness skin graft donor sites epithelialize by maturation of epidermal progenitor cells from dermal elements (eg, hair follicles). Therefore, donor sites can be harvested several times for patients who experienced large injuries to facilitate acute wound coverage and reconstruction, as long as there is sufficient thickness of dermis left behind to allow epithelialization. Areas with thick dermis, like the back, and/or many hair follicles, like the scalp, tolerate serial harvests well. When possible, patients are given the opportunity to select donor sites. However, rationing donor sites/skin when they are limited or to achieve a better aesthetic outcome (eg, scalp donor skin for face resurfacing) is often required. The recipient sites must be clean (ie, very low bacterial and fungal counts, no biofilm) and well-vascularized (ie, not tendon or bone). Grafts fail due to imbibition barriers (eg, seroma or hematoma beneath the graft), bacterial or fungal colonization/infection, and shear injury. Shear injury is prevented by the use of bolsters, splints, and postoperative immobilization.

### Dermal Templates

Dermal templates are biologic, biosynthetic, or synthetic matrices that facilitate more organized neovascularization and collagen deposition, replicate properties of dermis (eg, pliability), and enhance graft function and appearance. Dermal templates also aid burn reconstruction by sparing donor sites and minimizing recipient site scarring since the split-thickness skin grafts can be thinly harvested when applied onto well-vascularized dermal templates with less inflammation than that associated with prolonged open wounds. Importantly, dermal templates can be used to create a vascularized wound bed over healthy tendons and bones. By doing so, a skin graft can be used to resurface a wound that would otherwise require flap reconstruction. However, dermal templates require at least one additional procedure, need approximately 2 to 3 weeks of maturation to allow sufficient vascularization, and carry significant risks of infection during the maturation phase.

### Local Tissue Rearrangement

Local tissue rearrangements (eg, variations of Z-plasty and Y-V plasty, local flaps) exploit recruitable tissue adjacent to scar bands and geometry to lengthen the contracted area (**Fig. 8**). Introducing even relatively small flaps of pliable skin and subcutaneous tissue into thickened contracture (or, during the acute phase, a wound edge at risk of contracture) interrupts lines of tension, resulting in a de-escalation of scar pathophysiology and improvements in adjacent scar.[9]

However, these techniques are not well-suited for broad scars or major skin deficits, which require adding skin via grafts or regional or distant flaps. Local tissue rearrangements require undermining to recruit, advance, transpose, and/or rotate tissue into the defect after scar release. Ambitious undermining can result in ischemia to local flaps, particularly when they were created from areas grafted previously (ie, skin without native subdermal vascular plexus). Y-V plasty requires less undermining to achieve similar lengthening and is often preferred in such areas. Joints are best covered with flaps rather than skin grafts, when able, because grafts contract over the joint. One of the ways to deal with broader scar bands causing joint contracture is by using "kissing flaps," where 2 V-shaped flaps with their apices facing toward and overlapping one another in the midpoint of the band. Areas above or below the flaps that cannot be closed can be skin grafted. By doing so, the contracture is released, and the flaps reduce the chance of recurrent contracture.

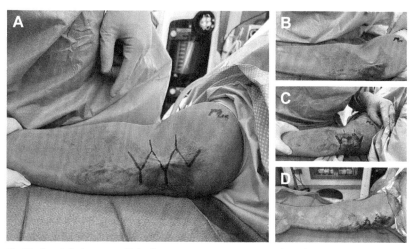

**Fig. 8.** Moderately long medial elbow contracture managed with running Y-V plasty. (*A*) Preoperative markings for running Y-V plasty; (*B*) preoperative image; (*C*) initial scar release and use of the "cut as you go" technique (ie, assessing V advancement potential before incising Y limbs); and (*D*) postoperative imaging demonstrating a more flap and long medial scar interrupted by healthy antecubital fossa skin.

### Tissue Expansion

Tissue expansion facilitates alopecia removal or soft-tissue recruitment in areas where there is insufficient tissue for local flaps; it may also be used to expand donor sites for free tissue transfer, as well as to expand donor skin when donor sites are limited. Tissue expansion is performed by temporarily implanting inflatable balloons beneath healthy, uninjured tissue that is gradually expanded with saline until the additional tissue is sufficient to close or cover the anticipated defect. Tissue expansion is commonly used for reconstruction of scalp, face, and neck deformities where matching skin color, texture, and flushing similarities generates better outcomes. Tissue expansion requires months of time commitment from patients and surgeons (eg, at least 2 operations, weekly visits for expansion), along with patience for complications, like infection and expander extrusion, which are common.

### Other Flaps

Advanced reconstruction options, like regional or free flaps and tissue transplantation, are used for burn reconstruction, particularly when vital structures need to be covered and excellent skin pliability is required. Flaps might include skin, fat, fascia, muscle, cartilage, and/or bone, depending on the functional and aesthetic needs of the recipient area. Fascial flaps (eg, radial forearm and temporoparietal fascia flaps) are thin and particularly useful for covering vital structures in areas that require good pliability (eg, back of hand) or lining facial structures (eg, nose). Muscle flaps can be used to fill large contour defects and cover exposed joints and orthopedic hardware (eg, patients with collocated burn and fracture). However, challenges with venous drainage after tangential or epifascial excision, need for additional skin autografts, and donor site morbidity limit the utility of muscle flaps in some situations. Composite tissue transplants for hand and face have also been performed in select cases.

## COMMON BURN RECONSTRUCTION PROBLEMS AND SOLUTIONS

Burn reconstruction is challenging given the extent and complexity of scar-related deformities, frequent major skin and soft-tissue deficits, and reliance on both healed and scarred skin for reconstruction procedures. However, despite the heterogeneity of burn injuries and the people who live with burn scars and contractures, there are common burn reconstruction challenges and procedures to address them.

### Head, Face, and Neck

Facial reconstruction is among the most challenging aspects of burn care but has the potential to markedly improve facial functions, body image, and satisfaction with appearance.[19]

### Eyelids

Eyelids have critical roles in protecting the cornea, conjunctiva, and globe and anchor facial appearance. Loss of eyelid function can occur by direct injury or by scarring of the areas around the eyelids, including the forehead, cheeks, and neck (ie, related cutaneous functional units), that result in cicatricial ectropion. For patients at risk of ectropion, the deformity can be mitigated with prophylactic tarsorrhaphy (ie, de-epithelialization of the lateral and/or medial upper and lower lids followed by suture closure) with care to maintain central pinhole vision.[20] Tarsorrhaphies are released once the scar has sufficiently matured (6–8 months) or when they are no longer tolerated by the patient.

The key step in evaluating patients with lid deformities is determining their ability to close the lids completely. Inability to close the eyelids and protect the cornea from exposure keratitis and ulceration is one of the few indications for early or urgent reconstruction. Bell's phenomenon (ie, palpebral-oculogyric reflex) protects the cornea even in the presence of ectropion by rolling the cornea up under the upper eyelid while asleep. Patients with normal upper eyelids can wait longer than those who do not without the risk of losing vision. Minor lid deformities that do not threaten corneal health generally improve with stretching, scar maturation, and nonsurgical scar management procedures (eg, ablative laser treatments).

Reconstruction of cicatricial ectropion typically involves scar release and division of scar tethers from periocular muscles followed by a skin graft, often a thick graft harvested from areas above the clavicles to maximize color match (eg, full-thickness graft from the neck or retroauricular area, thick split-thickness graft from the scalp) (**Fig. 9**).

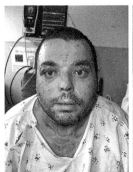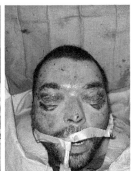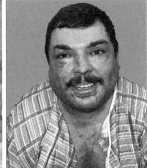

**Fig. 9.** Lower eyelid ectropion managed with bilateral scar release and thick skin autograft.

Ideally, eyelids from both eyes are not reconstructed simultaneously given that bolster dressings are used postoperatively for 3 to 7 days and edema is common, together resulting in obscured vision.

Another periorbital deformity commonly encountered is the medial canthal web, particularly when both the eyelids and nose are injured and/or grafted. Medial canthal webs are well-suited to local tissue rearrangements (eg, double opposing Z-plasty, 5-flap or jumping man plasty) with the goal to disrupt, reorient, and lengthen the scar. Lateral canthal webs occur less commonly but can also be managed adroitly with local tissue rearrangements (eg, del Campo transposition).

### Nose

Nose deformities are particularly challenging and generally require advanced reconstructions. Loss and contraction of the nasal ala—alar retraction—is the most common defect. Reconstruction of alar retraction requires recreation of both the cartilage and skin (eg, composite grafts from the helical root of the ear). Additional deformities include a shortened nasal tip and a wide nasal dorsum. Although numerous procedures have been described for these deformities (eg, staged paramedial forehead flap reconstruction, inferiorly based nasal turndown flap), they often rely on adjacent healthy tissue that may not be available.[21] For such cases and when total nose reconstruction is required (eg, restoration of nasal lining, cartilage, skin and projection), distant tissue and microvascular techniques are required. Custom nasal prostheses can provide a permanent solution for some patients with total nasal destruction or temporary satisfaction until patients are able to undergo serial reconstruction procedures.

### Lips

Common lip deformities include upper and lower lip ectropion, microstomia, loss of the philtral columns and dimple, and loss of the mental crease from destruction of fascial tethers to the mental protuberance. Lip ectropion are treated analogously to those of the eyelids but may also require neck contractures to be addressed when present. Microstomia is addressed by commissuroplasty, which aims to widen the commissure using buccal mucosa advancement and restoring the commissure to a line tangential to the medial limbus (ie, transition zone of the opaque sclera and clear cornea at the medial border of the iris). Philtrum reconstruction is generally performed once the upper lip length and projection is restored using a philtrum-shaped skin graft. Fat grafting can be used to soften mature scar and add volume beneath the skin to create better projection.

### Ears

Ear deformities can be relatively minor (eg, localized scar, lobule and/or helix adherence to the mastoid) and simply addressed with scar release and thick skin graft to restore optimal angle with the scalp or be more complex (eg, major cartilage loss). Complex ear deformities typically require cartilage grafts to recreate the helix, but adequate soft-tissue coverage can be problematic since the adjacent skin and temporoparietal fascia may also be scarred. In cases of ear loss or extensive destruction, autologous tissue reconstruction, porous polyethylene scaffold reconstruction, or custom prostheses can be considered.

### Other Areas of the Face

Efforts are made to avoid scar excision and partial face resurfacing with skin grafts, given their generally poor aesthetic results. Initial use of ablative laser treatments and local tissue rearrangements for hypertrophic facial scars has supplanted the need for routine scar excision and is a superior strategy for maintaining important landmarks. When major resurfacing is required, particularly to address skin deficits causing cicatricial and/or lip ectropion, attention should be paid to the grafting along facial subunits to optimize aesthetic outcome. Tissue expansion, regional or distant flap reconstructions, and even face transplantation can be used for more complex reconstruction needs.

### Neck

Neck contractures are common, frustrating sequelae of burn injury that can be particularly disfiguring and functionally limiting. The functional implications of neck contracture include not only limited range of motion but also eyelid and lip ectropion and poor oral competence. Neck contractures are addressed by scar release and wound closure (eg, skin graft with or without dermal template, regional or distant flap). Scar release generally includes incision of the scar, contracted platysma, and fascial tethers. Custom splinting and positioning aids that improve range of motion are required for months after release and reconstruction to mitigate the risk of recurrent contracture.[22] Stretching and range of motion exercise regimens usually begin about 1 week following neck release.

### Breast

Unique breast deformities include scarred breast mounds, absence of nipple-areola complex (NAC), and amastia. Between 9 and 12 years of age, thelarche begins through hormonal stimulation (ie, ovarian estrogen), with breast development reaching maturity 2 to 4 years later.[11] Injury to the breast bud and/or scar around the breast that occurs before complete breast development can restrict breast growth, lead to marked asymmetry, and/or displace the NAC. Breast reconstruction in girls should occur once there is bulging suggestive of breast development.[23] Typically, scar release to deep fascia and skin grafting are performed to allow unrestricted breast bud growth and prevent an entrapped breast (**Fig. 10**). Reconstruction of unilateral amastia should occur only once the contralateral breast growth is complete to achieve symmetry. Amastia is reconstructed with either implants and/or autologous tissue (eg, deep inferior epigastric perforator artery flap). Fat grafting, NAC reconstruction, and shared decision-making are critical to ensure that patients understand the rationale and options regarding reconstruction timing, staging, and type. Breast prostheses can be used temporarily or in lieu of reconstruction if preferred.

### Perineum

Perineal scar contractures or webs form in people who have scar across the genitalia, perineum, and/or proximal medial thighs. Perineal webs can limit range of motion, ambulation, make hygiene challenging, and can have significant effects on body image, clothing fit, intimacy, and sexuality. Large local tissue rearrangements (eg, multiple trapezoid flaps) (**Fig. 11**) and/or scar release and skin grafting or regional flap reconstruction (eg, internal pudendal artery perforator flap) can be used to address perineal webs. Scar that tethers the labia or scrotum and contractures of the penile shaft can be managed with scar release and skin grafting. Total penis, scrotal, and vulvar reconstruction techniques are more complex but well described, although limitations due to the availability of adjacent healthy tissue may force distant tissue-based reconstruction.

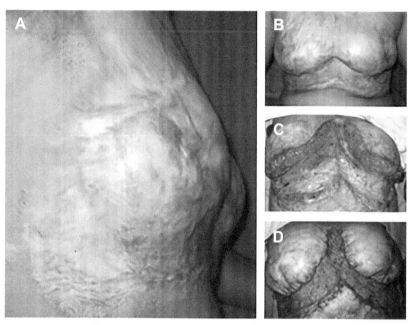

**Fig. 10.** Scar release of entrapped breast with skin autograft. (*A, B*) The entrapped breast before scar release. After freeing the breast tissue by incisional scar release (*C*), the inter-mammary cleft and inframammary folds are recreated (*D*). By doing so, the breasts are allowed their normal projection.

## *Upper Extremity*

The hands and upper extremities are commonly injured and, without excellent acute care, therapy, and timely reconstruction, can impact function and quality of life significantly.[24] Therapy efforts are focused on improving range of motion and preventing

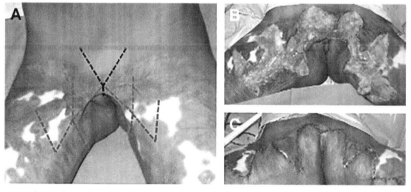

**Fig. 11.** Bilateral groin contractures released with local tissue rearrangements. (*A*) A preoperative photograph of the bilateral groin contracture. This was addressed with local tissue rearrangements (red and blue—double Z-plasties; black—Y-V plasty). (*B, C*) Scar release and closure after tissue rearrangements. Exercise, stretching, and nocturnal positioning regimens are required for a satisfactory outcome.

contractures in positions of rest (eg, arms adducted, elbows flexed, fingers flexed). When more than one joints are involved, contracture release should generally proceed from proximal to distal.

## Axilla

Axillary contractures present in 4 patterns (Kurtzman and Stern Classification): (1a) anterior *or* (1b) posterior axillary folds, (2) both folds with sparing of the axillary dome, or (3) both folds without sparing of the dome. Reconstruction is performed once range of motion has plateaued despite earnest exercise regimens and are designed to address each of these patterns (**Fig. 12**).[25] These include large tissue rearrangements (eg, running Y-V plasty, square flap, interdigitating trapezoidal flaps, transposition of chest or back tissue), central axis propeller flap when the dome is spared (**Fig. 13**), or scar release and skin grafting when the dome is not spared (**Fig. 14**). Patients must be prepared to continue stretching and range of motion exercises and adhere to splinting prescriptions for months after reconstruction.

## Elbow

Much like the axilla, contracture of the elbow can be caused by scar along the medial and/or lateral aspects of the elbow with or without spring of the antecubital fossa (see **Fig. 8**). Management of elbow contractures is analogous to the approaches described for the axilla. HO can affect any joint but is most common in the elbow and shoulder. Risk factors for HO include delayed wound closure, larger injury, and prolonged immobility.[26] Limitations of elbow and/or shoulder range of motion can limit upper extremity function significantly and compound disability related to concomitant hand contractures. Pharmacologic and/or surgical management of HO may be required if contracture is severe, refractory to therapy, and incompletely relieved with scar release and soft-tissue reconstruction. Serial examination of the hand should occur in patients

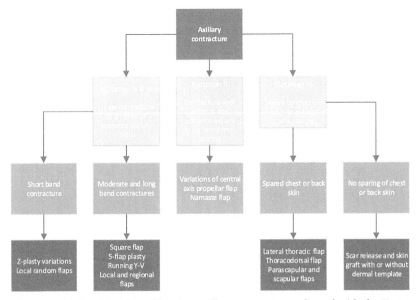

**Fig. 12.** Example algorithm for addressing axillary contractures aligned with the Kurtzman Classification.

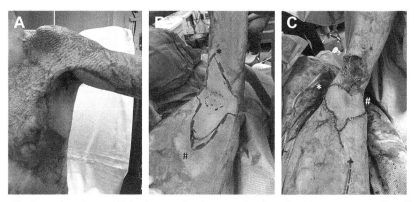

**Fig. 13.** Example of quadrilobed central axis propeller flap for Kurtzman type II axillary contracture. (*A*) Preoperative axillary contracture that includes the anterior and posterior axillary folds. The dashed red line in (*B*) outlines the quadrilobed central axis propeller flap before incision. (*C*) Position of the inset flap after its incision, elevation, and 90° rotation.

with significant elbow scarring and/or HO, given risk of ulnar nerve entrapment and neuropathy. The former can be relieved by scar release with extensive neurolysis.

### Wrist, Hand, and Fingers

Scar and contractures of the wrist, hand, and fingers can have a significant impact on functional recovery and quality of life. Contractures of the wrist typically occur on the dorsal surface and are readily treated with scar release and skin grafting. Volar contracture of the wrist results from keeping the wrist joint in a position of comfort during the acute phase of burn injury and is more difficult to manage and functionally disabling. Timely splinting can avoid this complication. Severe contractures may include shortened extensor tendons that require tenolysis for sufficient release. The defect created after scar release around the wrist may require staged reconstruction with a dermal template or flap coverage.

Given the specialized glabrous skin of the palm, all efforts during acute care are focused on supporting primary wound healing while maintaining range of motion, as skin grafting cannot replace the palmar fascial tethers or functions of the native

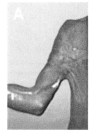
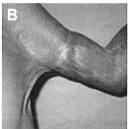
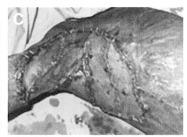

**Fig. 14.** Example of scar release and skin autograft for Kurtzman type III axillary contracture. (*A, B*) Anterior and posterior axillary fold contractures with obliteration of the axillary dome. (*C*) Axilla after scar release and skin sheet autograft. Complete shoulder abduction was limited by adhesive capsulitis and requires an exercise regimen and splinting strategy once skin autografts are stable.

palm.[27] When palmar contractures occur, they are best treated with scar release and skin grafting or regional flaps. Plantar donor sites are preferred when patients have pigmented skin for the best color match.

Web spaces are prone to contracture and are commonly treated with local tissue rearrangements (eg, variations of Z-plasty, 4- or 5-flap plasty) (**Fig. 15**). The key principles of web space release include: (1) provide adequate and appropriate skin to enable full range of motion, including sufficient dorsal hand and wrist skin if affected; (2) completely release contractures that restrict thumb or finger mobility; (3) restore palm width and the transverse metacarpal arch (for first web space contractures); (4) release the leading edge of the web contractures once the aforementioned principles are addressed; and (5) restore normal contour as able.[28]

Flexion contractures of the digits that cannot be resolved with therapy (eg, stretching, splinting, serial casting for children) require local tissue rearrangements. Scar release and skin grafting is performed if the contraction cannot be resolved with a local tissue rearrangement alone. Temporary Kirschner-wire fixation to immobilize the digit in extension is commonly performed with the aforementioned procedures (ie, 3–4 weeks). Flexion contractures of the proximal interphalangeal (PIP) joints may have been caused by injury to the extensor mechanism. The "burn claw" deformity occurs when there is hyperextension of the metacarpophalangeal joints from dorsal wrist and hand contracture in addition to PIP flexion deformity.[29] Surgical reconstruction of these deformities can be quite challenging, not only because of a lack of suitable dorsal skin coverage but also because of the need to reconstruct the extensor tendon mechanism and the scarred joints. PIP joint arthrodesis may be the best option for some patients, as this provides durable joint positioning in positions of function.[30] Lateral deviation of the border digits due to contracture band on their lateral aspects is difficult to correct surgically, especially when there is skeletal deformation due to long-lasting deformity. Prolonged buddy strapping following surgical correction can be helpful. Severe contractures of the fifth digit may warrant amputation if it obstructs the performance of daily tasks and reconstruction efforts would be unsatisfactory.

### Lower Extremity

Lower extremity deformities occur and are managed analogously to those of the upper extremity. Early and serial release of contracted toes in children is often required to

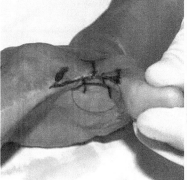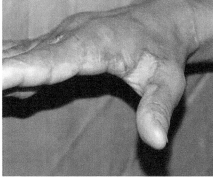

**Fig. 15.** Modified 5-flap or jumping man plasty for widening of first web space contracture. (*From*: Chen B, et al. The Modification of Five-Flap Z-Plasty for Web Contracture. Aesthetic Plastic Surgery. (2015) 39:922-926.)

facilitate adequate growth of the foot and toes themselves. Like fingers, longstanding toe contractures are often difficult to fully correct. A satisfactory toe position can be achieved with division of extensor tendons during reconstructive procedures without compromising ambulation. Plantar flexion deformity of the toes makes weight bearing very painful and places the dorsal surfaces at risk of friction- and pressure-related ulceration. Flexion deformities can be released by transverse incision and skin grafting. Most will need temporary Kirschner-wire fixation to maintain the position of the toes. Some joints are resistant to complete release if the contracture has been there for some time (eg, knee, elbow, shoulder). They can be released to a certain extent surgically and followed up with serial/progressive splinting or casting for more complete correction of the deformity.

The popliteal fossa is a particularly challenging location. Flexion contracture and chronic wounds are common and are often insufficiently managed with stretching, splinting, and ablative laser treatments alone. These generally require local tissue rearrangement (eg, square flap) and/or skin autograft. Using local flaps or minimally meshed skin autografts around the popliteal fossa during the acute reconstruction can mitigate some of the morbidity associated with popliteal fossa burn injuries (see **Fig. 1**).

## POSTRECONSTRUCTION SURGERY REHABILITATION

Surgery is not a substitute for engagement with rehabilitation regimens. The success of burn reconstruction and scar rehabilitation depends on the performance of well-planned and -executed surgical procedures and an effective postoperative rehabilitation plan that includes patient and therapy engagement. The rehabilitation plan (eg, immobilization technique and duration, splinting and exercise regimens, plans for staged procedures) should be developed with the patient and therapy team before surgery. Postoperative exercises are often initiated before surgery so that patients can be sufficiently habituated. This is particularly important for patients, often children, who developed contractures, in part, from insufficient stretching, split use, and range of motion exercises.

Although postoperative care regimens vary by surgeon, patient, and procedure, immobilization often occurs for 3 to 7 days postoperatively to facilitate wound healing and mitigate shear risk when skin grafts are used. Immobilization should be fashioned in positions that maximize function (eg, axillary splinting ≥110° of shoulder abduction, neck in mild hyperflexion, eyelids with traction sutures, finger extension after flexion contracture release). Once wound healing is not threatened, passive and active range of motion exercises are begun. Physical and occupational therapists are invaluable in helping patients achieve maximal function. However, patients must learn exercise regimens and perform them multiple times per day without supervision to be successful. Splints are typically used for weeks to months following contracture release, and positioning aids are used at night (eg, shoulder wedge to facilitate mild neck hyperextension when sleeping). Splints are removed for range of motion exercises and replaced afterward. As range of motion is restored, splints are often transitioned to nighttime use only.

## SUMMARY

Burn reconstruction, when integrated with diligent multidisciplinary care and rehabilitation, is incredibly rewarding, as patients experience marked improvements in their functional recoveries. Outcomes of burn reconstruction and scar rehabilitation should be patient-centered and include patient-reported measures that can be used for assessing individual recoveries and system-level benchmarking.[7,10] Successful reconstruction programs include strategies to track patient needs, range of motion and functional gains, timing of staged procedures, and key milestones in functional recovery.

## CLINICS CARE POINTS

- Apply principles of reconstruction during the acute phase to mitigate scar rehabiliation needs over the long-term.
- Ensure both patient and scar readiness prior to embarking on reconstructive procedures.
- Surgery is not a substitute for adherence to an exercise, stretching, and/or splinting program.

## ACKNOWLEDGMENTS

This work was developed under a grant from the National Institute on Disability, Independent Living, and Rehabilitation Research, United States (NIDILRR grant number 90DPBU0005). NIDILRR is a Center within the Administration for Community Living (ACL), Department of Health and Human Services (HHS). The contents of this manuscript do not necessarily represent the policy of NIDILRR, ACL, or HHS, and you should not assume endorsement by the Federal Government. The approach to and principles of burn reconstruction and scar rehabilitation presented here were furthered from the experience, work, and mentorship by Drs. Loren Engrav, Matthew Klein, David Heimbach, Nicole Gibran, Tam Pham, Gary Fudem, and Shankar Man Rai. Their patient-centered approach to holistic burn rehabilitation has been taught to many and described, in part, herein.

## REFERENCES

1. James SL, Lucchesi LR, Bisignano C, et al. Epidemiology of injuries from fire, heat and hot substances: global, regional and national morbidity and mortality estimates from the Global Burden of Disease 2017 study. Inj Prev 2020; 26(Supp 1):i36–45.
2. Goverman J, He W, Martello G, et al. The Presence of Scarring and Associated Morbidity in the Burn Model System National Database. Ann Plast Surg 2019; 82(3 Suppl 2):S162–8.
3. Gupta S, Wong E, Mahmood U, et al. Burn management capacity in low and middle-income countries: A systematic review of 458 hospitals across 14 countries. Int J Surg 2014. https://doi.org/10.1016/j.ijsu.2014.08.353.
4. Truche P, Moeller E, Wurdeman T, et al. The Plastic Surgery Workforce and Its Role in Low-income Countries. Plast Reconstr Surg Glob Open 2021;9(4):e3428.
5. Gupta S, Wong EG, Mahmood U, et al. Burn management capacity in low and middle-income countries: a systematic review of 458 hospitals across 14 countries. Int J Surg 2014;12(10):1070–3.
6. Sheckter CC. Unwinding the False Paradigm of Acute versus Reconstructive Management of Burn Injuries. Plast Reconstr Surg 2022;150(5):1124e–5e.
7. Luna Bs E, Sheckter CC, Carrougher GJ, et al. Self-reported health measures in burn survivors undergoing burn surgery following acute hospitalization: A burn model system national database investigation. Burns 2022. https://doi.org/10.1016/j.burns.2022.05.010.

8. Carrougher GJ, McMullen K, Amtmann D, et al. Living Well" After Burn Injury: Using Case Reports to Illustrate Significant Contributions From the Burn Model System Research Program. J Burn Care Res 2021;42(3):398–407.

9. Papp A, Berhanu A, Thomas MR, et al. Interrupting the seams: The principle of preventive burn reconstruction. Burns Open 2019;3:121–5.

10. Sheckter CC, Carrougher GJ, McMullen K, et al. Evaluation of Patient-Reported Outcomes in Burn Survivors Undergoing Reconstructive Surgery in the Rehabilitative Period. Plast Reconstr Surg 2020;146(1):171–82.

11. Fisher M. Pediatric Burn Reconstruction: Focus on Evidence. Clin Plast Surg 2017;44(4):865–73.

12. Finnerty CC, Jeschke MG, Branski LK, et al. Hypertrophic scarring: the greatest unmet challenge after burn injury. Lancet 2016;388(10052):1427–36.

13. Goei H, van der Vlies CH, Hop MJ, et al. Long-term scar quality in burns with three distinct healing potentials: A multicenter prospective cohort study. Wound Repair Regen 2016;24(4):721–30.

14. Huang S, Dang J, Sheckter CC, et al. A systematic review of machine learning and automation in burn wound evaluation: A promising but developing frontier. Burns 2021;47(8):1691–704.

15. Richard RL, Lester ME, Miller SF, et al. Identification of cutaneous functional units related to burn scar contracture development. J Burn Care Res 2009;30(4):625–31.

16. Ross SW, Malcolm J, Maitz J, et al. Fractional ablative laser therapy for the treatment of severe burn scars: a pilot study of the underlying mechanisms. Burns 2023. https://doi.org/10.1016/j.burns.2022.12.017.

17. Hultman CS, Friedstat JS, Edkins RE, et al. Laser resurfacing and remodeling of hypertrophic burn scars: the results of a large, prospective, before-after cohort study, with long-term follow-up. Ann Surg 2014;260(3):519–29 [discussion: 529-32].

18. Miletta N, Siwy K, Hivnor C, et al. Fractional Ablative Laser Therapy is an Effective Treatment for Hypertrophic Burn Scars: A Prospective Study of Objective and Subjective Outcomes. Ann Surg 2021;274(6):e574–80.

19. Friedstat JS, Klein MB. Acute management of facial burns. Clin Plast Surg 2009;36(4):653–60.

20. Klein MB, Ahmadi AJ, Sires BS, et al. Reversible marginal tarsorrhaphy: a salvage procedure for periocular burns. Plast Reconstr Surg 2008;121(5):1627–30.

21. King IC, Nikkhah D, Martin NA, et al. Nasal reconstruction in panfacial burns: useful techniques in challenging cases. Ann Plast Surg 2014;73(6):638–9.

22. Sabel J, Kristine P, Terken T, et al. The latest rendition of the ring neck collar formally known as 'Watusi. J Burn Care Res 2021;42(1):177–8.

23. Sadeq F, Cauley R, Depamphilis MA, et al. Reconstruction of Severe Burns to the Breast in Pediatric Patients: A 10-Year Experience. J Burn Care Res 2020;41(3):568–75.

24. Sterling J, Gibran NS, Klein MB. Acute management of hand burns. Hand Clin 2009;25(4):453–9.

25. Karki D, Mehta N, Narayan RP. Post-burn axillary contracture: A therapeutic challenge. Indian J Plast Surg 2014;47(3):375–80.

26. Levi B, Jayakumar P, Giladi A, et al. Risk factors for the development of heterotopic ossification in seriously burned adults: A National Institute on Disability, Independent Living and Rehabilitation Research burn model system database analysis. J Trauma Acute Care Surg 2015;79(5):870–6.

27. Fudem G, Dowlatshahi A, Francalancia S, et al. The Cinderella Layer and Fascia Tethers https://cinderellalayer.com. Accessed March 1, 2023.
28. Greyson MA, Wilkens SC, Sood RF, et al. Five Essential Principles for First Web Space Reconstruction in the Burned Hand. Plast Reconstr Surg 2020;146(5): 578e–87e.
29. Brown M, Chung KC. Postburn Contractures of the Hand. Hand Clin 2017;33(2): 317–31.
30. Klein MB. Burn reconstruction. Phys Med Rehabil Clin N Am 2011;22(2):311–25, vi-vii.

# UNITED STATES POSTAL SERVICE® Statement of Ownership, Management, and Circulation
## (All Periodicals Publications Except Requester Publications)

| 1. Publication Title | 2. Publication Number | 3. Filing Date |
|---|---|---|
| PHYSICAL MEDICINE AND REHABILITATION CLINICS OF NORTH AMERICA | 009 – 243 | 9/18/2023 |

| 4. Issue Frequency | 5. Number of Issues Published Annually | 6. Annual Subscription Price |
|---|---|---|
| FEB, MAY, AUG, NOV | 4 | $342.00 |

7. Complete Mailing Address of Known Office of Publication (Not printer) (Street, city, county, state, and ZIP+4®)

ELSEVIER INC.
230 Park Avenue, Suite 800
New York, NY 10169

Contact Person
Malathi Samayan

Telephone (Include area code)
91-44-4299-4507

8. Complete Mailing Address of Headquarters or General Business Office of Publisher (Not printer)

ELSEVIER INC.
230 Park Avenue, Suite 800
New York, NY 10169

9. Full Names and Complete Mailing Addresses of Publisher, Editor, and Managing Editor (Do not leave blank)

Publisher (Name and complete mailing address)

Dolores Meloni, ELSEVIER INC.
1600 JOHN F KENNEDY BLVD. SUITE 1600
PHILADELPHIA, PA 19103-2899

Editor (Name and complete mailing address)

MEGAN ASHDOWN, ELSEVIER INC.
1600 JOHN F KENNEDY BLVD. SUITE 1600
PHILADELPHIA, PA 19103-2899

Managing Editor (Name and complete mailing address)

PATRICK MANLEY, ELSEVIER INC.
1600 JOHN F KENNEDY BLVD. SUITE 1600
PHILADELPHIA, PA 19103-2899

10. Owner (Do not leave blank. If the publication is owned by a corporation, give the name and address of the corporation immediately followed by the names and addresses of all stockholders owning or holding 1 percent or more of the total amount of stock. If not owned by a corporation, give the names and addresses of the individual owners. If owned by a partnership or other unincorporated firm, give its name and address as well as those of each individual owner. If the publication is published by a nonprofit organization, give its name and address.)

| Full Name | Complete Mailing Address |
|---|---|
| WHOLLY OWNED SUBSIDIARY OF REED/ELSEVIER, US HOLDINGS | 1600 JOHN F KENNEDY BLVD. SUITE 1600 PHILADELPHIA, PA 19103-2899 |

11. Known Bondholders, Mortgagees, and Other Security Holders Owning or Holding 1 Percent or More of Total Amount of Bonds, Mortgages, or Other Securities. If none, check box ☐ None

| Full Name | Complete Mailing Address |
|---|---|
| N/A | |

12. Tax Status (For completion by nonprofit organizations authorized to mail at nonprofit rates) (Check one)
The purpose, function, and nonprofit status of this organization and the exempt status for federal income tax purposes:

☒ Has Not Changed During Preceding 12 Months
☐ Has Changed During Preceding 12 Months (Publisher must submit explanation of change with this statement)

PS Form 3526, July 2014 [Page 1 of 4 (see instructions page 4)]   PSN: 7530-01-000-9931   PRIVACY NOTICE: See our privacy policy on www.usps.com

---

| 13. Publication Title | 14. Issue Date for Circulation Data Below |
|---|---|
| PHYSICAL MEDICINE AND REHABILITATION CLINICS OF NORTH AMERICA | AUGUST 2023 |

| 15. Extent and Nature of Circulation | | Average No. Copies Each Issue During Preceding 12 Months | No. Copies of Single Issue Published Nearest to Filing Date |
|---|---|---|---|
| a. Total Number of Copies (Net press run) | | 126 | 134 |
| b. Paid Circulation (By Mail and Outside the Mail) | (1) Mailed Outside-County Paid Subscriptions Stated on PS Form 3541 (Include paid distribution above nominal rate, advertiser's proof copies, and exchange copies) | 81 | 90 |
| | (2) Mailed In-County Paid Subscriptions Stated on PS Form 3541 (Include paid distribution above nominal rate, advertiser's proof copies, and exchange copies) | 0 | 0 |
| | (3) Paid Distribution Outside the Mails Including Sales Through Dealers and Carriers, Street Vendors, Counter Sales, and Other Paid Distribution Outside USPS® | 29 | 30 |
| | (4) Paid Distribution by Other Classes of Mail Through the USPS (e.g. First-Class Mail®) | 13 | 11 |
| c. Total Paid Distribution (Sum of 15b (1), (2), (3), and (4)) | | 123 | 131 |
| d. Free or Nominal Rate Distribution (By Mail and Outside the Mail) | (1) Free or Nominal Rate Outside-County Copies included on PS Form 3541 | 3 | 3 |
| | (2) Free or Nominal Rate In-County Copies included on PS Form 3541 | 0 | 0 |
| | (3) Free or Nominal Rate Copies Mailed at Other Classes Through the USPS (e.g. First-Class Mail) | 0 | 0 |
| | (4) Free or Nominal Rate Distribution Outside the Mail (Carriers or other means) | 0 | 0 |
| e. Total Free or Nominal Rate Distribution (Sum of 15d (1), (2), (3) and (4)) | | 3 | 3 |
| f. Total Distribution (Sum of 15c and 15e) | | 126 | 134 |
| g. Copies not Distributed (See Instructions to Publishers #4 (page #3)) | | 0 | 0 |
| h. Total (Sum of 15f and g) | | 126 | 134 |
| i. Percent Paid (15c divided by 15f times 100) | | 97.62% | 97.76% |

* If you are claiming electronic copies, go to line 16 on page 3. If you are not claiming electronic copies, skip to line 17 on page 3.

PS Form 3526, July 2014 (Page 2 of 4)

| 16. Electronic Copy Circulation | | Average No. Copies Each Issue During Preceding 12 Months | No. Copies of Single Issue Published Nearest to Filing Date |
|---|---|---|---|
| a. Paid Electronic Copies | ▶ | | |
| b. Total Paid Print Copies (Line 15c) + Paid Electronic Copies (Line 16a) | ▶ | | |
| c. Total Print Distribution (Line 15f) + Paid Electronic Copies (Line 16a) | ▶ | | |
| d. Percent Paid (Both Print & Electronic Copies) (16b divided by 16c × 100) | ▶ | | |

☒ I certify that 50% of all my distributed copies (electronic and print) are paid above a nominal price.

17. Publication of Statement of Ownership

☒ If the publication is a general publication, publication of this statement is required. Will be printed ☐ Publication not required.
in the NOVEMBER 2023 issue of this publication.

| 18. Signature and Title of Editor, Publisher, Business Manager, or Owner | Date |
|---|---|
| Malathi Samayan - Distribution Controller   *Malathi Samayan* | 9/18/2023 |

I certify that all information furnished on this form is true and complete. I understand that anyone who furnishes false or misleading information on this form or who omits material or information requested on the form may be subject to criminal sanctions (including fines and imprisonment) and/or civil sanctions (including civil penalties).

PS Form 3526, July 2014 (Page 3 of 4)   PRIVACY NOTICE: See our privacy policy on www.usps.com

# Moving?

## Make sure your subscription moves with you!

To notify us of your new address, find your **Clinics Account Number** (located on your mailing label above your name), and contact customer service at:

**Email: journalscustomerservice-usa@elsevier.com**

**800-654-2452** (subscribers in the U.S. & Canada)
**314-447-8871** (subscribers outside of the U.S. & Canada)

**Fax number: 314-447-8029**

**Elsevier Health Sciences Division**
**Subscription Customer Service**
**3251 Riverport Lane**
**Maryland Heights, MO 63043**

*To ensure uninterrupted delivery of your subscription, please notify us at least 4 weeks in advance of move.

Printed and bound by CPI Group (UK) Ltd, Croydon, CR0 4YY

03/10/2024

01040467-0004